Health Informatics
(formerly Computers in Health Care)

Kathryn J. Hannah   Marion J. Ball
Series Editors

For other titles published in this series, go to
www.springer.com/series/1114

Jerry Stonemetz • Keith Ruskin
Editors

Anesthesia Informatics

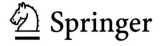 Springer

Editors
Jerry Stonemetz, MD
Clinical Associate
Anesthesiology and Critical Care Medicine
Johns Hopkins University
Baltimore, MD
USA

Keith Ruskin, MD
Professor
Anesthesiology and Neurosurgery
Yale University School of Medicine
New Haven, CT
USA

Series Editors
Kathryn J. Hannah
Adjunct Professor
Department of Community Health Science
Faculty of Medicine
The University of Calgary
Calgary, Alberta T2N 4N1, Canada

Marion J. Ball
Vice President, Clinical Solutions
Healthlink, Inc.
2 Hamill Road
Quadrangle 359 West
Baltimore, MD 21210, USA
and
Adjunct Professor
The Johns Hopkins University
School of Nursing
Baltimore, MD 21205, USA

ISBN 978-0-387-76417-7   e-ISBN 978-0-387-76418-4
DOI:10.1007/978-0-387-76418-4

British Library Cataloguing in Publication Data

Library of Congress Control Number: 2008930768

Printed on acid-free paper

Spinger Science+Business Media
springer.com

Foreword

Anesthesia Information Management Systems (AIMS) have been in existence for several decades, but their use in clinical practice has been very limited until recently. When initially developed, AIMS were primarily designed to replace paper records with an electronic form. Great debate ensued within the anesthesia community as to the value of these systems because of the concern that unedited data available in the system could place the practitioner at greater risk from a malpractice crisis. Yet, a growing body of evidence suggests that these concerns are unfounded; anesthesiologists and anesthesia departments have therefore become more accepting of this technology. In parallel, the healthcare industry has recognized that electronic medical records are a key element of improving patient safety and reducing error. Many insurers are discussing the development of incentives for implementation of electronic medical records. The recent implementation of pay-for-performance incentives has further enhanced the desire to implement AIMS because of the ability to document compliance with process measures (e.g., antibiotic timing). In this context, interest in adopting AIMS technology is growing within the anesthesia community, and numerous vendors have entered the field.

As anesthesiologists, we pride ourselves on our technologic savvy. Yet, the ability to purchase and implement an AIMS is new to most, and the expertise is limited to a handful of individuals throughout the nation. Jerry Stonemetz and Keith Ruskin have edited this multi-authored text, which includes most of these thought leaders to help the anesthesia community in all aspects of AIMS implementation from purchase through future implications. Drs. Stonemetz and Ruskin have been leaders in the field in different ways and have helped to define and push the field along from the perspectives of technology and the ability to improve billing and compliance. The authors of the individual chapters have established many of the standards and have helped to determine many of the benefits and shortcomings of this technology. Therefore, this extremely well-written book will be useful to a wide array of readers, from those interested in initially purchasing an AIMS, to those in the midst of implementing an AIMS, to those trying to utilize their AIMS to improve efficiency and safety. The case-based approach helps to frame this work in a very practical manner. Therefore, I anticipate that *Anesthesia Informatics* will both help anesthesiologists, anesthesia departments, and hospitals to purchase the ideal technology for their unique situations and help them to utilize it for the ultimate goal of improving patient safety and health-system efficiency.

Lee A. Fleisher, MD
Robert D. Dripps Professor and
Chair of Anesthesiology
Professor of Medicine and Critical Care
University of Pennsylvania School of Medicine

Adjunct Professor of Health Systems Informatics
Johns Hopkins University School of Medicine

Series Preface

This series is directed to healthcare professionals who are leading the transformation of healthcare by using information and knowledge to advance the quality of patient care. Launched in 1988 as *Computers in Health Care*, the series offers a broad range of titles: some are addressed to specific professions such as nursing, medicine, and health administration; others to special areas of practice such as trauma and radiology. Still other books in the series focus on interdisciplinary issues, such as the computer-based patient record, electronic health records, and networked healthcare systems.

Renamed *Health Informatics* in 1998 to reflect the rapid evolution in the discipline now known as health informatics, the series continues to add titles that contribute to the evolution of the field. In the series, eminent experts, serving as editors or authors, offer their accounts of innovation in health informatics. Increasingly, these accounts go beyond hardware and software to address the role of information in influencing the transformation of healthcare delivery systems around the world. The series also increasingly focuses on "peopleware" and the organizational, behavioral, and societal changes that accompany the diffusion of information technology in health services environments.

These changes will shape health services in the new millennium. By making full and creative use of the technology to tame data and to transform information, health informatics will foster the development of the knowledge age in healthcare. As co-editors, we pledge to support our professional colleagues and the series readers as they share the advances in the emerging and exciting field of health informatics.

Kathryn J. Hannah
Marion J. Ball

Preface

The seeds of this project were sown at a chance meeting between one of the editors (JS) and Marion Ball, PhD, at The Johns Hopkins University. Dr. Ball, who is arguably the matriarch of medical informatics, convinced us that we should take on the challenge of describing the components of the new field of Anesthesia Informatics. When Keith Ruskin agreed to participate as a co-editor, the vision for the content of this book began to materialize. Together, we were able to recruit international experts on each topic within the area of medical informatics in the perioperative setting. All of the authors have actually used the clinical systems discussed in this book, giving them real-world experience as well as expertise in the theoretical aspects of medical informatics.

This book is written with the practicing physician in mind. Although each of the authors has written a highly detailed, academically rigorous chapter, the goal was to make *Anesthesia Informatics* readable by a clinician with a problem to solve. For example, the chapters on communication in the operating room will be helpful to anesthesiologists who need to communicate important information to their staffs.

The editors are indebted to many people whose help was invaluable. Keith Ruskin would like to thank his wife Andrea and son Daniel, who understood why so many weekends were spent in front of a computer. He would also like to thank many of the residents and faculty in the Department of Anesthesiology at Yale University, who kindly read chapters and offered thoughtful opinions. Jerry Stonemetz wants to thank his wife Lysia and his three daughters Shey, Shannon, and Lyssa, who have always been so supportive of his endeavors and time spent away from home. He also wants to acknowledge the many faculty at The Johns Hopkins University who provided an environment of intellectual stimulation. Finally, we must acknowledge the impressive efforts of Tzipora Sofare, MA, an editor in the Department of Anesthesiology/Critical Care Medicine at The Johns Hopkins University. Without her efforts, this book would likely not have been completed. She converted rambling, ambiguous text into a book that is readable and quite informative. Thank you, Tzipora, for all of your help.

Jerry Stonemetz, MD
Clinical Associate
Department of Anesthesiology
  and Critical Care Medicine
Johns Hopkins Medical Institutes
Baltimore, MD
USA

Keith J. Ruskin, MD
Professor of Anesthesiology
  and Neurosurgery
Department of Anesthesia
Yale University School of Medicine
New Haven, CT
USA

Contents

Part B   Operating Room Management System

> **ORMS Case Scenario**—A case scenario that highlights concerns regarding efficiency, productivity, and patient safety between an ORMS and an EMR where integration and collaboration did not occur.
> Jerry Stonemetz

Part C   Mobile Computing, Education, and Simulation

> **Communication Case Scenario**—A case scenario that defines improved communication between providers and patients, utilizing all of the technology components available today.
> Keith Ruskin

Contributors

William D. Ankerstjerne, MECE, CWNE, ACDE, CCE
The Children's Hospital of Philadelphia, Philadelphia, PA, USA

R. Lebron Cooper, MD
Ochsner Health System, New Orleans, LA, USA

Christine Doyle, MD
Coast Anesthesia Medical Group, O'Connor Hospital, San Jose, CA, USA

Richard Epstein, MD, CPHIMS
Jefferson Medical College, Philadelphia, PA, USA

Ruth Fanning, MD
Stanford University, Palo Alto, CA, USA

Jeffrey Feldman, MD, MSE
Children's Hospital of Philadelphia, Philadelphia, PA, USA

David Gaba, MD
Stanford University, VA Palo Alto Health Care System, Palo Alto, CA, USA

Frank J. Gencorelli, MS
University of Miami, Miller School of Medicine, Miami, FL, USA

Gordon Gibby, MD
University of Florida, Gainesville, FL, USA

Michael Higgins, MD, MPH
Vanderbilt University School of Medicine, Nashville, TN, USA

Martin Hurrell, PhD
Informatics CIS Ltd., Glasgow, UK

Jonathan Kendler, MS
Wiklund Research & Design, Concord, MA, USA

Sachin Kheterpal, MD, MBA
University of Michigan Medical School, Ann Arbor, MI, USA

Viji Kurup, MD
Yale University School of Medicine, New Haven, CT, USA

Robert Lagasse, MD
Montefiore Medical Center, Bronx, NY, USA

Phillip Lane, MD, JD, MBA, MPH
Rush University Medical Center, Chicago, IL, USA

David Lubarsky, MD, MBA
University of Miami/Jackson Memorial Hospital, Miami, FL, USA

Jerrold H. May, PhD
The Joseph M. Katz Graduate School of Business, University of Pittsburgh
Pittsburgh, PA, USA

Alan Merry, MB ChB, FANZCA, FFPMANZA
University of Auckland, Auckland, New Zealand

Terri Monk, MD
Duke University Medical Center, Durham, NC, USA

Stanley Muravchick, MD, PhD
Hospital of the University of Pennsylvania, Philadelphia, PA, USA

Andrew Norton, MD, FRCA
Pilgrim Hospital, Boston, UK

Michael O'Reilly, MD, MS
University of Michigan Hospitals, Ann Arbor, MI, USA

Ravindra Prasad, MD
University of North Carolina School of Medicine, Chapel Hill, NC, USA

Christopher Reeves, MD, MBA
Johns Hopkins Medical Institutions, Baltimore, MD, USA

Mohammed Rehman, MD
Children's Hospital of Philadelphia, Philadelphia, PA, USA

David L. Reich, MD
Mount Sinai School of Medicine, New York, NY, USA

Melvin Reynolds, MIScT, MBCS
AMS Consulting, Ross-on-Wye, UK

Gil Ritchie, PhD
Greenville Hospital System, Greenville, SC, USA

Stephen T. Robinson, MD
Oregon Health and Science University, Portland, OR, USA

Keith Ruskin, MD
Yale University School of Medicine, New Haven, CT, USA

Nirav Shah, MD
University of Michigan Hospitals, Ann Arbor, MI, USA

William Spangler, PhD
Duquesne University, Pittsburgh, PA, USA

Paul St. Jacques, MD
Vanderbilt University School of Medicine, Nashville, TN, USA

Alia Stanciu, MBA
The Joseph M. Katz Graduate School of Business, University of Pittsburgh
Pittsburgh, PA, USA

Jerry L. Stonemetz, MD, MS
Johns Hopkins Medical Institutions, Baltimore, MD, USA

David Strum, MD
Queens University, Kingston General Hospital, Ontario, Canada

Laurence Torsher, MD
Mayo Clinic College of Medicine, Rochester, MN, USA

Luis G. Vargas, PhD
The Joseph M. Katz Graduate School of Business, University of Pittsburgh
Pittsburgh, PA, USA

Michael M. Vigoda, MD, MBA
University of Miami/Jackson Memorial Hospital, Miami, FL, USA

David Wax, MD
Mount Sinai School of Medicine, New York, NY, USA

Michael Wiklund, MS, PE
Wiklund Research & Design, Concord, MA, USA

Marisa L. Wilson, DNSc, MHSc, RN
University of Maryland School of Nursing, Baltimore, MD, USA

David Young, MD
Advocate Lutheran General Hospital, Chicago, IL, USA

Abbreviations

AACD	American Association of Clinical Directors
ACGME	Accreditation Council for Graduate Medical Education
ACL	Anesthesia Clinical Leader
ACS	American College of Surgeons
ACS NSQIP	American College of Surgeon's NSQIP
ADL	Archetype Description Language
ADT	admission/discharge/transfer
AIMS	anesthesia information management system(s)
ANSI	American National Standards Institute
AP	access point
APR DRG	all-patient refined DRG
APSF	Anesthesia Patient Safety Foundation
ARNP	advanced registered nurse practitioner
ASA	American Society of Anesthesiologists
ASTM	American Society for Testing and Materials
BPP	bin-packing problem
BSI	British Standards Institute
CAN	Controller Area Network
CASE	Comprehensive Anesthesia Simulation Environment
CCR	Continuity of Care Record
CDA	Clinical Document Architecture
CDC	Centers for Disease Control and Prevention
CDMA	code division multiple access
CDRH	Center for Devices and Radiological Health
CDSS	clinical decision support system(s)
CEN	Comité Européen de Normalisation (European Committee for Standardisation)
CENELEC	European Committee for Electrotechnical Standardization
CIMIT	Center for Integration of Medicine and Innovative Technology
CLSI	Clinical and Laboratory Standards Institute
CME	Continuing Medical Education

CMS	Centers for Medicare and Medicaid Services
CP	constraint programming
CPOE	computerized physician order entry
CPOM	Committee on Performance and Outcomes Measurement
CPT	current procedural terminology
CPU	central processing unit
CQI	continuous quality improvement
CRNA	certified registered nurse anesthetist
CTV	Clinical Terms Version
DAS	distributed antenna systems
DBMS	database management systems(s)
DDTF	Data Dictionary Task Force
DEA	Drug Enforcement Agency
DES	Data Encryption Standard
DICOM	Digital Imaging and Communications in Medicine
DL	Description Logic
D-MIM	Domain Message Implementation Model
DPC	doctor preference card
DRG	disease-related grouping
DSL	digital subscriber line
DSS	decision support system(s)
ED	emergency department
EIA	Electronic Industries Alliance
EMR/EHR	electronic medical record/electronic health record
EU	European Union
FDA	Food and Drug Administration
GEHR	Good European Healthcare Record
GMDN	Global Medical Devices Nomenclature
GS1 HUG	GS1 Healthcare User Group
GSM	global system for mobile communication
H&P	history and physical
HHS	US Department of Health and Human Services
HIPAA	Healthcare Insurance Portability and Accountability Act
HIS	hospital information system
HL7	Health Level 7
HMD	Hierarchical Message Description
HQ	HealthQuest
ICD	International Classification of Diseases
ICU	intensive care unit
IEC	International Electrotechnical Commission

IEEE	Institute of Electrical and Electronics Engineers
IHE	Integrating the Healthcare Enterprise
IHTSDO	International Healthcare Terminology Standards Development Organization
IOM	Institute of Medicine
IOTA	International Organization for Terminology in Anesthesia
IPM	Implementation Project Manager
IPPS	Inpatient Prospective Payment System
IP-RFID	Internet protocol–radio-frequency identification
IrDA	Infrared Data Association
ISO	International Standards Organization
IT	information technology
IV	intravenous
LAN	local area network
LCD	liquid crystal display
LOINC	Logical Observation Identifiers Names and Codes
MD PnP	Medical Device "Plug-and-Play" Interoperability Program
MDC	medical device communication
MDD	Medical Devices Directive
MDDL	medical device data language
MIB	Medical Information Bus
MOC	Maintenance of Competence
MRI	magnetic resonance imaging
MSH	Message Header
MSMC	Mount Sinai Medical Center
NHS	UK National Health Service
NIBP	noninvasive blood pressure
NIC	network interface card
NICU	neonatal intensive care unit
NPfIT	National Programme for Information Technology
NPO	nil per os, nothing by mouth
NSQIP	National Surgical Quality Improvement Program
OIG	Office of the Inspector General
OLAP	online analytical processing
OOAD	Object-oriented Analysis and Design
OR	operating room
ORMS	Operating Room Management System(s)
OSCE	Objective Structured Clinical Examination
OSI	Open Systems Interconnection
OWL	Web Ontology Language

P4P	Pay for Performance
PACS	Picture Archiving and Communication System
PACU	postanesthesia care unit
PAT	Preanesthesia Testing
PC	personal computer
PCA	patient-controlled anesthesia
PCD	patient care devices
PCEA	patient-controlled epidural anesthesia
PDA	personal digital assistant
PDF	portable document format
PEC	preoperative evaluation clinic
PGP	Pretty Good Privacy
PHI	protected health information
PICU	pediatric intensive care unit
PIM	personal information management
PKE	public key encryption
POC	point of care
POC-CIC	Point-of-Care Communications Industry Consortium
POP	point of presence
QA	quality assurance
RAID	redundant array of independent drives
RDBMS	relational database management system(s)
RDF	Resource Description Framework
RFI	request for information
RFID	radio-frequency identification
RFP	request for proposals
RIM	Reference Information Model
RM	revenue management
R-MIM	Refined Message Implementation Model
ROI	return on investment
ROM	risk of mortality
RSS	Really Simple Syndication
RTLS	real-time location services
SCIP	Surgical Care Improvement Project
SCIP	Secure Communications Interoperability Protocol
SDO	Standards Development Organization
SICU	surgical intensive care unit
SIGGAS	Special Interest Group for the Generation of Standards in Anesthesia
SLC	syringe-loaded cartridge
SNOMED	Systematized Nomenclature of Medicine
SNOMED CT	Systematized Nomenclature of Medicine-Clinical Terminology
SNOMED RT	Systematized Nomenclature of Medicine-Reference Terminology

SNOP	Systematized Nomenclature of Pathology
SOI	severity of illness
SP	standardized patient
SQL	Structured Query Language

TC	technical committee
TCAS	Traffic Alert and Collision Avoidance System
TDMA	time division multiple access

UK	United Kingdom
UML	Unified Modeling Language
UMPC	Ultra-Mobile PC
URAC	Utilization Review Accreditation Commission
US	United States
USB	universal serial bus

VHA	Veterans' Health Administration
VITAL	Vital Signs Representation
VoFI	voice over WiFi
VoIP	voice over Internet protocol

W3C	World Wide Web Consortium
WiFi	wireless fidelity
WLAN	wireless local area network
WLC	wireless LAN controller
WWAN	wireless wide area network

XML	Extensible Markup Language

Introduction

Originating in the late 19th century, anesthesia has often been cited as one of the greatest accomplishments in medicine, along with sanitation and antibiotics. With the advent of anesthesia, it became possible to explore the human body with surgery without being limited by time or tolerance of the patient. And, with the advent of anesthesia, surgery has become a never-ending evolution of manipulation of the body in an attempt to correct diseases, prolong life, or simply enhance personal appearance. Since the birth of the specialty, anesthesiologists have continuously pushed the envelope of technology. From exploration of different drugs for the induction of anesthesia to current efforts at enhancing patient safety and the recognition of anesthesia as the only specialty to provide a "six-sigma" improvement in patient safety, anesthesiologists constantly endeavor to expand our repertoire of tools to deliver a safe and effective anesthetic. The goal of this book is to explore and reveal methods of using computers and other informatic solutions toward further expanding the anesthesia repertoire. Typically, the authors of these chapters are evangelists and, as such, in their enthusiasm, may be biased that these tools are more important than is actually the case. Consequently, we have made every effort to identify existing examples of informatic solutions rather than simply present marketing hype.

Information technology has become an integral component of healthcare, and anesthesiologists have been at the forefront of the discipline of medical informatics for decades. Ironically, however, a neurosurgeon created the first anesthesia record. As a medical student, Harvey Cushing was administering anesthesia, and his patient died during surgery—not an uncommon occurrence. This fatality had a lasting effect on Cushing, and with the help of another medical student, Amory Codman, he created the first record of an anesthetic. Carefully documenting pulse and respirations, they demonstrated that retrospective review of these records could be useful in analyzing adverse outcomes during surgery and that such a review had the potential of standardizing the delivery of anesthesia to improve patient care.

Over 30 years ago, Anesthesia was one of the first specialties to actually explore computerization of the clinical episode. Early developments at Duke University demonstrated that the entire anesthetic event could be captured electronically. Gravenstein and his colleagues edited the first publication about computerized anesthesia records in 1987. Gravenstein points out that simply recording what happened does not allow us to analyze the quality of the anesthetic delivered.

Only through detailed analysis of volumes of raw data are we able to extrapolate the effective quality delivered. Ideally, this analysis will become simpler once the entire anesthetic experience is digitized.

By the end of 2006, anesthesia information management systems (AIMS) had penetrated less than 10% of the market. Polling of clinicians and hospital administrators over the past 20 years has led us to believe that the reason for this resistance to market acceptance can be summarized by three primary reasons. First, it is very difficult to improve on pen and paper. Having spent many years learning their craft, anesthesiologists may be reluctant to adopt any technology that distracts them from their primary job—caring for the patient. The early systems that were commercially available had to overcome this resistance through enhanced functionality that could unequivocally demonstrate their ability to reduce the amount of work necessary to create an anesthetic record. The new graphical user interfaces have contributed greatly to increasing the usability and acceptance of these computerized systems. Second, many continue to harbor a grave concern that the electronic footprint could be used against us as a liability. We feel that we have addressed this concern in these pages. Finally, we believe that the pivotal reason why AIMS have not been aggressively adopted is that, as an industry, AIMS vendors have failed to demonstrate any significant return on investment to the customer. And despite how fervent the anesthesiologist may be to implement an AIMS, the real decision typically lies in the hands of the hospital administrator who signs the purchase order for these expensive systems. Therefore, we have spent considerable time in this text clearly demonstrating how an AIMS, which captures the acute care event, so rich in clinical data, can be an investment that provides an improvement in patient care, analysis of the delivery of an anesthetic, a critical component with which to guide process improvement, and a valuable tool that can be utilized toward cost-saving measures.

In their infancy, computerized anesthesia systems were referred to by the acronym ARK, which stood for automated record keepers (and, in some cases, anesthesia record keepers). This acronym actually became the foundation for the name of the first commercial vendor—Arkive. As with most early leaders in any field, this company advanced the technology but fell victim to insufficient sales to warrant a sustainable business in a market that was just too slow to adopt the new technology. As other vendors entered the field, they frequently attempted to distinguish themselves from their competitors by increasing the functionality and breadth of their offerings by expanding into the preoperative arena and, hence, considered themselves more than simply "record keepers." This enhanced functionality was reflected primarily by a change in the acronym to AIS (anesthesia information system) and AIMS (anesthesia information management system). So, what is the proper acronym for these systems? Even our contributing authors could not universally agree. The topic generated some early discussions among us that were interesting and provided the energy to motivate all involved toward finishing their contributions. As with most democratic initiatives, the majority ruled in this instance, and we standardized to AIMS, which will be used throughout this publication.

We have carefully identified and enlisted as contributing authors individuals whom we felt were nationally and, in some cases, internationally recognized for their knowledge and expertise in the areas discussed. Given the guidance and challenge by our publishers at Springer, we began to create a publication that would have broad appeal to anyone interested in Anesthesia Informatics as well as to those who would have a proclivity for reading a book on clinical information systems.

A wealth of information is available to any clinician with access to a desktop or handheld computer. Online literature searches and journal articles, continuing medical education, and clinical guidelines are just a few of the many resources available that will allow any physician to practice more effectively. The rapid growth in variety and quality of online medical information offers physicians an unprecedented opportunity to use information technology for both education and patient care. This information can be accessed through laptop computers, handheld devices, and Blackberries, each of which has become small, faster, and easier to use. As well, modern medical education has changed significantly over the past decade. In the past, most training programs relied on a curriculum that exposed trainees to specific subject areas at specific times during the training period. Modern training programs now rely on a competency-based curriculum in which trainees are required to meet specific educational goals. In response to these changes in educational philosophy, nearly every medical school and residency training program has had to change its curriculum. Many institutions have begun to adopt medical simulation as an integral component of their educational programs. Although these systems are not yet a mandatory component of residency training programs, many large institutions have begun to train their residents using simulation. Although the role of simulators in medical education is widely acknowledged, their utility for evaluating clinical skills remains controversial, and anesthesiologists are frequently asked to participate in the decision to purchase a simulator and to serve as a part of the simulation team.

We understood that our mission was to create a book that covers the essentials of clinical systems specific to the field of Anesthesia that would include discussions of the evolving collection of information systems that capture the anesthetic experience as well as other important areas, such as communications, security, education, and simulation. We agreed that it would delve into the area of Operating Room Management Systems (ORMS), given the close overlap and potential integration between these two clinical realms. The book also includes sections on Communications and Computer Simulation. These are relevant and necessary because anesthesiologists have participated, if not taken the lead, in these two areas.

One of the primary tenets that we as a group espouse is the use of standards going forward. Nowhere is this more evident than in the simple acronym—AIMS—that we use to describe the clinical systems that encompass our specialty. And, unless a higher standards body can demonstrate a more ubiquitous term, we hope that we are partially responsible for establishing this as a universally accepted standard acronym. If this is our only accomplishment, we will obviously be disappointed. As you will see upon perusing this text, we are advocating many standards—in terminology, functionality, usability, and decision support. Our desire is to educate practicing anesthesiologists about the possibilities for standardization that currently exist, so that they can help to convince vendors that adoption of these standards is necessary.

As you peruse this book, you will read about rationale for an AIMS that encompasses better patient preparation (Chapters 9 & 10), reduction of errors (Chapter 11), improved charge capture (Chapter 14), decision support (Chapter 15), process improvement (Chapter 16), and operating room efficiency (Chapter 22). You will read about opportunities to improve workflow and reduce wasted effort. We will discuss our perspective on the rationale for purchasing an AIMS in the larger context of a hospital's overall goals of reducing expenses, increasing revenue, and demonstrating that they are providing quality care on a case-by-case basis. This latter demonstration will become a requirement for reimbursement as third-party payers pursue value-based purchasing.

As with all editors, our challenge was to create a publication that would be up-to-date and not obsolete by the time of publication. Given the relative dearth of published material regarding Anesthesia Informatics, we have relied on expert opinion and, where feasible, report on real-life situations and experiences. Consequently, we feel we have succeeded in our effort to create a publication that is relevant and pertinent, and we hope that you agree. We are confident that this book will be a valuable reference for anyone already using clinical systems, considering the purchase of these tools, or just curious about the potential of anesthesia-related systems.

Finally, we have employed real-life examples of implementations and utilization to demonstrate how AIMS may be of value and, more importantly, how you as a customer can better prepare for this significant change to your work environment. We have made every effort to elucidate the rationale for why these systems are essential. It is our hope that once you have read this publication, you will have a better understanding of both the possibilities and the limitations of implementing an AIMS and that you will be equipped with a clear idea of why you should be advocating implementation of an AIMS at your facility. We are confident that you will be a better-informed customer after you have read this book and will continue to use it as a reference tool once you make the decision to go digital.

Jerry Stonemetz, MD
Clinical Associate
Department of Anesthesiology
    and Critical Care Medicine
Johns Hopkins Medical Institutes
Baltimore, MD
USA

Keith J. Ruskin, MD
Professor of Anesthesiology
    and Neurosurgery
Department of Anesthesia
Yale University School of Medicine
New Haven, CT
USA

Part A
The Anesthesia Information
Management System

Informatic Case Scenario

Imagine practicing medicine in an environment where access to patient information is as transparent as the ability to access your banking information via your Web-based bank account. This is a common analogy cited in advocating for the advancement of electronic health records. Although this vision has practically become a cliché, we are far removed from its reality in today's clinical world.

What are the real advantages of moving to an electronic environment for anesthesia? Since the beginning of the capture of the anesthetic episode with printed documents, espoused by Codman and Cushing, we have become accustomed to capturing all vital-sign data and many other details of the delivery of anesthesia. The paper record now defines our billing records, our legal protection in the event of an adverse event, and a practical burden while providing care to our patients. However, the utilization of these paper records to improve patient safety, understand practice patterns, or even predict patient behavior has not been realized at most institutions. Clearly, translating data from a paper record into a useful database or reporting tool requires additional manpower and is impractical in today's cost-conscious healthcare environment.

What if, instead, the clinical episode were captured electronically and all relevant data elements were captured in a database that would allow collation of data and comparison of events across institutions? Would that improve care and patient safety? We do not really know the answer to this question, except that intuitively, we believe this to be a logical deduction that continues to propel us toward universal acceptance of electronic medical records. Acute care represents one of the most probable areas where capture of electronic data will actually translate into improved care. The ability to capture comprehensive data elements in a paper record is relatively impossible, especially in those situations where the care provider is taxed with delivering intensive care, such as with trauma or large, invasive procedures. Our collective perception is that electronic records for the anesthetic episode will facilitate better data collection, providing opportunities to learn from our experiences that are not currently possible. Unfortunately, as an industry, AIMS vendors have done a poor job of illustrating the true value of their systems and the return on investment that they could deliver to the real customer of these systems—the hospital.

Would the clinician's ability to provide a safer, more refined anesthetic be improved if he had immediate exposure to past anesthetic records, key components of previous anesthetic experiences, relevant patient data such as previous labs, EKGs, and other diagnostic tests? We believe it would. According to the 2005 Sentinel Event analysis by The Joint Commission, over 60% of Sentinel Events ascribed to anesthesia were secondary to inadequate preoperative evaluation. Surely, access to pervasive patient data would improve this situation. Comparison of anesthetic management within an anesthesia department is essential for an effective Quality Improvement process, and proper management is currently a significant resource drain for most departments with paper records. Prevention of drug errors in anesthesia represents one of the key areas in which we need to focus our attention as a specialty. Pretending that we do not need improvement in this arena is simply ignoring all evidence to the contrary. Decision support available to us preoperatively, intraoperatively, and postoperatively will begin to define our specialty and dramatically improve care. The scenarios cited, above in which the clinician has immediate access to up-to-date information are possible in an era of paper records, and only incorporating AIMS technology will provide the methods with which to move our practices into the era of fully transparent electronic medical records. And now, the case scenario.

At the "University," a group of motivated, dedicated practitioners formed a Coalition to shepherd an aggressive implementation of the ultimate solution, an informatic system that would deliver the safest, most effective anesthesia possible. They arranged for dedicated IT support to either develop or enhance existing clinical applications to provide transparent access to all clinical data. In concert with hospital administration, the Coalition was able to effectively require that any commercial vendor's application must provide access to data and a binding commitment to facilitate integration with other clinical systems. Even beyond the basic clinical system utilization, this Coalition also worked with leadership from the ASA, other world anesthesia societies and standards bodies, and the Centers for Medicare Services to create an alternative-practice environment. One of the key missions of the Coalition was to analyze how best to provide safe, comprehensive anesthesia care to an aging and rapidly expanding population.

Based on evidence gathered through safety research, it was clear that the patients must be engaged in their care. Excluding them and their responsibility had been demonstrated to lead to less than the best possible outcomes. Consequently, the first phase for the informatic system was the creation of a personal health record to which patients had access and for which they had some accountability in maintaining their health information. Access to these data was made available online so that patients could update their health records directly, and any tests or results from studies performed could be appended to the health record and immediately viewed by the appropriate providers. Additionally, one of the key goals of this effort was the ability to store data as discrete elements as opposed to images of information (as was the limitation of the standard technology previously in place). Obviously, the goal of implementation of this health record was to eliminate the loss of critical information and the resultant redundant ordering of tests or delays in delivery of care or treatment. To avoid creating duplicate volumes of data in massive databases, the health record was designed such that data from disparate systems were viewable as thumbnails within the electronic record, similar to the way HTML documents are viewed over the Internet.

The second phase of the informatic system was to alter the method in which care was delivered by facilitating a proactive approach, rather than the reactive approach being practiced. For example, once a patient was scheduled for surgery, the system would begin prompting the collection and analysis of data and forwarding alerts and action items to appropriate entities rather than waiting for someone to request information. With the completion of a Web-based questionnaire in the surgeon's office, combined with demographic and clinical information from the patient's health record, a rules-based engine in the AIMS module of the system began a triage of testing and evaluations of patients determined by the comorbidities of the patient and the surgical severity of the scheduled procedure. Determination of the necessity of cardiac, pulmonary, or other system evaluations was calculated and forwarded to the anesthesia preoperative team for authorization. Once tests were ordered, results were automatically made available to the patient's record, and notification of the preoperative team allowed for analysis and decisions far in advance of the day of surgery, further eliminating delays and cancellations. Specific instructions tailored to the surgery and the patient were provided to the patient and made part of the health record. Consequently, preoperative care plans were customized rather than applied in a shotgun manner.

On the day of surgery, patient registration and check-in was smoother and easily facilitated rapid preparation of surgical patients. One immediate benefit noted by the coalition was a significant improvement in patient satisfaction because patients were not required to come to the hospital 2 hour in advance in order to be ready for surgery. Rather than arriving at the hospital at 5:30 a.m. for the first case, patients could arrive at 7 a.m. and be ready to be seen by the physicians within 15 minutes of arrival. This later arrival time was made possible because the extensive nursing and anesthesia preoperative assessment had been completed as part of the preoperative preparation, and the nurses and physicians who were meeting patients for the first time were simply reviewing and verifying information rather than completing forms or electronic records. The preoperative process became focused on patient care rather than on chart creation. The physician not only had access to the health record, preoperative tests, and consultations, but also had immediate availability to any previous anesthesia records, regardless of the institution at which the patient had had the previous surgery.

Ultimately, the real value of this new informatic system was to seamlessly allow collection of patient clinical data into a large database for analysis and benchmark comparisons. Working with the hospital's IT department, the anesthesia department was able to set the standard for demonstrating compliance with the initiatives of the Surgical Care Improvement Project and The Joint Commission's Core Measures. This group was able to effectively demonstrate that they were delivering the highest quality patient care and allowed the hospital to become recognized as one the leading healthcare institutions in the world.

Chapter 1
Rationale for Purchasing an AIMS

Jerry Stonemetz and Robert Lagasse

The editors of this book assume that its readers either have recently made the decision to purchase an AIMS or are contemplating a purchase soon. The material presented in this book is intended to be a resource for facilities as they attempt to revise current workflow and behavior to become more facile in their electronic documentation. However, it is reasonable to ask why these systems are important or even necessary. Is it appropriate to risk expending large amounts of resources—both capital and human—and to potentially alter the entire workflow of an organization? What factors make this decision relevant for an institution, and how will an organization realize a return on investment (ROI) as a result of this decision? These questions and others must be addressed at the beginning of the decision-making process. The goal of this chapter is to provide some answers.

Advocates of electronic medical records argue that simply creating a printed record from the digital system is passé. If the only expectation is to capture vital-sign data from patient monitors and turn these data into a printed record, then AIMS do not justify their expense. However, nowhere else in healthcare do they make more sense than in the acute care arena, where patients are connected to a myriad of monitors and clinical information changes rapidly and dramatically. Computerized systems should be capable of collecting vital-sign data and collating patient information faster, better, and more comprehensively than any practitioner could hope to do using paper records while simultaneously providing a high level of care to the patient. The need for this capability is essential in a world where anesthesiologists' coverage is being expanded from the ICU, ED, and ORs to more remote areas. Nevertheless, the real customers of an AIMS will actually be the hospital and the administrator who controls the purse strings for the purchase of such systems. Clearly, any rationale for the purchase of these expensive systems must include a compelling ROI, the potential for which must be recognized by the administrators.

Although AIMS technology was proposed over 20 years ago, its adoption has been slow.[1,2] Concerns over behavior change, costs, and legal implications have been recognized as primary deterrents in migration to electronic records. With advances in computational power, ease of use, and commodity pricing of hardware, many of these concerns have diminished. All the while, clinicians have intuitively recognized that electronic records could potentially provide value and improve

J. Stonemetz, K. Ruskin (eds.) *Anesthesia Informatics*,
© Springer Science+Business Media, LLC 2008

patient safety. The directors of the Anesthesia Patient Safety Foundation (APSF), a patient safety–focused group sponsored primarily by the ASA, have gone on record to state "The APSF endorses and advocates the use of automated record keeping in the perioperative period and the subsequent retrieval and analysis of the data to improve patient safety."[3] Ironically, it was the ability to retrospectively review and analyze adverse patient events in an effort to improve patient safety that prompted Cushing and Codman (as medical students) to create the first anesthesia record.[4]

Described by some as the "black box" or flight recorder for anesthesiology, AIMS have been recognized and advocated as a method by which to provide better tools to analyze adverse events and near misses, and to provide a global repository of outcomes data that may help to shape future safety efforts.[5] Properly configured and implemented, an AIMS should facilitate the collection of accurate and comprehensive clinical data, thereby representing the anesthetic management of a given patient. From these data, it should be easier for institutions to demonstrate compliance with regulatory requirements, better charge capture of professional fees, and clinical competency through performance measurement. However, the importance of proper configuration and deployment of an AIMS in order to realize these benefits cannot be overemphasized. The medical literature and popular press illustrate this point with examples of clinical systems that have failed miserably and, in some cases, even resulted in patient harm.[6]

Return on Investment

All AIMS purchases must be evaluated in terms of their ROI to aid the customer's decision-making process. Essentially, the ultimate question is: Will this system save money or increase revenue in a manner that will allow the customer to realize a substantial return on the purchase price and the ongoing manpower and support costs? Few studies that actually evaluate ROIs are available in peer-reviewed journals. Some information is obtainable from business journals and from the chief financial officer or the chief information officer of an institution. It is essential that a customer understand the ROI models and be certain that the projected payback is real, and not simply sales hype.

ROI models have been applied to AIMS purchases, particularly computerized patient records and computerized physician order entry systems.[7] As a recent editorial argues, however, hospital administrators (customers) must be able to evaluate their return in more ways than solely the classic financial models.[8] This argument is based on the belief that AIMS will provide more transparent access to patient data, decision support, alerts, and improved patient care, with decreased effort associated with delivery of that care. As Dr. Frisse points out, "To the healthcare professional, the true ROI may be measured in terms of ease of use, total expended effort, and satisfaction with the results achieved."[8] Therefore, organizations should fully appreciate the implications of deploying an AIMS and understand the compelling arguments that support the decision to purchase such a system.

The contributors to this text obviously are evangelists of AIMS and truly do believe that these systems help to deliver better patient care and, just as importantly, help to document that better care was delivered.

Current projections suggest that AIMS have penetrated ~7% of their potential market, but that market penetration is expected to grow to 25% prior to 2010. The reasons given for this projection are varied but primarily focus on the diffusion of innovation[9] and the necessity of hospitals to effectively manage OR costs and revenue. According to the 2005 Frost & Sullivan report, 4908 surgical services were operating in the US in 2003.[10] Total costs of surgical services were $183 billion, or $37 million per surgical service on average, which amounts to an average cost per surgery of $18,380. Therefore, if a surgical service were to implement an AIMS and realize even a 1% reduction in costs, this would equate to a savings of ~$370,000 per year and result in a recovery of the implementation expense within 2–3 years.[10] In actuality, Frost & Sullivan believe that effective implementation of electronic clinical information systems may be able to generate nearly a 5% reduction in costs, or over $1.86 million annually. Additionally, most of these systems improve charge capture, resulting in increased reimbursement and a more rapid recovery of the cost of implementation. The ability to improve reimbursement and reduce expenses will be further detailed elsewhere in this text. Therefore, in the remainder of this chapter, we will focus on the other intangible factors that we feel will have an equally important role in driving the increasing market penetration of AIMS.

Information Technology to Improve Safety

The report issued in 2000 by the Institute of Medicine, *To Err is Human: Building a Safer Health System*, brought national attention to patient safety and prompted coordinated efforts at reducing errors.[11] In addition to the unnecessary deaths, errors were responsible for $17–29 billion in financial losses. The IOM report called for a concerted effort at creating tools, protocols, and research studies to enhance the science behind patient safety. The 2001 follow-up report, entitled *Crossing the Quality Chasm: A New Health System for the 21st Century*, called for increased focus on six healthcare goals, referred to by the acronym STEEEP: safety, timeliness, effective, efficient, equity, and patient centered.[12] This report specifically indicated that electronic systems could support quality improvement and potentially eliminate errors through computerized physician order entry, automated reminders, clinical decision support, and an alignment of financial incentives for both patients and practitioners.

An outstanding example of using an AIMS to improve patient safety was recently demonstrated by Kheterpal et al.;[13] they were able to review a large data set of anesthesia cases and correlate some specific variables to the development of renal failure postoperatively in patients who were not expected to develop this complication. This type of study is a great example of the power of a database of clinical information that is meaningfully tied to outcomes.

Core Measures

Various government agencies, such as The Joint Commission, the Leapfrog Group, the Institute for Safe Medication Practices, and the Institute for Healthcare Improvement, began to advocate adoption of electronic clinical information systems toward reducing errors at the point of care. In 1997, The Joint Commission initiated the collection of outcome measurements, referred to as ORYX data. Starting in 2002, hospitals were required to report specific "core" measures that were collected and compared with those of other hospitals. Beginning in 2004, in collaboration with the Centers for Medicare and Medicaid Services (CMS), The Joint Commission defined these core measures as hospital quality measures, and both organizations required them for comparative analysis.[14] Today, all hospitals are clearly focused on capturing and improving these core measures. Most hospital administrators who must operate within budgeted dollars to purchase new clinical information systems are becoming keenly interested in using these expensive electronic systems to capture and report core measures. Therefore, in addition to reducing costs and increasing reimbursements, AIMS can help hospitals to capture critical data elements necessary for reporting to regulatory and accrediting agencies. In fact, CMS has begun to reimburse physicians and hospitals for reporting quality data through the Physicians Quality Reporting Initiative and the Reporting Hospital Quality Data for Annual Payment Update programs, respectively.

As Dr. Mark Frisse eloquently describes, electronic records must be able to provide a better environment for improving patient safety and enhancing workflow.[8] National efforts at improving patient safety and demonstrating that each institution is a highly reliable organization have become status quo.[15] Seven years after the IOM's shocking revelation that our healthcare system is not perfect, leaders have finally accepted the reality that we must focus on process improvement and safer patient care. As we attempt to achieve demonstrable improvements, most will attest that paper-based efforts are too imperfect and too cost prohibitive.

Surgical Care Improvement Program

Subsequent to the IOM reports noted earlier, additional attention has been directed toward reducing surgical errors and improving outcomes. Primary among these efforts is the Surgical Care Improvement Project (SCIP), a national partnership of organizations under the auspices of both the CMS and the Centers for Disease Control and Prevention (CDC) that is focused on improving surgical care, with a goal of reducing postoperative complications by 25% nationally by 2010.[16] Toward this end, the SCIP initiative primarily assesses major outcomes such as surgical-site infections; postoperative sepsis; and respiratory, cardiovascular, and thromboembolic complications.[17] The SCIP initiative was patterned after the National Surgical Quality Improvement Program (NSQIP)—a successful risk-adjusted database of perioperative outcomes that contains over one million surgical encounters.

With these data, the Veterans' Health Administration (VHA) was able to compare performance among all VHA hospitals using standard surgical outcomes. Merely by capturing the relevant data and providing comparative analysis, the VHA was able to improve the performance levels of its hospitals.[18] Private hospitals and surgical groups became interested in this effort and created the American College of Surgeon's NSQIP (ACS NSQIP) program. However, it remains to be seen whether the private-sector hospitals involved in this subsequent effort will be able to reproduce the VHA's results. The primary difference is that unlike private hospitals, the VHA uses a standardized EMR in all of its hospitals. One standardized system facilitates comprehensive data collection for surgical encounters at each institution and allows for comparison between hospitals. In NSQIP's first 10 years, the 30-day postoperative mortality for major surgery decreased by 27%—from 3.1% in 1991 to 2.2% in 2002. An even more dramatic decline was seen in postoperative morbidity. The number of patients undergoing major surgery in the NSQIP who experienced one or more of 20 predefined postoperative complications decreased from 17.8 to 9.8% over 10 years. At the same time, the median length of stay declined by 5 days. It is unlikely that there has been a better demonstration of the value of electronic health records. The combination of an increased focus on reporting of core measures, SCIP initiatives, and better risk assessment is clearly leading to a scenario where paper records will be inadequate. Unless all hospitals adopt electronic records with standardized nomenclature and semantics, it will be a long time before we are able to achieve a real impact on patient safety and improved surgical outcomes.

Outcome Analysis and Performance Improvement

At the Long-term Outcome Workshop sponsored by the APSF in September 2004, Dr. Robert Lagasse suggested that EMR systems may be able to enhance our ability to link intraoperative events to short- and long-term outcomes but that this effort is currently hindered by the "relative lack of sound risk-adjustment models to assess outcomes independent of the many underlying variables that can affect them."[19] Studies have demonstrated that patients with more extensive comorbid conditions and more complex surgical procedures may have different surgical outcomes than those with less severe conditions or simpler procedures;[20] however, an effective predictive model that correlates readily available patient data with hard outcomes such as length of stay, total costs of care, and mortality has not been identified. Prediction of outcomes based on risk-adjustment models was first demonstrated by Charlson.[21] The ASA Physical Status Classification inadequately predicts perioperative outcomes primarily because of a lack of consideration of surgical factors as confounding variables.[22] Khuri and the group[23] responsible for the VHA NSQIP study were able to demonstrate better predictive values with a system based on preoperative classification of comorbid conditions and ASA Physical Status.

Unfortunately, the capture of preoperative medical conditions continues to occur predominately in paper format and is often fragmented, thus limiting its usefulness.

Capture of this information into an AIMS that is made available to anesthesiologists allows for more proactive assessment and management of surgical patients. Chapter 9 includes a more comprehensive discussion of this model and a description of the positive value of gaining access to those data. Ideally, a fully implemented AIMS that commences the moment a patient is scheduled for surgery would allow better assessment of surgical patients, possibly segregating the preoperative management into different care pathways that are dependent upon risk stratification. Again, this function is literally impossible in the current "paper world."

Without an AIMS, the ability to adequately establish and monitor clinical effectiveness and quality improvement may be severely hampered. Handwritten anesthesia records poorly reflect the true incidence of adverse intraoperative events that are linked to mortality,[24] whereas an AIMS may be able to establish the causes that led to the adverse event which would otherwise be unknown.[25] Unfortunately, current AIMS without sophisticated decision support systems typically require a degree of self-reporting of adverse events, and as such, actual occurrence rates may be underreported and potentially underestimated.[26] Vigoda et al.[27] were able to demonstrate that use of interventions such as education, workflow integration, and individual feedback dramatically increased the compliance rate of comprehensive documentation. Their findings showed that improved user interface designs are critical to enhanced documentation. Continual feedback from users to the vendors of AIMS should ultimately facilitate the ease of documentation and thoroughness of record completion.

National Patient Safety Goals

All anesthesia departments and, ultimately, all anesthesiologists are compelled to participate in a formal process improvement plan if they currently staff an accredited facility. Primarily under the oversight of The Joint Commission or other accrediting organizations, such as the Accreditation Association for Ambulatory Health Care or the American Accreditation Association of Ambulatory Surgical Facilities, healthcare facilities must demonstrate a well-documented effort at quality improvement. These efforts include (a) identification of errors and other patient care concerns and (b) methodology to address and correct these concerns. The inability to correlate paper documentation to actual events has led to modification of the accreditation process and prompted The Joint Commission to adopt unannounced surveys with "tracer methodology" in an attempt to drive measurement of indicators closer to patient encounters. In 2003, The Joint Commission also began to publish National Patient Safety Goals based on reported sentinel events.[28] In particular, specific safety goals that are applicable to an anesthesia practice concern the following:

- Goal 1—patient identification ("time-out"), using two patient identifiers
- Goal 2—effective communication among care providers (read-back provisions on orders, "do not use" list of abbreviations, effective handoff communication)
- Goal 3—medication safety (labeled syringes, standardized drug concentrations)

- Goal 7—reduced healthcare-associated infections (use of hand hygiene, reporting of loss of function secondary to infection as a sentinel event)
- Goal 8—medication reconciliation (accurate list of all medications at every phase of care)
- Goal 13—as a safety strategy, encouragement of patients to be active participants in their care (define means for patients and families to report concerns)
- Goal 15—identification of patient safety risks inherent in the patient population

All of these patient safety goals have been facilitated through the application of AIMS. For example, in an attempt to reduce wrong-site surgery and improve communication, each procedure should be preceded by a "time-out" during which the surgeon, OR staff, and anesthesia provider pause to verify the correct patient, surgical site, objective of the surgery, and availability of equipment required. Documentation of compliance is critical to compliance with Joint Commission standards. More important, an AIMS makes this information available to all interested parties so that deficiencies can be corrected prior to the final time-out. Electronic records have the ability to provide this functionality and to credibly document the actual timing of the time-out (Fig. 1.1).

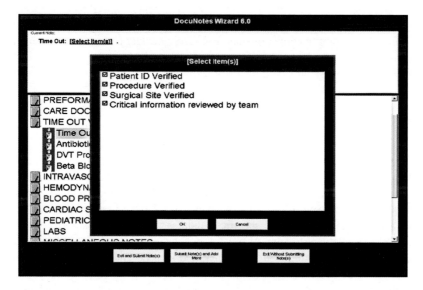

Fig. 1.1 Time-out checklist (screen shot courtesy of DocuSys, Inc., Mobile, AL)

Adverse Events

In addition to documenting actions required for Joint Commission compliance, anesthesia departments must demonstrate that they participate in an active program for evaluating and responding to adverse events. Obviously, any sentinel event will require a detailed analysis and performance of a root-cause analysis; however, many adverse events may be considered "near misses" and consequently serve as a means of identifying potential risk and system problems (Goal 15). Capture of specific events during an anesthetic is facilitated by an AIMS. For example, instances of difficult airway management can be documented and collated as a report made available to the department chairman or compliance officer. Occasional difficulty with airway management is to be expected, but chronic recurrence, particularly with one specific provider, may indicate that the provider has a competency problem or that a system problem exists, such as inadequate equipment or inadequate preoperative evaluation.

Maintenance of Certification in Anesthesiology

As part of their Maintenance of Certification in Anesthesiology, anesthesiologists who are certified by the American Board of Anesthesiology after 2000 are required to provide documentation of ongoing self-assessment and lifelong learning, continual professional standing assessment, and periodic self-directed assessments of practice performance and quality improvement; they must also regularly undergo an examination of cognitive expertise. In the paper world, coordinating, tracking, and documenting compliance with these requirements entail significant manpower and an additional burden to most anesthesia departments. An AIMS can automatically generate an accounting of the number of each type of case, procedures performed, and complications encountered. The management of this information remains the purview of the department, and illustrating capture of these data is essential to the American Board of Anesthesiology.

Committee on Performance and Outcomes Measurement

The ASA has recognized the crucial role of performance improvement and has taken a leadership role in establishing guidelines for its members. The Committee on Performance and Outcomes Measurement (CPOM) was created to establish guidance and leadership in this area (ASA Bylaws 7.162). In accordance with the ASA's strategic plan, one of the specific mandates for CPOM was:

Create a mechanism to support practice management programs, improve communications and marketing of the specialty, and identify and promote professional opportunities. (Goal 2)

Within this goal, *Objective 2.5* further stipulated, "Develop a mechanism for measuring performance and clinical outcomes." With consideration of this objective, a national database for reporting adverse perioperative outcomes was created. Although the CPOM feels that this type of clinical repository will eventually become a mandate (particularly after the VHA NSQIP demonstrated improved care across their entire network of hospitals), the costs of this data collection and analysis can be prohibitive. As the entire industry moves toward collection of discrete data elements of patient care and outcomes, the rationale will become compelling to develop a national database of performance measures to be maintained by the ASA. The ASA CPOM has already established Guiding Principles for the Development of Performance Measures. We believe that the ASA will continue to take a lead in establishing the role of AIMS in this national database by setting standards for data capture, semantics, and ontology of care events; in fact, the ASA has charged at least two of its committees to begin formulating the standards required to establish a national database for anesthesia. Chapters 6 and 7 of this book discuss data standards for interfacing to other systems and monitors. Chapter 6 specifically discusses the efforts of the Data Dictionary Task Force, which was initially sponsored by the APSF as a subsidiary organization of the ASA and has evolved into the International Organization for Terminology in Anesthesia.

Pay for Performance

Growing frustration at the inability to substantially reduce errors has begun to force payers to seek value-based purchasing through pay-for-performance (P4P) initiatives aimed at inducing healthcare providers to do a better job. Concerned that the insurance industry may develop payment incentives without proper guidance, several physician groups initiated discussions regarding appropriate parameters for establishing incentive programs. In 2004, a conference of 250 physicians and medical managers was convened under the auspices of the Johns Hopkins University and a for-profit organization known as American Healthways. From this conference, a consensus statement was proposed that included design principles for metric attributes, data collection, and incentives. Foremost among these design principles was the necessity to have measures based on scientific evidence, with the least data collection burden. The consensus statement was adopted by the ASA House of Delegates in 2006 as the Principles for Quality Incentive Programs in Anesthesiology. In this document, the ASA states that (a) performance incentive programs must be designed to allow their adoption with minimal administrative burden and cost and (b) electronic clinical records are desirable in this regard. However, the current level of market penetration would make this suggestion too restrictive to be a prerequisite for participation.

Examples of potential P4P measures that meet the recommended criteria include:

1. Timing and choice of antibiotics
2. Maintenance of normothermia for colorectal surgery
3. Maintenance of perioperative serum glucose at or below 200 mg/dL during cardiac surgery
4. Appropriate use of perioperative beta blockade

These measures reflect processes that are directly under the control of anesthesiologists. It is fairly easy to envision how an AIMS could assist in the documentation and reporting of these measures. An AIMS may also be necessary to ensure that evidence-based process measures are continually linked to the best possible outcomes. Along those lines, the ASA CPOM has proposed that the mere use of an AIMS be promoted as a P4P measure.

Physician Quality Reporting Initiative

Through the Physician Consortium for Performance Improvement (Consortium) that was first convened in March 2000, the American Medical Association (AMA) is a major force in the development of performance measures for physicians. The Consortium comprises more than 100 national medical specialties, the Agency for Healthcare Research and Quality, and the CMS, among others. As put forth in 2000, the original mission of the Consortium was to improve patient health and safety by developing evidence-based clinical performance measures that enhance quality of patient care and that foster accountability. The Consortium's mission changed dramatically in 2006, when the AMA signed a pact with Congress, called the Joint House–Senate Working Agreement. In this document, the AMA promised to develop 140 physician performance measures covering 34 clinical areas. It also agreed that in 2007, doctors would voluntarily report three to five performance measures and would receive additional payment to offset the burden of collecting the data. As a result of this agreement, the President of the US signed the Tax Relief and Health Care Act of 2006, which established the Physician Quality Reporting Initiative under the CMS.[29] Of the 74 current performance measures, only one measure applies to anesthesiologists: timely administration of antibiotics within 60 minutes before incision (see Chap. 14). Provided anesthesiologists achieve an 80% compliance with reporting this measure, they would be entitled to a 1.5% bonus payment on all Medicare payments over the time period that the measure was reported. Effective July 1, 2007, the initial incentive program was designed to run only the latter half of the year and typically represented less than a $10,000 bonus for most groups. Many physicians have questioned the rationale of attempting to change their systems to capture this information and report the appropriate CPT Category II codes for such a nominal reimbursement. AIMS users should be able to easily incorporate these changes into their systems with minimal data collection burden.

As pay-for-reporting evolves to P4P with set compliance goals, AIMS functions will also evolve. For example, to be compliant with measures of perioperative antibiotic administration, AIMS can incorporate prompts to remind anesthesia providers of the need for antibiotic dosing, appropriate antibiotic selection, and timely redosing.[30,31] These simple AIMS prompts can also affect a hospital's bottom line. In 2006, hospitals received a 0.4% increase in their market basket update if they reported certain performance measures, among which was the administration of perioperative antibiotics. In 2007, amendments to the Deficit Reduction Act increased this 0.4%–2% of the market basket update. Additionally, in ongoing efforts to link quality to payment, CMS has proposed that in 2008 hospitals not be allowed to bill Medicare for hospital-acquired conditions, such as postoperative wound infections.

One of the founding principles of P4P is that the incentive to improve quality measures exists only where a gap between actual practice and ideal practice exists. Once the majority of anesthesiologists demonstrate compliance with a measure, it will likely be retired as an incentive measure. Without the use of an AIMS, it is unclear how any anesthesia group could possibly adapt to what may be a rapidly changing landscape with frequently evolving measures.

Measuring Quality

Since the eye-opening report by the IOM, healthcare providers and hospitals have become as concerned as healthcare consumers about who in fact is providing quality healthcare. This concern has led to critical evaluations of the relationship between processes of care and healthcare outcomes by a wide spectrum of stakeholders, including patients, healthcare providers, researchers, politicians, the media, and others.[32] These same groups are seeking comparisons of healthcare outcomes, identification of best practices, and public accountability. One of the most common methodologies of comparing providers uses risk-adjusted mortality rates. Organizations (such as the Leapfrog Group and Healthgrades.com) that publish performance ratings often use this methodology to compare hospitals and physicians.[33, 34] However, as demonstrated in a recent review article, risk-adjusted mortality rates are poor indicators of quality of care.[35]

Quality Metrics

The focus on measuring quality has gained increased importance as payments become aligned with reportable measures that are thought to demonstrate quality. Much of this effort has arisen primarily because consumers and the government perceive that healthcare organizations have not risen to the challenge of improving safety and quality. As reported by the Medicare Payment Advisory Commission to Congress in 2004, Medicare beneficiaries, mirroring trends in care for the rest of the population, face "significant gaps between care known to be effective and the care delivered," especially where patient safety issues are concerned.[36] Currently, we predominately use reporting metrics to quantify healthcare entities into percentiles of quality providers. Pronovost et al.[37] commented in an editorial in *JAMA* that tracking progress in patient safety is an elusive target. In that article, they describe many of the problems and dilemmas associated with reporting measures and how surveillance bias could arbitrarily cause the illusion that one provider has a higher frequency of poor measures than another provider. They also provide a new measurement model that incorporates a culture survey into the calculations and primarily asks: how often are patients harmed, how often do we learn from our mistakes, and has a safe culture been created?

Information Technology to Measure Quality

As we filter through the various policy changes that will occur in the next few years, healthcare providers will be tasked with an ever-expanding set of clinical performance measures to quantify and qualify demonstration of quality and safety. These tasks will essentially be impossible with a paper-based clinical record. As the science of safety expands, providers are becoming increasingly aware of the integration between safety and the organization where the care is rendered. Simply focusing efforts on identifying and quantifying errors has not optimized the safety of our patients.[38] As a result, Rozich et al.[39] have proposed the use of "trigger tools" to measure and detect events related to patient harm. This methodology (a) identifies adverse events in the medical record that are ultimately linked to patient harm and (b) may provide a wider view of potentially problematic areas on which to focus attention. In the context of an AIMS, it is possible to establish trigger tools within the normal collection of monitoring data that provide real-time alerts and indications of clinical scenarios that may lead to harm. Advancing the interaction between an AIMS and the user should lead not only to a safer environment, but also to documentation that can demonstrate action and reaction to patient safety concerns as they occur.

Conclusion

We are convinced that AIMS are here to stay and that one can either embrace the technology and help to shape it or vainly try to avoid the changes that are on the way. AIMS are likely to follow a similar adoption pathway as other technologic advances such as pulse oximetry and capnography, with eventual inclusion into standards of care. With George W. Bush's mandate that the American people need to be served by electronic records by the year 2014, he established a new office within the Department of Health and Human Services—the Office of National Coordinator for Health Information Technology—to promote and coordinate the movement toward total adoption of electronic records. All healthcare providers will one day be using them. Certainly, the AIMS of 2014 will be far different from the commercial versions available today, but the goal may be the same: automatic capture of the processes of care provided so that anesthesiologists can focus primarily on the patient. Subsequent chapters of this text will include illustrations of how

AIMS will provide various opportunities for a return on the capital and behavioral investments. None may be more important than the ability to rapidly and effectively demonstrate that your practice, group, or hospital is providing the highest quality care possible. This capability, from our perspective, represents the single greatest potential rationale for purchasing an AIMS.

Key Points

- Purchase of any information technology requires close scrutiny of the ROI; however, good clinical systems may improve the delivery of healthcare in ways that are not easy to analyze.
- Information technology has been recognized as a key method by which to improve healthcare, and now measurement and reporting of core measures are essential.
- The SCIP initiative has been incorporated into essential performance reporting and is relatively impossible without an AIMS.
- Outcome analysis and performance improvement have become essential components of all departments. The use of an AIMS is critical for these functions.
- The ASA has recognized the movement to AIMS and is developing guidelines for future development, primarily through the Committee on Performance and Outcome Measures.
- P4P has been implemented and will continue to expand. Without an AIMS, groups will not be able to meet the reporting requirements in a cost-effective manner.
- The practice of measuring quality is associated with challenges but will continue to remain a focus of consumers and healthcare purchasers. AIMS hold the promise of enhancing the ability to truly measure quality.

References

1. Gravenstein JS. The automated anesthesia record. Int J Clin Monit Comput 1986; 3:131–4
2. Klocke H, Trispel S, Rau G, et al. An anesthesia information system for monitoring and record keeping during surgical anesthesia. J Clin Monit Comput 1986; 2:246–61
3. Anesthesia Patient Safety Foundation. APSF endorses use of automated record keepers. APSF Newsletter 2001; 16(4):49. http://www.apsf.org/resource_center/newsletter/2001/winter/02ARK.htm. Accessed December 18, 2007
4. Beecher HK. The first anesthesia records (Codman and Cushing). Surg Gynecol Obstet 1940; 71:689–93
5. Bierstein K. Anesthesia information systems...Where awareness is good! ASA Newsletter 2007; 71(3):37–9
6. Koppel R, Metlay JP, Cohen A, et al. Role of computerized physician order entry systems in facilitating medication errors. JAMA 2005; 293:1197–203

7. Kaushal R, Jha AK, Franz C, et al. Return on investment for a computerized physician order entry system. J Am Med Inform Assoc 2006; 13:261–6

8. Frisse ME. Comments on return on investment (ROI) as it applies to clinical systems. J Am Med Inform Assoc 2006; 13:365–7

9. Rogers EM. Diffusion of Innovation, 5th ed. New York: Free Press, 2003

10. U.S. High Acuity Care Information Systems Markets. N07D-48. Palo Alto, CA: Frost & Sullivan, 2006

11. Institute of Medicine. Corrigan J, Kohn L, Donaldson M, eds. To Err Is Human: Building a Safer Health System. Washington, DC: National Academy, 1999

12. Institute of Medicine. Committee on Quality of Health Care in America. Crossing the Quality Chasm: A New Health Care System for the 21st Century. Washington, DC: National Academy, 2001

13. Kheterpal S, Tremper K, Englesbe M, et al. Predictors of postoperative acute renal failure after noncardiac surgery in patients with previously normal renal function. Anesthesiology 2007; 107:892–902

14. Facts about ORYX for hospitals, core measures, and hospital core measures. http://www. jointcommission.org/AccreditationPrograms/Hospitals/ORYX/oryx_facts.htm. Accessed June 15, 2007

15. Institute for Healthcare Improvement. IHI Innovation Series white paper. Improving the Reliability of Health Care. Boston, MA: Institute for Healthcare Improvement, 2004

16. Surgical Care Improvement Project. http://www.aha.org/aha/issues/Quality-and-Patient-Safety/scip.html. Accessed June 15, 2007

17. Bratzler DW, Hunt DR. The surgical infection prevention and surgical care improvement projects: National initiatives to improve outcomes for patients having surgery. Clin Infect Dis 2006; 43(3):322–30

18. Khuri S, Daley J, Henderson WG. The comparative assessment and improvement of quality of surgical care in the Department of Veterans Affairs. Arch Surg 2002; 137:20–7

19. APSF Long-term Workshop on Outcomes. http://www.apsf.org/assets/Documents/APSF_LTO_Wkshop_Report.pdf. Accessed December 18, 2007

20. Daley J, Henderson WG, Khuri SF. Risk-adjusted surgical outcomes. Annu Rev Med 2001; 52:275–87

21. Charlson ME, Pompei P, Ales KL, et al. A new method of classifying prognostic comorbidity in longitudinal studies: Development and validation. J Chronic Dis 1987; 40:373–83

22. Macario A, Vitez TS, Dunn B, et al. Hospital costs and severity of illness in three types of elective surgery. Anesthesiology 1997; 86:92–100

23. Khuri SF, Daley J, Henderson WG, et al. The National VA Surgical Risk Study: Risk adjustment for the comparative assessment of the quality of surgical care. J Am Coll Surg 1995; 180:519–31

24. Sanborn KV, Castro J, Kuroda M, et al. Detection of intraoperative incidents by electronic scanning of computerized anesthesia records. Comparison with voluntary reporting. Anesthesiology 1996; 85:977–87

25. Thrush DN. Automated anesthesia records and anesthetic incidents. J Clin Monit Comput 1992; 8:59–61

26. Benson M, Junger A, Fuchs C, et al. Using an anesthesia information management system to prove a deficit in voluntary reporting of adverse events in a quality assurance program. J Clin Monit Comput 200; 16:211–7

27. Vigoda M, Gencorelli F, Lubarsky D. Changing medical group behaviors: Increasing the rate of documentation of quality assurance events using an anesthesia information system. Anesth Analg 2006; 103(2):390–5

28. National Patient Safety Goals. http://www.jointcommission.org/PatientSafety/NationalPatient SafetyGoals/. Accessed December 18, 2007

29. Medicare Physician Quality Reporting Initiative Fact Sheet. http://www.cms.hhs.gov/PQRI. Accessed June 20, 2007

30. O'Reilly M, Talsma A, VanRiper S, et al. An anesthesia information system designed to provide physician-specific feedback improves timely administration of prophylactic antibiotics. Anesth Analg 2006; 103:908–12
31. Wax DB, Beilin Y, Levin M, et al. The effect of an interactive visual reminder in an anesthesia information management system on timeliness of prophylactic antibiotic administration. Anesth Analg 2007; 104(6):1462–6
32. Jacobson B, Mindell J, McKee M. Hospital mortality league tables: Question what they tell you—and how useful they are. Br Med J 2003; 326(7393):777–8
33. Leapfrog Group. http://www.leapfroggroup.org/home. Accessed June 25, 2007
34. Healthgrades.com. Web site: http://www.healthgrades.com/. Accessed June 25, 2007
35. Pitches D, Mohammed M, Lilford R. What is the empirical evidence that hospitals with higher-risk adjusted mortality rates provide poorer quality care? A systematic review of the literature. BMC Health Serv Res 2007; 7:91
36. Medicare Advisory Commission focuses on quality of care, patient safety. Qual Lett Healthc Lead 2004; 16(4):10–1
37. Pronovost P, Miller M, Wachter R. Tracking progress in patient safety. JAMA 2006; 296(6):696–9
38. Rozich J, Haraden C, Resar R. Adverse drug event trigger tool: A practical methodology for measuring medication related harm. Qual Saf Health Care 2003; 12:194–200
39. Resar R, Rozich J, Classen D. Methodology and rationale for the measurement of harm with trigger tools. Qual Saf Health Care 2003; 12(Suppl II):ii39–ii45

Chapter 2
The Vendor–Customer Relationship

Stanley Muravchick

No off-the-shelf solution exists for electronic anesthesia record keeping and perioperative information management. Every AIMS is installed in a unique environment of equipment and hardware, software and network parameters, interconnected databases, and clinical workflow. Every vendor's AIMS, regardless of how highly developed and mature it is at the time of sale, requires reconfiguration and customization to meet the needs of the customer's administrative and clinical end users. Therefore, every AIMS implementation project should have a designated Anesthesia Clinical Leader (ACL)—a clinically experienced physician or certified registered nurse anesthetist, who can accurately anticipate the extent to which the vendor's software must be modified to suit the users and to what extent the users must be asked to change their workflow patterns to accommodate the AIMS software. Assuming that adequate resources have been allocated for technical support of the AIMS, these decisions and the extent to which they are supported and adopted by the other users become the primary determinants of successful AIMS implementation and operation. Continuing cooperation and clear channels of communication between the vendor and the customer are necessary to optimize the "goodness of fit" between the vendor's product and the needs of the customer. Several basic areas that must be considered are discussed in detail in the following sections.

Adapting to the Clinical Environment

After the contract for AIMS implementation has been signed, the vendor's and the institution's implementation teams meet to define roles and develop contact information and meeting schedules. The vendor's hardware expert should survey every workstation location to identify equipment in use, data port availability and configurations, and electrical and network connectivity. Availability of AIMS driver software (digital data interfaces) must be confirmed for every input device and physiologic monitor included in the AIMS installation. The vendor's hardware expert must devise a hardware-mounting solution at each anesthetizing location and, working with the ACL, ensure that it is compatible with the customer's clinical workflow requirements. The customer's Implementation Project Manager (IPM)

J. Stonemetz, K. Ruskin (eds.) *Anesthesia Informatics*,
© Springer Science+Business Media, LLC 2008

advises the vendor's installation and implementation team regarding the institution's security processes for personnel and equipment, the layout of the OR suite and recovery areas, and times during which anesthetizing locations and equipment can be accessed without disrupting the OR schedule.

Changing Customer Workflow to Fit the AIMS

Clinical workflow patterns and requirements can be defined and, if necessary, modified only by the customer, ideally through the ACL. Even with a well-designed AIMS, resistance to change by clinicians can be formidable. To have a successful implementation, the customer must inform the vendor of workflow details such as how surgical patients will be identified and how their account numbers will be confirmed before initiating the AIMS. Is the data manually obtained from the hospital chart, transferred electronically from the OR scheduling database, or optically scanned from an encoded wristband? The customer must decide what computer workstations will be used for reviewing and completing the anesthesia preoperative assessment and how and where the anesthesiologists will review records and complete missing data elements prior to record closure. Is a paper copy of the anesthesia record needed by the institution? If so, how and where will it be generated, are specific format requirements dictated by the institution, and who will pass the hardcopy on to those providing postoperative patient care?

Other important considerations include an assessment of anesthesia-related clinical workflow in ambulatory surgery areas, obstetric floors, ICUs, and off-site anesthetizing locations such as endoscopy and radiology suites. Rarely does the anesthesiologist have significant control over these work environments. Even finding a place to install an AIMS workstation may be a challenge, and physiologic monitoring equipment in these areas may not be compatible with, or accessible by, the AIMS. If available from the vendor, a cart-based mobile AIMS computer system configuration, with or without attached physiologic monitoring devices, may be the best choice for locations where delivery of anesthetic care often moves from one procedure room to the next. However, this approach is substantially more expensive than a fixed workstation and requires that the customer provide reliable wireless network access to the AIMS server, secure overnight storage, and define responsibility for physical maintenance and recharging of battery packs. It may also require that the ACL engage in extensive discussion and negotiation with the radiologists, cardiologists, obstetricians, and nursing personnel, who must also accommodate the changes in their working environment that are created by the installation of an AIMS.

Changing the AIMS to Fit the Customer's Workflow

The IPM and ACL communicate the customer's expectations to the vendor with regard to integration of the AIMS-related workflow into existing clinical practice patterns. Most AIMS vendors offer user-selectable, subspecialty-specific (e.g., out-patient, pediatric, cardiac) screen templates for which lists of drugs, fluids, and procedure documentation comments can be configured by the subspecialist anesthesiologists themselves. This adaptability makes the AIMS appear more user friendly and promotes end user "buy in" to the transition from paper record to AIMS through an increased sense of control over change. However, it also requires a substantial contribution of time and effort by the various end users to establish consensus regarding the preferences of the anesthesia providers.

Modifications of the AIMS that go beyond selectable templates and drop-down lists to produce truly different versions of the AIMS, even if agreed to by the vendor, can be expected to generate expensive increases in implementation time and human resources. Excessive customization and modification increases the difficulties associated with training end users and adequately training IT support personnel to provide AIMS troubleshooting, maintenance, and software upgrades. It may also produce unintended adverse consequences with regard to overall AIMS stability, leading to delays and disruption of the implementation schedule.

If extensive configuration changes or user-selected options are considered essential by the ACL, it may be practical to identify a secure nonclinical demonstration site for installation of a prototype AIMS workstation and a test server. A test system requires that the institution make available a complete anesthesia delivery and physiologic monitoring system that will not be available for clinical use for several months. Alternatively, the vendor's AIMS test workstation may be able to provide a demonstration mode that generates simulated physiologic data, a less-desirable but still valuable approach. Regardless of how the AIMS test system is assembled, it should facilitate evaluation of trial configurations and extensive testing of the user input devices (keyboard, mouse, scanner) and digital data interfaces. In this way, the ACL and IPM can review and revise, if necessary, all versions and options within the clinical and administrative interfaces before AIMS user training and full AIMS implementation.

Adapting to the Customer's Information Systems Environment

Given the complexity of an AIMS, the vendor must be familiar with the customer institution's existing monitoring and anesthesia delivery equipment; its network and server capabilities; and its IT policies, procedures, and maintenance resources. The vendor may need to accommodate a variety of software operating systems within the user's institution, including versions specialized for handheld wireless devices.[1] In turn, the customer should expect the vendor to provide functional diagrams of all hardware and software components, including servers and network hardware, that will be required for the completed AIMS, as well as bandwidth requirements for both hardwired and wireless network access.

At a minimum, an AIMS must receive patient admission/discharge/transfer (ADT) information and surgical schedules, but typically, an interface also exists with the laboratory testing information system. Therefore, the customer should expect the AIMS vendor to provide the necessary data interfaces with these essential existing institutional databases and to consult with the institution's interface specialists or other software vendors as needed. Although most medical data streams use some variety of the industry-standard Health Level 7 (HL7) data format, subtle differences are associated with how data elements are transmitted by different applications. For example, medical record and patient account numbers may be generated by the ADT system with a fixed number of digits but subsequently "stripped" of leading zeroes by the interface when shared with other applications to simplify printing of identification documents.

In consultation with the customer's IPM and ACL, the vendor's implementation team must also specify to the customer's IT personnel how each interface should be configured to "filter" data flow, limiting AIMS data inflow to those elements needed for perioperative care. For example, which preoperative laboratory results should be displayed for each patient and for what time period prior to surgery? Which ADT elements are essential to generate professional services billing statements, and which should be masked to protect patient confidentiality? Troubleshooting and "tweaking" these interfaces can be difficult and time consuming, but it is incumbent upon the vendor to test and verify the accuracy and reliability of interface data transfer for each element needed by the AIMS.

Most essential interface capabilities may already be included in the AIMS software, but some may require the vendor to write a custom interface. Once created and tested, the interfaces between information systems are usually managed by the institutional interface engine already in use by the customer. The essential interfaces for ADT, surgical scheduling, and laboratory data should function in real time; i.e., they should update the AIMS whenever a data transaction occurs in any connected database, rather than through a batch process that occurs once or twice per day.

Most AIMS are Microsoft Windows based and therefore require substantial knowledge of security and database integrity issues of the Microsoft operating system workstation, including routine updates and security patches for both servers and workstations. By sharing and clarifying institutional IT procedures, the customer partners with the vendor in this process of adapting an AIMS to the institutional information system environment. IT departments of large academic institutions and many community hospitals have an established process for adding extra clinical workstations or establishing new user groups on existing networks. Most expect that the personal computer at each AIMS workstation will be initially configured using the customer's standard workstation image. The customer can provide the AIMS vendor with the exact operating system configuration and the applications for remote workstation access and "malware" protection that are currently supported by its IT personnel. These applications are installed under site licenses, and updates are tested and remotely distributed to the workstations by the customer's IT personnel according to a maintenance schedule.

Installation of other institution-supported clinical applications, such as computerized physician order entry or perioperative nursing documentation, to the AIMS workstation should be carefully considered. The ability to access routinely used applications from a single workstation will be a convenience appreciated by the customer's clinical end users. However, the installation of multiple large applications on a single personal computer may require upgraded hardware and will add complexity to the implementation and troubleshooting process, thereby allowing greater probability of unanticipated software incompatibility and system malfunction. Rarely will the vendor be able to provide the customer with examples of proven AIMS reliability at other installation sites that have an identical set of workstation applications. Even if successfully installed, each additional application generates an incremental requirement for workstation downtime because of server reboots and software upgrades and patches. Nevertheless, if the opportunity exists to set up and thoroughly test a demonstration system before full AIMS implementation, it may be reasonable to use AIMS workstations, preferably those outside the OR, for other clinical purposes.

The customer must also review institutional policies with regard to allowing clinical end users access to the Internet from clinical workstations. Some potential benefit is gained by the ability to quickly obtain medically related information from the Web, but Internet access also introduces opportunities for user distraction and data corruption. Protecting the AIMS installation from Internet-based security threats requires isolation of the AIMS servers and workstations behind the institution's firewall. It also requires that the customer and the vendor cooperate with regard to installation of compatible third-party programs to protect the AIMS from viruses, worms, and other sources of application or data corruption that may come from other sites—even those inside the customer's firewall. The customer's IT personnel should also establish a defined disaster and data recovery plan should the AIMS servers be physically damaged. Finally, only the customer can provide the vendor with an accurate picture of institutional and departmental priorities regarding sharing of compliance and regulatory documentation and billing information, estimates of future needs for AIMS expansion, and expectations regarding expanded integration with other databases within the institution.

Cooperating to Realize the Full Potential of an AIMS

Training the Users and Going Live

The importance of selecting appropriate training paradigms for the various AIMS end users cannot be overstated—it remains the most fundamental determinant of eventual user acceptance.[2] Vendors usually provide estimates of the hours of individual and group training that are required for proper training on their AIMS and recommendations regarding the preferred training modality, either in a classroom setting or one-to-one setting at a simulated clinical workstation. Training of technical staff, especially those who provide network and server support, is the responsibility of the vendor and should be explicitly included in the AIMS contract.

The vendor should also train the system administrator to manage the perioperative database and provide administrative personnel with instruction for generating standard and custom reports. Customers should ask for both digital and hardcopy versions of user and administrator manuals for future reference.

The primary role of the end user will determine the best training modality for each user group as well as where the emphasis of the training sessions should be placed. Administrators or billing personnel need to learn how to review completed anesthesia records and will wish to extract information through report generation. Anesthesia providers need to quickly and correctly identify the patient and access existing clinical data, enter additional perioperative data, and open and close the anesthesia record. Nonanesthesia clinician end users such as perioperative nurses or surgery residents may need only rudimentary AIMS training so that they can review perioperative patient information. Also, some group-specific requirements such as completion of attestations of medical direction and supervision are highly important to attending anesthesiologists but do not apply to other anesthesia providers (e.g., residents in training and nurse anesthetists). Additional in-depth training and troubleshooting exercises should be optionally available for a few superusers in each of the user groups. These are individuals who volunteer to champion the AIMS, facilitate the go-live process, and act as an ongoing training resource for their colleagues after go-live. Superusers should have in-depth familiarity with AIMS software, a willingness to assist in decision making regarding configuration changes, and advanced diagnostic skills obtained through the vendor's training process.

Most large institutions already have nursing- or IT-based software training personnel and facilities that are available to train clinical end users of the institution's medical software systems. Working with the vendor, the customer's IT training resource can coordinate the scheduling, content, equipment, and facilities needed for classroom-style sessions. Ideal for administrative and support personnel, classroom sessions are even more effective if they feature hands-on learning with individual workstations that run a training version of the AIMS application. However, the demands of the surgical schedule often make it difficult to relieve clinicians of their OR responsibilities for scheduled classroom sessions. Therefore, unless it is feasible to have off-hour (weekend or evening) classroom instruction, it may be unrealistic for the customer to rely solely on this training modality for a large anesthesia group. Even with these accommodations, some end users will miss all classroom sessions because of vacation, illness, or other commitments.

Other training options for anesthesia providers include unscheduled open, or drop-in, training sessions. An AIMS demonstration system with computer-generated vital signs can be set up for access throughout the workday in a location close to the OR. However, this training modality requires a considerable time commitment and virtually continuous availability of the vendor's trainers or a customer's system champion for at least several days and perhaps a week. Open sessions can be further supplemented by Web-based tutorials that are particularly valuable if some of the customer's clinicians are based at satellite hospitals or move among multiple locations. With a Web-based training system, clinicians can participate in training as their schedule permits. However, providing Web-based content requires substantial vendor support and is not particularly effective for users with limited computer expertise or for advanced training in troubleshooting. Hardcopy "cheat sheets," such as laminated pocket-sized cards that describe the basic keystrokes needed to identify a patient and complete and close an automated anesthesia record file, can be of great value for all anesthesia providers, regardless of their training modality or skill level.

AIMS training in any mode must accommodate the varied skills and attitudes that users bring to the process. Some users are highly computer literate, but others may not be as computer savvy and require additional instruction and encouragement. In addition, timing is important. Concepts and techniques acquired during training are quickly forgotten if they are not immediately reinforced by clinical experience. Training new residents or student anesthetists to use an AIMS is especially challenging because they have not yet acquired a frame of reference for how the AIMS process relates to clinical workflow. Nevertheless, all end users must master basic troubleshooting skills such as confirming the connection to the network and rebooting the workstation. In addition, all "trained" anesthesia providers should be required to demonstrate the ability to generate an anesthetic record that meets departmental standards for accuracy, completeness, and regulatory compliance.

For the AIMS go-live event, the vendor must provide on-site support personnel during normal working hours and rapid-response assistance by telephone or pager during off hours. Therefore, scheduling an AIMS go-live concurrently with other institutional priorities such as The Joint Commission inspections or other large IT implementations should be avoided. Availability of training and implementation resources may actually dictate the customer's preferred approach to go-live. If available customer or vendor resources are not sufficient to train all support staff and end users within a short time span and provide go-live assistance at all anesthetizing locations, an incremental approach, with small user groups trained sequentially in synchrony with the planned sequence for go-live, may be necessary. Even a vendor with limited resources can intensively train a small number of end users who can then function as teachers for those to be trained later as the AIMS is more widely implemented. This train-the-trainers approach also provides the customer with enthusiastic superusers and additional AIMS advocates within the department.

Enhancing User Access

To meet federal regulations designed to protect the confidentiality of patient information, access to an AIMS workstation requires authentication of user identity and confirmation of access privileges. This process can be accomplished with a variety of input devices, including keyboard, magnetic or optical scanning, or biometric identification. Transition from a paper anesthesia record to an AIMS can be facilitated if the vendor is willing to configure the AIMS to use the identification devices and processes already employed at the customer's institution (e.g., for restricted area access or the use of drug or scrub suit dispensers). Sharing the institution's active directory or similar user database can also minimize the administrative workload associated with keeping AIMS user lists current, especially in large departments with active training programs. Additionally, it facilitates immediate and coordinated termination of privileges for employees upon their departure or termination.

Including Additional Informational Databases

Additional interface capability for data exchange may be seen as essential by the ACL and IPM. Because developing custom interfaces is expensive and time consuming, all new interfaces must be implemented through a process that budgets their development costs and defines responsibility for demonstrating proper functionality. Nevertheless, sharing data from the institution's emergency department, blood bank, or computerized physician order entry system may greatly facilitate timely transfer of vital signs, allergies, medications, and difficult airway status. An interface with the institution's pharmacy system permits both drug utilization cost analysis and a mechanism by which to provide detail regarding the use of controlled substances. An interface with the institution's perioperative services or materials management database can be used to log and track the use of disposables, providing both inventory control and charge capture. Similarly, data exchange through interfaces or by integration with the software used for perioperative nursing documentation can minimize redundant keyboard entry for basic patient demographics and synchronize the timing of tracked events, such as entry into the OR, antibiotic administration, and the performance of the patient safety time-out. Academic institutions will have considerable interest in establishing a physiologic data warehouse that can be used to store and organize data for purposes of clinical research. The value of an AIMS for single-site[3] and for multi-institutional collaborative research[4] is now clearly established.

Expanding an AIMS to Nontraditional Sites

The complexity of AIMS implementation increases significantly in non-OR anesthetizing locations or facilities and usually requires innovative and flexible solutions. The scheduling of procedures that require anesthesia care in off-site locations may not follow the same process that is used for scheduling surgical procedures, and clinical workflow is often characterized by intermittent anesthesia care interspersed with intervals without billable activity. The vendor must configure the AIMS to deal with discontinuous anesthesia billing time if the customer expects that the AIMS will be used in such locations. In particular, obstetric services with a large number of emergency or add-on patients may reveal the shortcomings of the patient identification process used by an AIMS. Similar situations exist in endoscopy suites and cardiac electrophysiologic and catheterization laboratories.

Maximizing Clinical Efficiency

An AIMS could be used to provide automated interservice communication to optimize patient care, e.g., by alerting the anesthesia pain service when a patient with an epidural is ready for postoperative care. An AIMS could also be configured to query the physiologic database in near real time to identify significant variations from acceptable limits and then to warn clinicians using automated paging. Other back-end, real-time processes might search the AIMS database for documentation completeness or missing attestations and then page the attending anesthesiologist to provide the missing data[5] or alert the anesthesia provider immediately when data are lost or other internal AIMS inconsistencies develop.[6]

Once implemented, each AIMS also offers ample opportunity for customization and integration with ancillary software modules that can perform tasks beyond those initially intended by the AIMS vendor, including procedure and diagnosis coding and specialized billing functions using unique business rules preferred by the customer's institution.[7,8] Custom enhancements to an AIMS might also include "clinical contexting," which permits access to all patient-related data from a single workstation and integration of AIMS physiologic data flow with "expert system" software that supports real-time clinical decision making.

Applying Innovative Technology

Many computer-based peripheral technologies that are quickly adopted in the retail or industrial environment are slow to be incorporated into medical systems such as AIMS. Bar-coded packaging, radio-frequency identification for object and patient tracking and location, voice recognition user interfaces, and heads-up graphic display projection are only a few examples of technology with great potential for use within an AIMS. The feasibility has already been established of automated real-time tracking of IV drug administration with barcoding and digital imaging for confirmation of drug dosage, as well as crosschecking for unwanted drug interactions.[9] With cooperation between vendor and customer, application of advanced programming techniques such as object-oriented analysis could also broaden the range of activities supported by an AIMS to new areas of education and research.[10]

Vendors of medical information systems can justify the investment of funds required for the research and development of these techniques and technologies only when a compelling business case for their development has been demonstrated.

As in other areas, the adoption of these technologies is driven by customer demand rather than by vendor initiative. Physicians in particular tend to be conservative and slow to change their routine clinical practice unless compelled to do so by regulatory or financial considerations. However, the greater the awareness of AIMS customers of the potential benefit of these technologies and the more strongly their availability is requested during contract negotiations with vendors, the sooner innovation will be a common feature of AIMS and other complex medical information systems.

Working Together for Mutual Benefit

Contracts

Contracts define terms and specify what is expected of both parties with regard to costs and deliverables. Regardless of verbal assurances, it is unrealistic for the customer to assume, or for the vendor's salesperson to imply, that any hardware, intellectual property, or services not specifically included in the contract should be provided by the AIMS vendor without additional charge. Many large institutions already have a master contract with an AIMS vendor that is largely devoted to defining terms and legal remedies related to contractual obligations. For purchase of an AIMS, a supplemental contract details software, hardware, installation, pricing, and dates and terms of delivery and completion. The final payment can be made contingent upon meeting the acceptance criteria itemized in the contract, and it is not unusual for the entire contractual payment schedule to be linked to achievement of specific installation milestones.

Although regulations are dynamic and each institution is different, the Sarbanes-Oxley Act and other federal and state requirements have created a general acceptance of the fact that financial relationships between institutional employees and the AIMS vendor must be completely and freely disclosed. Conflict-of-interest policies that preclude employees or faculty members from exerting influence on financial decisions if they have a significant direct or indirect financial interest in the vendor are almost universal. For example, if an anesthesiologist has received honoraria or research support from an AIMS vendor, that person may not be involved in the selection of the AIMS vendor or in contract negotiations without full disclosure of potential conflicts to all parties.

Negotiating and Accepting Compromise

The modification of well-established clinical workflow patterns, the physical disruption, and the training required for AIMS implementation often make it a lightning rod for complaints and criticism directed at the vendor. The ACL and

IPM must articulate the most important customer expectations with regard to the final appearance and functionality of the clinical and administrative user interfaces and the AIMS database. They also must communicate those expectations clearly to the vendor well in advance of the AIMS go-live event. Such communication can be accomplished with a contractual document such as a list of acceptance criteria that, if met, confirm to both vendor and customer that AIMS implementation is complete and acceptable. Acceptance criteria also help to clarify the customer's concept of which essential functions must be provided by the AIMS in order to go, and to stay, paperless.

Given the complexity of an AIMS and the extent to which it must fulfill many future needs of many parties within the institution, it may also be helpful to add a scope-of-project document as an appendix to the contract for an AIMS purchase and implementation. This jointly authored document should list, in succinct terms, what features, services, or warranties are, or are not, included in the initial contract between vendor and customer. Items that may typically be included or excluded in a scope-of-project document include annual retraining of personnel, installation of future AIMS software upgrades, automated physician concurrency tracking, customized clinical research reports, and periodic revision of wording in compliance-related documentation. It is unfair to the vendor for the customer to assume that functionality or services not specified as deliverables in either the acceptance criteria or scope-of-project documents will nevertheless be supplied by the AIMS vendor.

Codevelopment of AIMS Enhancements and Upgrades

Most early AIMS were installed in academic medical centers that had in-house informatics expertise and well-established IT infrastructures. The academic centers also had administrative staff and established policies to handle financial relationships between medical center employees or school of medicine faculty and the private sector. Therefore, many intellectual property partnerships were formed between academic centers and the AIMS industry.

However, community medical centers also offer ample opportunities for the customer and vendor to work together to advance general recognition of the advantages of an AIMS and to continually refine and improve the ability of an AIMS to contribute to high-quality, cost-effective perioperative patient care. One example of enhanced collaboration is using an AIMS to generate a score that is predictive of a patient's risk of nausea and vomiting and to recommend customized prophylactic therapy for this anesthetic complication.[11] A second example is for a center to serve as a vendor's demonstration site and thereby gain prestige in the community and an advantageous position with regard to the vendor's product development process. Any costs associated with hosting site visits from prospective AIMS customers are assumed by the vendor, including compensation for the time required by physician and support staff who might be asked to "meet and greet" visitors to their institution.

Establishing a Formal Agreement for Product Development

The vendor and the customer can share their knowledge, experience, and innovative concepts for mutual benefit in several other ways. It may be useful to both parties if the customer organizes a voluntary group of users or superusers who can meet on a regular basis once the AIMS implementation is complete. The group can review the strengths and weaknesses of the final installed product and make suggestions for improvements to be included in subsequent upgrades. The vendor receives valuable feedback regarding the performance of the product, and the customer gains a clear and consistent channel of communication with the vendor to facilitate the incorporation of desired improvements in future product upgrades.

Another option, particularly at academic medical centers, is to establish a formal, vendor-funded entity within the customer's institution to advance the AIMS concept. The best interests of the academic centers dictate that intellectual property rights and patent arrangements should be contractually negotiated to control, monitor, and potentially profit from any joint efforts in software development. A perioperative informatics center or similar think-tank concept can be created within an anesthesiology department that compensates participating faculty, directly or indirectly, for time and effort spent in ongoing AIMS development. In return, the vendor, especially if small, obtains cost-effective and focused access to substantial clinical information system user expertise that exists among a customer's faculty and staff. Initiatives for envisaging new products or innovative aspects of AIMS functionality can be presented by the vendor or by the customer; ideas may be highly product specific or more general proof-of-concept proposals. Peer-reviewed publications that are based on AIMS-derived data or experiences by faculty who participate in a vendor-supported perioperative informatics center enhance awareness of the viability of the AIMS concept and the credibility of the vendor's claims regarding the clinical and financial benefits of their product.

To protect the proprietary information that must be shared in this process, participating members of the customer's faculty or clinical staff should expect to be asked to sign a nondisclosure or confidential disclosure agreement. These legal contracts, widely used in IT relationships, create a confidential relationship between the parties to enable them to share certain information and concepts during the development process while protecting the business interests of the vendor from competitors. The contract can be binding upon the vendor, the customer, or both, depending on the exact circumstances of the cooperative relationship.

Conclusion

Every AIMS installation, regardless of the maturity the product, occurs in a unique environment and therefore requires extensive configuration and customization. Hence, maximizing the chances for successful implementation and long-term use of an AIMS requires close cooperation between the vendor and the customer's implementation manager and anesthesia clinical leadership. Cooperation in the areas of full disclosure of information system priorities and policies, hardware and software environment, contractual expectations, and training modalities is particularly important. Collaboration between vendor and customer after AIMS implementation can be informal and voluntary or can be defined contractually, with financial compensation by the vendor in return for sharing the customer's clinical experience and expertise. Collaboration permits further mutual benefit in the areas of system refinement, additional functionality, application of new technology, and the development of advanced clinical software systems for decision support, risk management, education, and clinical research.

Key Points

- Every AIMS installation is unique and reflects the cooperation of the vendor and customer.
- To be successfully implemented, the AIMS must be modified to suit the customer's workflow, and the customer must adapt workflow patterns to the AIMS.
- AIMS training is a major responsibility shared by both customer and vendor.
- A "scope-of-project" document protects the vendor.
- An "acceptance criteria" document protects the customer.
- Collaboration between vendor and customer with regard to innovation and product development is mutually beneficial.

References

1. Krol M, Reich DL, Dupont J. Multi-platforms medical computer systems integration. J Med Syst 2005; 29: 259–70
2. Quinzio L, Junger A, Gottwald B, et al. User acceptance of an anaesthesia information management system. Eur J Anaesthesiol 2003; 20:967–72
3. Benson M, Junger A, Fuchs C, et al. Use of an anesthesia information management system (AIMS) to evaluate the physiologic effects of hypnotic agents used to induce anesthesia. J Clin Monit Comput 2000; 16:183–90
4. Jost A, Junger A, Zickmann B, et al. Potential benefits of Anaesthesia Information Management Systems for multicentre data evaluation: Risk calculation of inotropic support in patients undergoing cardiac surgery. Med Inform Internet Med 2003; 28:7–19
5. Spring SF, Sandberg WS, Anupama S, et al. Automated documentation error detection and notification improves anesthesia billing performance. Anesthesiology 2007; 106:157–63
6. Vigoda MM, Lubarsky DA. Failure to recognize loss of incoming data in an anesthesia record-keeping system may have increased medical liability. Anesth Analg 2006; 102:1798–802
7. Okamura A, Murayama H, Sato N, et al. Automated anesthesia billing by electronic anesthesia record keeping system. Masui: Jpn J Anesthesiol 1999; 48:903–8

8. Reich DL, Kahn RA, Wax D, et al. Development of a module for point-of-care charge capture and submission using an anesthesia information management system. Anesthesiology 2006; 105:179–86

9. Merry AF, Webster CS, Mathew DJ. A new, safety-oriented, integrated drug administration and automated anesthesia record system. Anesth Analg 2001; 93:385–90

10. Bicker AA, Gage JS, Poppers PJ. An evolutionary solution to anesthesia automated record keeping. J Clin Monit Comput 1998; 14:421–4

11. Junger A, Hartmann B, Benson M, et al. The use of an anesthesia information management system for prediction of antiemetic rescue treatment at the postanesthesia care unit. Anesth Analg 2001; 92:1203–9

Chapter 3
Request for Information/Request for Proposals

Richard H. Epstein

Selecting an AIMS is a complex process that requires careful consideration not only by the anesthesiology department, whose work flow will be dramatically affected by the choice, but also by the IT department of the hospital. In addition, input from stakeholders who use other hospital information systems (e.g., Medical Records, Pharmacy, Lab, Nursing, Biomedical Engineering) should be solicited because the deployment of the AIMS likely will impact these areas in some way.

Many IT directors and Chief Information Officers are biased and push for a single-vendor solution for their hospital information system (HIS), rather than a multivendor, best-of-breed approach. From their perspective, dealing with one generally large vendor greatly simplifies IT issues related to communication, contracts, support, and maintenance. However, anesthesia department chairs should insist that due diligence be exercised in the selection process and that the final decision not be made on the basis of convenience, but rather on considerations of the system that will generate the maximum benefit to both parties: the institution *and* the anesthesia department.

It is not necessarily true that integrating the AIMS offering of a specific HIS vendor with its other perioperative HIS products (e.g., OR scheduling and case-cart management, ICU system, physician ordering system, EMR, financial management system, etc.) will be any easier than doing so with a third-party AIMS. The principal reason for this lack of seamless integration is that the AIMS database usually does not share fields with the vendor's other HIS databases. In some cases, the HIS vendor has simply purchased a third-party system or entered into a marketing agreement with another company. Thus, interfacing with the vendor's AIMS or a third-party AIMS is functionally equivalent. In the case of the large HIS vendors, separate development teams work on the various products, each with priorities driven by their primary customers. One cannot always count on close integration or even cooperation among these teams. Another potential problem is that the AIMS offered by the large vendor may not have been widely deployed. Consequently, the product may lack maturity, and the vendor may lack experience in the practical implementation of the system. Thus, a strong case can be made by an anesthesia department to purchase the AIMS that best meets its clinical and business needs rather than simply accepting whatever AIMS is offered by the hospital's principal HIS vendor.

J. Stonemetz, K. Ruskin (eds.) *Anesthesia Informatics*,
© Springer Science+Business Media, LLC 2008

The purpose of this chapter is to provide a methodology that anesthesia departments can use to evaluate and compare AIMS products. It is essential to recognize that it is only during the selection and negotiation process that the institution will have any leverage with respect to delivered functionality, service requirements, custom modifications, data conversion, and remedies for noncompliance with contract terms. Failure to specify terms and expectations in writing will likely lead to disappointment when oral promises that were made by the AIMS sales team remain unfulfilled. Unfortunately, a customer receiving a system that does not meet expectations is more the rule than the exception when it comes to the purchase of any complex software solution. It is not always the case that the sales team lied in an effort to close the deal; in many cases, the fault can be traced to the salesperson's lack of understanding of the potential client's needs or his inadequate knowledge of the delivered functionality of the product. Thus, it is important to specify in considerable detail the requirements that the AIMS must meet. The two main tools that should be used by the customer to specify the requirements that their AIMS should meet – the request for information (RFI) and the request for proposals (RFPs)—are described in this chapter.

Defining AIMS Requirements

It is not adequate to state, "We want to replace our manual anesthesia record," for the benefits of the AIMS will transcend the mundane chore of charting in the OR. The AIMS has evolved far beyond the early formulation of these products as automated record keepers (see Chaps. 14–17) and are increasingly being used for such purposes as ensuring billing and regulatory compliance, measuring and enhancing pay for performance initiatives, and providing decision support.

It is important to carefully consider the other HIS products with which the AIMS will interface, a process that is usually implemented through the Health Level 7 (HL7) communication protocol. The statement by a vendor that "we are HL7 compliant" is inadequate assurance that integration among systems will be successful; the devil, as always, is in the details. Specific information must be requested from vendors as to the systems with which their AIMS has been successfully interfaced, the types of HL7 messages that they are able to process, and any limitations or additional hardware or software requirements necessary to implement the interfaces. Although transferring data between two systems is usually straightforward, expertise is required to configure the inbound and outbound interface engines so that data fields are formatted and mapped correctly. Such configuration almost always entails support from vendors of both the transmitting and the receiving software. It is strongly suggested that the other vendors' costs to configure their part of the interface be determined early in the process because the expense will contribute to the overall project budget.

Almost every hospital has an OR scheduling system, and the ability to receive scheduling messages and updates into the AIMS should be a high priority. Otherwise, surgical case information will have to be manually entered into the AIMS, creating the potential for inaccurate or out-of-date data. Most hospitals have separate admission/discharge/transfer (ADT) systems into which demographic and insurance data and other information related to the specific patient encounter are entered, including medical record and account numbers. An interface is required to keep the AIMS data synchronized with this reference source. An interface between the AIMS and the hospital lab system is also highly desirable so that preoperative and intraoperative labs can be brought into the AIMS, where they can be reviewed easily and correlated with clinical and physiologic events. If the anesthesia group is using a billing system, the ability to send information to that system is another potential benefit of automation and should be considered as part of the system specification. The information may flow through an outbound HL7 interface or through separate reporting software that queries the AIMS database for billing data.

A decision should also be made regarding the desired direction of each interface. In a one-way interface, information flows either to or from the AIMS, whereas in a two-way interface, information flows in both directions. Bidirectional interfaces are generally more difficult to implement and are often deferred until a later phase of the project. Consultation with IT personnel is recommended if a flow out from the AIMS is being considered. For example, the ADT system may be used as the definitive source of patient information, feeding multiple systems, and a workflow in which a change in spelling of the patient's last name in the AIMS that updates the ADT system may not be allowed.

A major difference between an AIMS and most other HIS products is that extensive communication with diverse monitors acquiring real-time patient data is required. Thus, it is important to generate a list of all such devices from which one wants the AIMS to acquire data, along with the model, software version, and the presence or absence of communication ports. Examples include physiologic monitors, capnographs, anesthesia machines, ventilators, etc. Each device will require that a specific software driver be installed in the AIMS to interpret the data being transmitted, along with a specially designed cable; therefore, it is critical to ensure that the vendor supports the particular device. Care should also be taken to verify that the monitor is capable of sending out a signal, especially if older equipment is in use. Consultation with the biomedical engineering department of the hospital is strongly recommended, and it may be necessary to engage the vendor of the monitor as well. Even though a device may have what appears to be a communication port, the internal hardware for this port may be absent, necessitating that the device be replaced or upgraded to communicate with the AIMS, expenses for which must be factored into the overall AIMS budget.

All current AIMS products send their data back to databases that are stored on a centrally located computer over the hospital's internal network. Such networks may be hardwired (i.e., the AIMS workstation located in the OR is connected by a cable to a network port), wireless (i.e., the AIMS workstation transmits and receives data over the air to an access port), or hybrid (i.e., some locations are wired, and some are wireless). All AIMS products can be safely assumed to support wired connections, but specific questions must be asked regarding the capability of the vendor's product to work in a wireless environment. It should be determined whether a dedicated network is required by the vendor's AIMS (e.g., it requires more bandwidth than is available on the hospital's wireless network), because considerable costs may be incurred in providing this capacity. It is also important to know what will happen if the network goes down in the middle of a case. Will the system continue to function locally until the network is restored, or will the record be aborted, resulting in the need to convert to a manual record? Will any data be lost?

In defining the AIMS specification, the customer should develop a list of all locations where dedicated workstations will be installed (e.g., each OR and procedure room where anesthesia care is provided) and whether or not support in remote locations (e.g., MRI, CT, cardiac catheterization lab, etc.) is required. It is often desirable to provide mobile workstations for areas where cases are done less frequently, and the number required should be determined. Several additional standby workstations should be identified that can be immediately pressed into service should equipment problems occur in another location. Because some development and testing will likely be needed, asking for additional licenses to be provided without charge for such purposes is recommended.

Another consideration is whether or not any existing electronic systems will be replaced by the new AIMS. These might include quality assurance systems, preoperative anesthesia evaluation systems, and billing systems. If so, such requirements must be included in the AIMS specification. A similar consideration concerns reports that are generated for the department or hospital that use data from systems being replaced by the AIMS. The customer should specify whether the vendor is expected to rewrite or to assist in the rewriting of these reports using data from the new system.

Because the AIMS will be deployed on the hospital's internal network, it will likely be necessary to install certain software on those workstations (e.g., antivirus, antispam, remote support software, physician order entry systems, browsers, etc.). The hospital's IT department should be consulted to determine what software is required as part of its standard installation. In many institutions, consistency among workstations is required by use of standard operating system images and log-on profiles. It is important to specify that the AIMS product must be compatible with the operating system and any software required by hospital IT to be installed on the workstation. For example, if IT requires a certain security product to be present on every workstation and the vendor's AIMS will not operate correctly when that product is present, a major hurdle will be encountered regarding the ability to deploy that AIMS. Another barrier to product selection would be if the hospital supports only the Microsoft Windows 2000 operating system on workstations and the AIMS requires Windows XP.

In the specifications, it should be clear that the vendor's AIMS must meet privacy and security requirements of HIPAA. The vendors' interpretation of what security and privacy features must be in their AIMS may be quite different from those required by the privacy officer at the customer's institution. It must be remembered that the hospital is responsible for HIPAA compliance—not the vendor, who is outside the jurisdiction of the regulation. It is recommended that the hospital's privacy officer be contacted to determine the specific requirements that must be met by software products that handle protected health information (see Chap. 19).

Request for Information

Currently, at least a dozen vendors offer AIMS products, and sorting through the features, limitations, advantages, and disadvantages of each can be a daunting task. Although professional and trade shows (e.g., annual meetings of the ASA and the Healthcare Information and Management Systems Society) are good places to see all of the systems in one venue, the decision should not be based on the marketing presentation of the product or the friendliness of the sales team. Likewise, the slickness of the vendor's Web site is not an indication of how well the AIMS will perform or the reliability and responsiveness of the vendor. Because everyone's needs are different, a formal approach is recommended to gather basic information about the systems, with particular focus on those areas that are absolute requirements.

We recommend a two-stage approach. In the first step, an RFI is created and sent to all vendors whose AIMS the department wishes to consider (Fig. 3.1). If earlier in the selection process, some vendors were dismissed out of hand for a variety of reasons, it is not be necessary to send the RFI to all of them. In the second step, described in the next section, a formal RFP is submitted.

The RFI is a short document in which vendors are asked to respond briefly to a series of questions to define the high-level functionality of the product. The document is also designed to separate delivered functionality from marketing hype and promotional material. Evasive or nonresponsive answers from the vendor or failure to follow specific instructions for completion of the RFI are signs of potential problems down the road. An additional benefit of the RFI is that issues and costs that the customer may not have thought of will likely arise from the responses.

In the RFI, the customer should provide the vendors with basic information about their facility (e.g., type of hospital, number of anesthetizing locations, cases per year, basic network description). The deadline for the response (typically ~2 weeks) should be specified, along with any requirements as to how the responses are to be provided. A table format submitted electronically is recommended because this configuration allows the customer to cut and paste the vendors' responses into one table to facilitate comparison.

Once the responses are returned and analyzed, vendors who do not meet the basic requirements can be dropped from consideration. Clarification may need to be requested from some vendors if their answers are not adequate. This is a good time for the customer to consult with colleagues who have installed the AIMS products that are being considered. If several sources provide negative feedback regarding promised functionality that was not delivered, support issues, system unreliability, etc., the customer should proceed with caution. Site visits to institutions that are currently running the products under consideration are also very helpful

The Department of Anesthesiology at XYZ Hospital is seeking to purchase an anesthesia information management system (AIMS) and is requesting information from potential vendors. XYZ is an academic medical center with approximately 50 anesthetizing locations that perform approximately 40,000 cases per year. The system will be running on a 100 MB/s Ethernet backbone, with 802.11g wireless access required.

You must complete this form electronically by entering your answers into the cell adjacent to each question and returning the file to jsmith1@xyz.edu. Responses returned in a different format will be rejected. **The deadline for return of the RFI is mm/dd/yyyy hh:mm. Responses received after this deadline may be rejected.**

General Questions	
How many facilities are *currently* using your AIMS for patient care?	
How many facilities of your AIMS are in progress, or under contract, awaiting the start of installation?	
What is the typical range of time from start of installation to first use in the OR for actual clinical care?	
Please enter any explanatory comments pertaining to this section, including items that are planned or are under development.	
Network Questions	
Will your system *currently* run on a wireless network? Indicate the number of installations in which wireless access has been implemented.	☐ Yes ☐ No # _____
What are the bandwidth requirements for wireless access?	
Is a dedicated wireless network for the AIMS recommended? That is, a network that is separate from the general hospital wireless network.	☐ Yes ☐ No
Will your system run locally if the network goes down? That is, will the system continue to work if the connection to the server is broken?	☐ Yes ☐ No
Please enter any explanatory comments pertaining to this section, including items that are planned or are under development.	
Interface Questions	
Will your system currently accept a live HL7 feed from an ADT system to populate patient demographics? If no, is this functionality anticipated and when?	☐ Yes ☐ No
Will your system currently accept a live HL7 feed from an OR scheduling system? If no, is this functionality anticipated and when?	☐ Yes ☐ No
Will your system currently accept a live HL7 feed from a lab system? If no, is this functionality anticipated and when?	☐ Yes ☐ No
Does your system have an outbound HL7 capability?	☐ Yes ☐ No
Please enter any explanatory comments pertaining to this section, including items that are planned or are under development.	
Security Questions	
Are IDs and passwords maintained within the AIMS?	☐ Yes ☐ No
Can IDs and passwords be maintained outside of the AIMS (e.g., X.500, active directory, etc.)? If yes, provide details.	☐ Yes ☐ No
Is a requirement to use strong passwords configurable in the AIMS?	☐ Yes ☐ No
Are password expiration criteria configurable within the AIMS?	☐ Yes ☐ No
Please enter any explanatory comments pertaining to this section, including items that are planned or are under development.	
Server Requirements	
What are the minimum server requirements (CPU, hard disk size, operating system) for a facility of our size?	
What are the recommended server requirements (CPU, hard disk size, operating system) for a facility of our size?	
What is the minimum number of servers required for a facility of our size?	
How many servers are recommended for a facility of our size?	
Please enter any explanatory comments pertaining to this section, including items that are planned or are under development.	

Fig. 3.1 Example request for information for an AIMS

Workstation Requirements		
What are the minimum workstation requirements (CPU, hard disk size, operating system, touch screen) for a facility of our size?		
What are the recommended workstation requirements (CPU, hard disk size, operating system, touch screen) for a facility of our size?		
Can additional workstations be added without vendor intervention (after purchase of additional workstation licenses)?	☐ Yes	☐ No
Please enter any explanatory comments pertaining to this section, including items that are planned or are under development.		

Patient Monitor Interfacing		
Can your system *currently* interface with ____ physiologic monitor model _____, software revision _____?	☐ Yes	☐ No
Can your system *currently* interface with _____ gas monitor model _____, software revision _____?	☐ Yes	☐ No
Can your system *currently* interface with _____ (other) monitor model _____, software revision _____?	☐ Yes	☐ No
Can your system *currently* interface with _____ model _____ anesthesia machine?	☐ Yes	☐ No
Please enter any explanatory comments pertaining to this section, including items that are planned or are under development.		

System and User Support		
Is a 24-hr hotline available for user problems?	☐ Yes	☐ No
Is a 24-hr hotline available for system/technical problems?	☐ Yes	☐ No
Is an account manager/contact person assigned to each facility?	☐ Yes	☐ No
Please enter any explanatory comments pertaining to this section, including items that are planned or are under development.		

Application Issues		
Is the system *currently* certified to run under Windows 2000? If yes, indicate the number of sites where implemented.	☐ Yes	☐ No
Is the system *currently* certified to run under Windows XP? If yes, indicate the number of sites where implemented.	☐ Yes	☐ No
Is the system *currently* certified to run under Windows Vista? If yes, indicate the number of sites where implemented.	☐ Yes	☐ No
Can drug libraries *currently* be imported into the system from external files?	☐ Yes	☐ No
Can the authorized user list *currently* be imported into the system from external files?	☐ Yes	☐ No
Does the system *currently* support ICD9 diagnosis coding?	☐ Yes	☐ No
Does the system *currently* support CPT procedure coding?	☐ Yes	☐ No
Please enter any explanatory comments pertaining to this section, including items that are planned or are under development.		

Database Requirements		
Does the system utilize a proprietary vendor database?	☐ Yes	☐ No
Can the system *currently* run using ORACLE as the database? If yes, indicate the number of sites where implemented.	☐ Yes	☐ No
Can the system *currently* run using an MS SQL Server as the database? If yes, indicate the number of sites where implemented.	☐ Yes	☐ No
Please enter any explanatory comments pertaining to this section, including items that are planned or are under development.		

Facility IT Support Requirements	
Indicate the category and number of FTE IT resources required for the implementation team.	
How many and what category of IT FTE resources are expected for support of an application at a facility of our size?	
Please enter any explanatory comments pertaining to this section, including items that are planned or are under development.	

Cost Estimate	
Note: These can be ballpark estimates necessary for budgeting, and vendors will not be held to exact values.	
What is the approximate cost per installed workstation, including required hardware (excluding cost of servers)?	
What is the approximate cost for system configuration (if additional to per-workstation cost)?	
What is the approximate cost of the yearly maintenance contract and other yearly charges?	
Please enter any explanatory comments pertaining to this section.	

Please include printed brochures, instruction manuals, specification sheets, and any other information that you feel will be of use to us in making our evaluation and send to: John Smith, MD; XYZ Hospital; 100 Main Street, Suite 1234; Anywhere, USA. Following receipt of the requested information, a formal Request for Proposal will be sent to qualifying vendors.

at this point, because additional issues may surface that must be resolved in the selection process. We recommend reducing the field to three to five AIMS vendors from whom a formal proposal will be requested.

Request for Proposals

The second step of the evaluation process involves sending out an RFP. The RFP is a formal document, often including sections with legal contract language, in which vendors are asked to provide a firm bid for the purchase of their fully specified system. Because this document is the basis for the contract that is ultimately written, the RFP should be created with great attention to detail and should cover every aspect of the project, even those that may be deferred until later. The RFP should be formulated in such a manner that it is possible to determine the cost of deleting various components from the bid.

An outline of items to include in an RFP for an AIMS system is provided in Fig. 3.2. The customer should ask the hospital's IT department if it has an RFP template or a recent RFP for another HIS system, because such documents will be helpful in covering general aspects of the proposal, especially any legal language that is typically included. It is also worthwhile to consult with representatives of the hospital's material management department or other department responsible for executing software contracts, because they may provide additional legal language that must be inserted into the RFP.

As much information about the hospital as is necessary for the vendors to have a full understanding of IT infrastructure, requirements, and expectations should be communicated in the RFP. For the vendors to accurately specify hardware requirements, they need to know details about operational processes, surgical volume, number and location of ORs, monitors, anesthesia machines, etc. Because some of this information is confidential or proprietary, the RFP should include clauses forbidding the vendor to disclose or use any of this information outside the scope of preparing the RFP. The vendors need to know all deadlines and timetables, and it is important to specify exactly how they are to respond to the request. They should be required to adhere to the format specified by the customer and encouraged to be succinct in their responses.

The RFP will repeat many of the questions listed in the RFI. However, the replies by a vendor to the RFP are formal assertions of how their AIMS functions—assertions for which they can be held accountable. If a sales representative has promised that the system will do x, y, or z, and these functions are important, the customer should be certain that these promises are addressed in the RFP.

It is important to remember that the vendor's bid is based on the RFP, and any missing items that are subsequently requested will likely be added to the final cost. It is generally better to overspecify system requirements in the RFP and then back them out at the time of contract negotiation rather than try to insert them later. For example, if 30–35 workstations are needed, the requested quote should be based on the larger number, along with a breakdown of costs if workstations are added or subtracted.

REQUEST FOR PROPOSALS

INTRODUCTION
- ☐ Description of the hospital organization
- ☐ Description of the project scope
- ☐ Description of the functional requirements of the AIMS
- ☐ A vision of what the AIMS is expected to provide
- ☐ List of all locations where AIMS is to be installed
- ☐ Description of modules needed in each location (if applicable to AIMS)
- ☐ A calendar of events related to the RFP and contract award process
- ☐ Deadlines for submission
- ☐ Vendor on-site presentation requirements, if requested
- ☐ Anticipated decision dates

VENDOR REQUIREMENTS
- ☐ Costs of all items either expressly or implicitly specified in the RFP
- ☐ Details regarding how RFP is to be completed and to whom it is to be sent
- ☐ Number of copies to be submitted
- ☐ Instructions on how RFP response should be formatted and organized
  - ○ Must follow specified format or proposal may be rejected outright
  - ○ Responses should be straightforward
  - ○ No promotional or advertising material should be included
  - ○ Request that section numbering in this RFP be maintained in responses to allow referencing to the corresponding RFP questions
- ☐ A separate Technical and Financial Proposal is sometimes requested

References
- ☐ Contact information for at least three facilities that use the same equipment with the same size and complexity as that under consideration

Project Specifications
- ☐ Detailed architectural and functional diagrams of all software components for complete system
- ☐ List of system requirements and details on how the AIMS meets them
- ☐ Description of software update processes
- ☐ Description of software requirements
- ☐ Description of hardware requirements (workstation and servers)
- ☐ Description of OR workstation installation process

Interfaces
- ☐ A listing of all interfaces by name and data to be passed between them
- ☐ Indication as to whether interfaces are one-way or bi-directional

Other
- ☐ Warranty, maintenance contract, and service terms (including technical and user support availability, response times, and equipment replacement)
- ☐ Amount of user and system administrator training hours provided in bid
- ☐ On-going support/maintenance FTE requirements
- ☐ Legal terms and conditions related to the RFP

Software Modules
- ☐ Cost breakdown by workstation and module and additional cost incurred by adding or subtracting workstations or modules

HIPAA Questionnaire
- ☐ Hospital IT likely has a detailed questionnaire to incorporate.

Fig. 3.2 Example of items to include in an RFP for an AIMS

Finally, we suggest that a list of scenarios that describe unusual events be included in the RFP and that the vendor be asked to explain how its system will handle the problem. A list of some sample scenarios is presented in Fig. 3.3. The true test of an AIMS is not how it performs when everything is working according to plan, but how it performs when various components (including humans) malfunction.

Important aspects of the RFP should be incorporated into the final contract by reference and/or as specific line items in the contract. Doing this will provide legal protection if the vendor fails to meet its representations.

Evaluating the RFP

The process of collating and analyzing the vendors' responses to the RFP can be quite time consuming, given the length of the document and the replies. It is helpful to specify a response format such that the answers can be cut and pasted to allow comparison among the vendors for each question. Financial information is easiest to process in a spreadsheet format, where equivalent pricing can be determined and compared. In some instances, clarification may be required if a vendor's answers are incomplete or unclear. It is unlikely that any one vendor will meet all of the requirements spelled out in the specification document; rather, the shortcomings must be balanced and weighted according to their importance to the department. It is beyond the scope of this chapter to recommend how this weighting should be accomplished, but the final decision will involve a tradeoff between features, functions, and cost.

It may be possible to exclude some of the vendors from further consideration after reviewing their RFPs. Those still being considered should be invited to make a formal presentation on-site to the committees charged with making the final recommendation. Typically, the customer task force includes a group making a technical assessment (usually with heavy IT representation), a group making a financial/business assessment (including department and hospital administrators), and sometimes a group making a functional assessment (end users). During these presentations (which typically take between one-half and one full day), the vendor is given the opportunity to present a product demonstration and a summary of its technical and financial proposals. We recommend that the vendors be provided with a list of the topics that they should cover at the technical and financial presentations. They should be prepared to answer questions from the committees, some of which may be submitted in advance. Scoring sheets may be used to measure how each vendor meets the requirements. For the product demonstration, if included, we recommend use of a standardized script for each vendor (sent to them in advance), in which they are asked to demonstrate specific functions of their system. This method permits a fair comparison of the products, as opposed to a contest in which the vendor with the slickest presentation team wins.

After the completion of the vendor presentations, the various individuals involved in the final decision-making process should meet to consider the material

---

Scenarios Describing Unusual Events

The following scenarios describe events that may occasionally arise and cause problems with the ordinary functioning of your AIMS. Please respond in detail to the questions asked. If a particular problem is not addressed by the current software release, but an update is scheduled for release in the future, please indicate as such, along with the anticipated date of delivery to the production environment.

1. A patient arrives in the OR, but ADT interface is down and the patient is not found. The remainder of the network is operational. How does the patient get entered into the AIMS? Can the AIMS be used for this patient, or must the provider revert to paper? What is your recommended approach to this problem?

2. A patient's OR record is recorded, but just prior to printing the hard copy of the anesthesia record, the network goes down and the network printers are inaccessible. Is it possible to attach a local printer to the workstation (assuming that the workstations have the necessary printer drivers) and print the record in the OR from the local copy of the anesthesia record?

3. An anesthesia resident goes to see a patient on the floor with a wireless tablet PC, but the signal from the wireless access point cannot be received in the patient's room. The patient was loaded from the network before the resident left the anesthesia workroom, and the resident has already started the evaluation. Can the resident complete the evaluation offline and then have the data written back to the network when a working access point   is reached?

4. An anesthesia resident is using a wireless tablet PC while seeing a patient when the signal to the wireless access point is lost. Can the evaluation and data be sent back to the server when a working access point is reached?

5. In the ED, an anesthesia resident sees a patient who has not yet been admitted (medical record not yet assigned). Can a preoperative evaluation be completed using the resident's wireless tablet PC, assuming that all of the network components are working? How will this information be connected to the patient once the patient is admitted and the information flows through the ADT interface? What is your recommended approach to this problem?

6. A workstation goes down in the middle of recording a case, and the hardware is replaced. Will the record of the case prior to the malfunction be retrievable from the network, assuming that all components of the network are functional?

7. Halfway through a procedure, a resident realizes that he has selected the wrong patient. How is this error corrected?

8. The hospital mistakenly assigns a new medical record number to a patient who is already in the system. How does the person completing the preoperative evaluation call up the old record so that the previous information can be transferred to the new encounter?

9. The anesthesia attending forgets to document his presence during the emergence from anesthesia. Until what period of time can he go back in and add this note to the record? Is a mechanism in place to append the record with this note after it has been closed?

10. The anesthesia record is printed from the OR to the PACU's network printer, but when the resident arrives, the hard copy cannot be located. How is another copy printed?

11. A "John Doe" trauma patient arrives in the ER and is immediately taken to the OR to control bleeding from a gunshot wound to the chest. No information about the patient is available. Can your AIMS be used to record the anesthesia record? Describe the steps in your system that would be required to begin recording data on the patient.

Fig. 3.3 Scenarios describing unusual events

provided by the vendors and the evaluations from the on-site presentations. From this meeting, the winning AIMS should be selected. The vendors should be notified of the decision as promptly as possible so that contract negotiations are initiated with the selected AIMS vendor. A discussion of that process is beyond the scope of this chapter, but it can be quite time consuming to conclude the final deal. The customer may wish to select a second choice in case a contract cannot be negotiated successfully with the winning vendor.

Conclusion

A formal approach to the evaluation of AIMS products based on a written specification of the requirements of the department of anesthesiology is recommended. Selecting an AIMS from a particular vendor simply because that vendor already has another major HIS implemented at the hospital may not result in the best choice. It is much more prudent to pick the product that best meets the various needs of the institution and the anesthesiology department. Distributing a short RFI to AIMS vendors whose products are to be considered is an effective method of narrowing the field to several candidates whose systems are to be evaluated in greater detail. The RFI process also generates material that can be used to formulate a more comprehensive RFP. The vendors to be further evaluated (typically three to five) are then sent a formal RFP in which the desired system is fully described, requirements specified, and details of the proposal process enumerated. Comparing the responses of the vendors, the specific functionality of their systems, and the costs will inform a rational basis for selecting finalist vendors who will then be asked to make a presentation on-site. Based on the RFPs, the vendor presentations, and additional information, such as site visits and feedback from colleagues who use the systems under consideration, the best possible AIMS choice can be made.

Key Points

- All AIMS requirements should be defined, especially those related to interfacing with other HIS products such as lab, scheduling, or ADT systems.
- All of the patient monitors with which the AIMS must communicate should be specified, and the capacity of these monitors to transmit data should be verified.
- Network requirements should be defined, and any required upgrades to the environment should be identified.
- The user should request a demonstration that the AIMS is compatible with other software (e.g., antivirus, remote management software) that must be installed on the AIMS workstations as part of the standard hospital image.
- The user should ask specific questions relating to how the product meets HIPAA and institutional security and privacy requirements.

Chapter 4
Implementation of an AIMS

Gilbert Ritchie and Stephen T. Robinson

As the chapter titles of this book imply, use of an AIMS within an anesthesia service affects far more than the intraoperative anesthesia record, although that is the use most visible to clinicians. When implemented well, an AIMS has the potential to positively affect almost every process—clinical and business—related to anesthesia delivery. The opposite is also true. When poorly implemented, an AIMS can degrade these same processes, leading to system failures, with lost clinical efficiency, poor-quality records, and the associated lost investment of time, money, and opportunity.

The risk of failure may be reduced by defining specific goals and outcomes that the AIMS is to achieve. Ideally, departmental and hospital leadership defined these goals and outcomes when the decision was made to acquire an AIMS, and once defined, they guided its selection or specifications. Those same goals and outcomes should also guide the implementation. Typical goals for use of the AIMS include:

- Supporting clinical processes and improving clinical efficiency
- Supporting quality improvement initiatives
- Supporting the administration in managing utilization of ORs, personnel, and supplies
- Supporting business processes such as billing
- Supporting clinical research by automatically collecting data in a manner that can be efficiently retrieved

Most institutions arrive at an AIMS implementation from one of two purchase pathways: the institution issues a Request for Information and/or a Request for Proposal followed by an evaluation of responses (see Chap. 3), or the institution works with a vendor who has an integrated system of which the AIMS is a part. For example, an institution may use a vendor's surgical information system and may sole-source the same vendor's AIMS because of its integration with the surgical system. Both approaches have merits and pitfalls, and the implications of each approach are profound. For example, the Request for Information/Request for Proposal approach, followed by a clinical evaluation of the top contenders and eventual selection of the "best of breed" may support most of the goals stated above; however, as it is not integrated with a surgical information system, some information may be duplicated between the two (e.g., patient medications and allergies, surgical event times). Interfaces can overcome the duplication, but with increased cost and complexity. This approach also tends to help the institution focus on its expectations of product performance, obtain a more detailed contract, and create the team necessary for implementation. In contrast, a vendor with an integrated system may have a less mature AIMS that does not support the anesthesia processes as well as the "best of breed," but data are less likely to be duplicated. Having a single vendor simplifies the process of identifying who has ownership of technical problems and will frequently be the default choice of the Chief Information Officer at an institution.

Generally, most benefits of an AIMS cannot be realized until all of the components are in place. Regardless of how one intends to use the data from an AIMS, these data must be collected and stored reliably, and the system must include most, if not all, relevant cases to provide a valid picture. Specific advice on AIMS implementation follows. The phases of implementation are divided into planning, testing, deployment, and transition to maintenance. Finally, life-cycle issues are discussed at the end of the chapter.

Planning

As expected with all complex projects, careful planning is the most important step to optimizing the efficiency of implementation. Vendors usually provide institutions with a project plan or statement of work that may define project steps, milestones, timelines, deliverables, and mutual resources required for the project. Although a valuable guide from which to start, it may require greater detail and expansion, depending on the scope of the implementation. Because of the project complexity, implementation must be viewed as an iterative process, even with the best of planning. For the purposes of this chapter, AIMS planning has been divided into the following areas: project personnel, scope, configuration, process, network and hardware, security, testing, and deployment.

Project Personnel

A diverse team is required to implement an AIMS. Although many potential variations are possible, the following roles are recommended to optimize the chances of success:

- Project Executive
- Project Manager
- Clinical Manager
- System Administrator
- Network Representative
- Biomedical Engineering Representative

One individual may assume multiple roles. Stakeholder groups that are not listed here, such as Perioperative Nursing, Quality Resources, and Billing, may require representation at various points in the project. Building a team of clinical users, often referred to as *superusers*, allows for high-quality input for clinical performance and creates an invaluable group to assist with testing and implementation. Finally, the AIMS vendor will play a role in all the above-named functions.

Although not typically a hands-on position, the Project Executive has the role of champion and provides oversight to the project. This individual should have the authority to push through institutional barriers that may impede the progress of the project. The Project Executive is the lead person to assess if the project is remaining on course and to help to redirect the project if it deviates from its budget or goals. At the extreme, this is the individual who will play a pivotal role in deciding whether the project should receive additional resources or be terminated. Advising and supporting the Project Manager is a crucial part of the Project Executive's job. The Project Executive must be able to provide guidance through the bureaucracy when unexpected needs arise, as they generally do. Often, the Executive's greatest contribution is to prevent relatively small requirements from stopping the project. For example, if installation of additional hardware is required, the Executive must obtain the necessary resources from the appropriate department in a timely manner.

The Project Manager is responsible for overseeing the project details and must stay aware of all aspects of the project and work closely with all the groups that have a stake in the project. The Project Manager is responsible for marshalling the resources required to complete the project. Ideally, the Manager will possess a mix of clinical and technical expertise, although the individual need not be a clinician or a technical professional. Most important, the manager should possess leadership and organizational skills. The vendor may have its own Project Manager to marshal its resources as well, but the vendor's Manager should not substitute for the institution's Manager. Rather, the two should work closely together.

The Clinical Leader is especially important if the Project Manager is not a clinician. The Clinical Leader helps to ensure that the clinicians' requirements for performance are adequately supported by the AIMS, assists the team to elicit and understand the clinical processes that are supported by the AIMS, and helps the key clinicians in each area to understand the capabilities of the AIMS. The Clinical Leader ensures that when different sites have similar processes, the AIMS configuration is consistently applied. Ultimately, this individual helps to determine when the AIMS requires modifications or when a clinical process should be changed.

The System Administrator is a key technical person for the project. This individual will be the institutional expert on the AIMS software and will support software that may simplify deployment and maintenance (e.g., remote installation and diagnostic software, database maintenance and backup software, and server performance monitoring software). This role requires technical knowledge and skills in database maintenance and server/network system management. The System Administrator may be a member of either the hospital's IT department or anesthesia services, depending on the level of support and resources available within each department, and must have an understanding of the clinical procedures and processes documented by the AIMS.

A Network Representative is another key technical role for AIMS implementation. AIMS applications depend on a responsive network to communicate data between the client workstations and the servers, making network planning critical to AIMS implementation. High network availability and reliability are required. The Network Representative will help to fit the AIMS network requirements into the existing structure where possible and identify areas necessary for expansion within the infrastructure to meet the robust requirements of an AIMS. As a mission-critical clinical tool, an AIMS may require a higher level of support than that to which the institution is accustomed. For example, the inability to access lab results for 10 minutes may seem a minor inconvenience, but in a busy ambulatory surgical center, a 10 minutes delay because a patient's preoperative assessment is not available would cause a major disruption.

Biomedical Engineering plays a key role in mounting workstations and connecting the patient monitor data cables to the workstations in the OR. The ergonomics of workstation mounting can be a major factor in the successful deployment of the intraoperative documentation component. If the institution's IT department lacks experience with clinical environments, Biomedical Engineering can prove to be an important ally in helping IT personnel to understand the unique needs of a particular setting. Biomedical Engineering can also help to troubleshoot communication issues between the patient monitors and the workstation.

The roles described above should be organized into teams with specific tasks:

- Core implementation team
- Configuration team
- Training team
- Support team

The primary task of the *core implementation team* is to see the project through to successful completion. It plays both leadership and oversight roles in the project. This team should include representatives of the main implementation entities and must develop connections to groups that are necessary to implement the product and groups that will be users of the product or its output. These connections facilitate efficient access to critical resources and help to identify previously unrecognized needs, problems, challenges, or stakeholders. Examples of resources can range from strategically locating servers to simply obtaining priority to run wire to activate a network junction. It is important that the core team be large enough to include representation of key players but not too large so as to be unwieldy or prevent meetings because of conflicts. One strategy is to have a smaller core team that always meets, while other key players only participate in meetings when their needs are being addressed or when their expertise is required. Core team members typically include the Project Manager, the System Administrator, the Network Representative, and a representative from Biomedical Engineering. Others may participate in these meetings as needed—e.g., managers of the clinical areas where AIMS components are being deployed.

The task of the *configuration team* is critical to a successful AIMS implementation. The vendor may provide extensive support for configuration, but the institution must provide its own resources to ensure that the system is configured properly to meet the institution's needs. The configuration task is described in detail in a later section of this chapter. The institution's configuration team should consist of the System Administrator, who will implement or manage the software configuration, and anesthetists and/or anesthesiologists who practice in the areas where AIMS components are to be deployed. For example, most AIMS enable the user to select from various case types at the beginning of a procedure so that drugs, events, and comments that are typically documented in that type of procedure are preloaded for ease of documentation. Practitioners who are familiar with special areas must work with the System Administrator to confirm the vendor's configuration or to build an appropriate configuration for those cases. The System Administrator or another individual, preferably a clinician familiar with the capability of the AIMS, must oversee these configurations to help to maintain maximum consistency among them. Similarly, staff members who perform the preanesthesia evaluation in the clinic should be engaged in configuring that AIMS component, so that the result will be compatible with the production environment of the clinic, capture the necessary data, and support the downstream processes.

The task of the *training team* is to plan and provide for user training. Although the vendor may provide trainers during initial deployment, the institution will have to provide for its own ongoing training. Institutions should identify front-line clinicians for this purpose and ensure that they receive extensive training from the vendor so that they can train others. These superusers may be involved in training at initial deployment as well. Because superusers receive extensive initial training, they can be valuable resources for the configuration team.

Once deployed, an AIMS will require a *support team* to manage new user registration, configuration refinements, and troubleshooting services. Members of this team are typically the System Administrator, the Biomedical Engineering representative, superusers, and others who have been delegated authority to manage various aspects of the system.

Scope

Scope defines the AIMS functions, where these functions are to be deployed, the number of workstations at each location, and the number of licenses required for each software component. It is common for customers to refer to these features as "deliverables," leaving the term "scope" to the vendors. The scope may include the requirements and responsibility for hardware, software, interfaces, training, and implementation timelines. While scope refers to the details of the project, it should not be confused with the broader concept that the product must be fundamentally functional. In other words, a lab interface must be explicitly included in the contract if it is to be part of the scope, whereas the ability to add a new drug to the system probably does not.

An understanding of existing clinical and business processes and how the AIMS is to support them is required to establish the project's scope. The project scope should be defined sometime during the procurement process and detailed in the contract between the institution and the vendor, with appropriate deliverables included by the institution's leadership. If the implementation process identifies any missing essential capabilities, it is critical to add them as quickly as possible. This process includes ensuring that adequate resources and funding from the institution are made available.

Both clinical and nonclinical functions and locations should be considered in the scope. In addition to the obvious clinical locations, such as the ORs and the preanesthesia clinic, some challenging and nonobvious clinical locations must also be considered, such as the labor rooms and the MRI suite. The nonclinical functions of billing, management reporting, and quality assurance will likely require installation in the nonclinical locations where support and managerial staff execute those functions.

If the vendor is expected to provide some custom features or components, the scope should identify and define these features. It is important to emphasize that an AIMS cannot do everything, and defining a realistic scope will help to ensure a successful implementation and minimize the need for vendor-provided custom features. Not only are custom features expensive, they also may not be supported in future versions of the vendor's software.

Configuration

AIMS are configurable, and much of the functionality specific to an institution may be achieved through configuration, which the institution can control, rather than through customization, which is accomplished by the vendor through code development or modification. The same understanding of clinical and business processes that contributes to scope definition is required for the configuration task. For example, understanding how patients arrive in preop holding, move to the OR, and then move to the PACU or ICU is necessary to plan and configure the AIMS components that may be deployed in those areas. Only then can the system be designed so that patient information flows in a way that supports the care and clinical processes. Usually, the institution is responsible for the configuration, but it is important to define the vendor's level of configuration support. Some components may be difficult to configure without substantial vendor support.

Process

AIMS implementation provides a valuable opportunity to evaluate clinical processes. In a meeting with the core team, all of the stakeholders, both clinical and business, should describe how they currently perform their tasks. This discussion will help to clarify how the AIMS should be implemented and the impact that the AIMS will have on each group, and the results of this discussion may be wide ranging. Some findings will lead to improvements independent of the AIMS product. For example, gathering together all of the surgery clinic schedulers may reveal how some clinics manage patient data more efficiently than others. Often, opportunities for the AIMS to support or enhance existing processes will be identified. Other information will reveal ways to optimize the AIMS configurations. In some instances, the AIMS will be less robust than the current process, but it is important to acknowledge the existing drawbacks and ensure that the advantages gained with the new system compensate for the limitations. An AIMS may provide opportunities to redesign some existing processes. The potential to eliminate paper will certainly create opportunities. For example, billing sheets can be eliminated, and the process of capturing charges redesigned. Similarly, the communication of preanesthesia evaluation information to the anesthesia team need not be limited to the transfer of paper. In fact, with an AIMS, the preanesthesia evaluation can be made available to others in addition to the anesthesia team for care planning; this may not have been previously possible.

Beware—an AIMS will not fix broken processes. Applying an AIMS component in a broken process without redesigning the process will ensure failure. If the underlying causes for failure are not discovered and fixed, deploying an AIMS will not resolve them.

Variable processes may be difficult to accommodate with an AIMS. For example, an institution may have a preanesthesia assessment outpatient clinic where most of the assessments are made; however, a different process is required for inpatient assessments. The former can be accomplished with fixed workstations hardwired into the network, whereas the latter may require mobile workstations that are either episodically connected to the network or wireless. Therefore, appropriate uploading of data should be ensured. This type of variability can even occur in areas that serve similar functions. For example, one preoperative area may have generous space for computers, while another site may be crowded and require an alternative solution.

New processes will also be required for an AIMS. The process of registering new users, inactivating terminated users, and managing users' access to system components must be developed. Once the system is deployed, a process by which to modify system configurations must be developed. As mentioned before, implementation is an iterative process, and controlling the configuration is important to ensuring that improvements are implemented without compromising data integrity.

Network and Hardware

Acquisition of hardware and expansion of networks are not the purposes of an AIMS, but they are essential for its implementation and are required to achieve the desired functionality of the system. Network and hardware planning should address the servers, workstations, patient monitors, interfaces, and test environment.

Network

An AIMS requires a reliable data network, and all locations in which AIMS components are to be used should be served by the facility's data network. Reliability is defined by network availability. Network outages should be very infrequent, and when they do occur, they should be brief. Ideally, the selected AIMS can tolerate infrequent, brief, episodic network outages without losing data or crashing. The Network Representative should guide the core team through any network issues.

At the beginning of the project, a survey should be conducted to assess network availability at the planned locations. Generally, one network connection will be required for each workstation. In patient-care locations that require monitor capture, an additional connection may be required if the monitors are to be connected directly to the network rather than to the workstation. A plan must be developed for areas that lack adequate connection. If a wireless network is being considered for part of the system, its signal strength and available data rates should be assessed. The vendor should specify the minimum recommended data rate.

Hardware

It is convenient to classify AIMS hardware components into the "back-end" hardware—servers and interface computers that are not located in the clinical areas—and the "front-end" hardware—the workstations that clinicians, managers, and others will use. On the back end, the AIMS may utilize one or more servers: a database server, a file server, and perhaps others. For small installations, a single computer may perform multiple server functions. In larger installations, separate computers may be provided for separate server functions. Sophisticated server installations may even have clustered servers to improve performance and/or reliability. The vendor will specify minimum requirements for the servers, or at least provide advice based on the scope of the planned deployment. The facility's IT department and the System Administrator, with advice from the vendor, should guide the core team on server size and performance recommendations. While these decisions are being made, plans for system expansion and longevity should also be made, with consideration for the annual case volume and the megabytes of data that each case will generate on average.

The vendor may support a "thin-client" model of deploying applications, e.g., using Citrix to run instances of client applications on the server with input from the client workstation. The alternative model, "thick client," has the applications installed on the client workstation. Both methods have their pros and cons. The thin-client model is usually easier for IT to support because the AIMS applications are not actually running on the client hardware. However, the applications may not perform adequately unless they are deployed as thick clients. The system may be deployed with a mixture of both models. The system administrator and the IT department, with input from the vendor, should make recommendations regarding this choice.

Server locations should be planned carefully, taking physical security, power reliability, and network reliability into consideration. Many facilities have a secure server room with uninterruptible and/or backup power available. Data backup hardware should be incorporated in the back-end hardware plan as well.

Another back-end group of components are the interfaces. Common interfaces include the following:

- *Admission/discharge/transfer (ADT)*. Typically, an AIMS receives ADT transactions, possibly filtered by patient location, through an interface. This method alleviates staff from having to enter all the patient demographic data and thus improves data reliability. Reliability of information is especially important for the patient's account number if a hospital charge interface is also planned. In our experience, many staff members do not know which field on the printed key plate is the patient's account number.
- *Hospital charges*. An AIMS may send anesthesia-based hospital charges to the hospital billing system to be added to the patient's account. In planning for a hospital charge interface, a process for auditing the interface to ensure that charges accurately flow from the AIMS to the billing system and a process for managing and resubmitting charges that are rejected by the billing system must be developed. Typically, rejections are due to erroneous account numbers, which can be minimized if account numbers are communicated through an ADT interface.
- *Laboratory*. Test results may be received into the AIMS to be included in the intraoperative record, or possibly as part of the preanesthesia evaluation. As intraoperative lab results are frequently required *stat*, the interface details must be carefully planned to ensure that results will be delivered in a time frame compatible with intraoperative care.
- *Surgery schedule*. Patient and case information may be received into the AIMS, populating a number of fields in the record that would otherwise have to be entered by clinical users.
- *Others*. Other interfaces may include clinic scheduling, ancillary results such as electrocardiographic or radiology reports, with or without actual direct access to the image, nonsurgery consults, and billing interfaces for professional fee charges.

An interface consists of two sides: a user side, which is provided by the facility, and a vendor side. Consider the ADT interface. The facility typically has a dedicated interface engine—a computer that is dedicated to feeding data from various sources to other systems. The interface engine is the user's side of the ADT interface. The AIMS vendor may provide a dedicated computer on their side of the ADT interface. Vendors and users typically specify that the data communication between the two computers be formatted as Health Level 7 (HL7) transactions. HL7 defines a set of transaction types and fields that supports communication of many types of health data, including ADT, lab results, and charges. Vendors have designed interface software to process HL7 transactions. To specify the interface, the vendor typically requires the user to map the ADT data elements to HL7 transactions and fields. Similarly, the vendor will map the same transactions and fields to their database tables. A vendor who offers an integrated set of clinical systems (e.g., surgery, scheduling, and anesthesia) may not require some interfaces because most of the data would be native to the shared database. However, it is important to avoid the assumption that the presence of two systems from the same vendor means that they are automatically integrated or even that they have an existing interface.

When planning the back-end hardware, facilities should provide for a test environment, which may consist of a single server and perhaps an interface computer. The test environment will be critical for testing software upgrades, backup processes, and new configurations before they are deployed on the primary servers. The test environment may also be useful for troubleshooting problems and allowing the institution to test other systems, such as a new lab system, against the existing program. The plan should also include use of back-end hardware for data queries and data backup. Regularly updating data on an additional server not only helps to protect the data, but enables the data to be queried. For complex queries, this type of configuration will ensure that clinical throughput to the production database is not inappropriately impacted. Mission-critical applications such as AIMS are particularly vulnerable to major, complex queries that affect point-of-care performance and response times.

Front-end hardware planning includes determining the number of workstations on which the AIMS client software will be installed (if configured as thick clients) or from which the software will be accessed (if configured as thin clients). Some locations may require or may benefit from special hardware. For example, the intraoperative workstations may require touchscreens and/or special serial data interfaces to the patient monitors. Many touchscreen technologies are available, and it is important to choose them carefully. It is best to have durable touchscreens that can be used with gloved hands or a stylus. One-milliliter syringe plungers can be used as convenient, disposable styluses. Depending on whether mobility is required, table-type computers may be necessary for preanesthesia evaluations. A plan should exist to support data entry for preoperative and postoperative evaluations of inpatients. The data entry may be accomplished by allowing ward and ICU computers to have access to these modules via Citrix, remote access, or a thick client. The core team must select what is best for the installation, with advice from the vendor. For components being purchased in large quantities, it is best to construct one working system and ensure that it is equipped, mounted, and functioning as desired before committing to a large purchase. Adequate time must be allocated for this process to ensure that purchasing and installing the hardware do not delay the project.

Within the ORs, computers are typically mounted on the anesthesia machines. Special consideration for the ergonomics of those mounts is required, because the workstation is being inserted into a heavily instrumented work area, with much of the equipment being critical, life-support devices. The core team should work with the facility's Biomedical Engineering department and the vendor to determine the best options for mounting to the anesthesia machines. On which side of the anesthesia machine should the workstation be mounted? One advantage to mounting on the left side (typically over the CO_2 absorber) is that the anesthetist can interact with the workstation without turning away from the patient. A disadvantage is that if an attending anesthesiologist is supervising the anesthetist, the attending and anesthetist must trade places so that the attending can interact with the workstation, e.g., when the attending enters attestations regarding participation and electronically signs the record. Mounting on the right side of the anesthesia machine reverses the aforementioned advantage and disadvantage. Other factors, such as the placement of the other equipment, may also influence the decision. If the choice is not obvious, the project team may want to try each option and then consider feedback from front-line users, because if the ergonomics are clumsy, it may jeopardize the success of the deployment.

The patient monitors themselves must be evaluated to determine their compatibility with the AIMS. Some uniformity of monitors and anesthesia machines is advisable to reduce the in-house support costs. The greater the variety, the more difficult it will be for Biomedical Engineering to troubleshoot monitor-to-workstation interface issues and replace workstations.

The vendor will specify how the monitors and anesthesia machines will connect to the AIMS. Most monitors and anesthesia machines can send digital data serially through a port, such as an RS232 port, which is the same kind as that on modems and personal computers. However, because multiple devices are interfaced to the AIMS within each OR, the vendor usually requires a more elaborate interface scheme than simply connecting a personal computer to a modem or printer. Although many configurations are possible, two basic variants exist. One uses a communication multiplexer that combines several serial data streams from monitors into a single data stream to the AIMS workstation, similar to the way in which a USB hub connects a mouse, external disk drive, and printer to a personal computer (Fig. 4.1). Another technique interfaces the monitors through a communication multiplexer to the network and then to the server, with the AIMS workstation also connecting via the network to the server (Fig. 4.2). Regardless of how the system is set up, it is necessary to carefully identify, in advance, what equipment is necessary and where it will be located.

If AIMS applications are to be deployed on bedside computers in the PACU or preop holding, the mounts for those computers should also be determined. Options

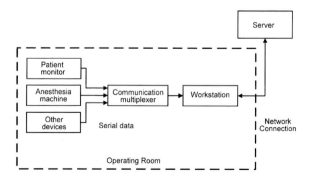

Fig. 4.1 Typical AIMS configuration in which the monitor data are stored on the local workstation and then flow to the central server for final storage

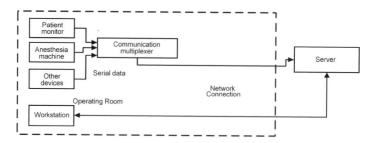

Fig. 4.2 Typical AIMS configuration in which the monitor data flow through the network to the central server for final storage. The workstation then accesses and shares these data for display when necessary

include wall-mounted computers, mobile carts, and tablets. Finally, if AIMS components are to be deployed on existing computers, their compatibility with the vendor's requirements, their ability to run the applications efficiently, and their ability to be maintained by the AIMS software support team should be assessed.

The project team should consider if applications that are not part of the AIMS are to be installed on OR and other AIMS workstations. One obvious candidate is software that accesses hospital and patient information, e.g., lab data, patient images, EMRs, and the surgery schedule. Increasingly, these data are accessed via a Web browser. However, access to Web browsers may also tempt staff with inappropriate distractions during patient care. Proxy servers can be used to disallow access to inappropriate Web sites or to allow only selected Web sites to be accessed. Access to other information, such as the facility's paging service, paging directory, and clinical protocols, may also be important. The clinical utility of each application or information source should be balanced against its potential for distraction.

Security

The network on which the AIMS relies has a security layer that prevents unauthorized access. Similarly, the AIMS has its own security features that limit unauthorized access to AIMS applications and patient data. AIMS security may be considered along three dimensions: application security, database security, and data backup. Application security is implemented by limiting the physical locations at which AIMS applications are deployed and by limiting the users who can access those applications. The clinical applications, such as intraoperative documentation and the preanesthesia evaluation, should be accessible by all anesthetists and anesthesiologists. However, the nurses in the preanesthesia clinic may need access only to the preanesthesia evaluation application. Nonclinical applications, such as management components, quality assurance, etc., may require more restrictive access to protect sensitive data and analysis.

In that AIMS data can be accessed through the AIMS applications or directly from the database; the database must be secured as well. One noteworthy way to realize a return on the AIMS investment is to extract data directly from its database for analysis that may not be available from the vendor's components. By using third-party software such as Microsoft Access or other database tools, data can be extracted directly from the AIMS database. However, granting users direct access to the AIMS database must be considered carefully. Only those with the need to access such data for management or research should be granted access. Furthermore, such access must be restricted to read-only.

The vendor should have full access to the AIMS database and file servers in order to support the customer in troubleshooting problems. As the vendor's access is remote, special precautions are required to prevent the servers from being visible to the public. Most facilities have a data security officer who can advise the core team on how to grant the vendor the necessary access, while fulfilling the institution's obligations under HIPAA.

Finally, to protect the data within the database and file server against loss or corruption, a data backup strategy must be developed and implemented. Typically, the database and file servers are completely backed up weekly or on some other regular schedule, and they are incrementally backed up nightly. Incremental backups copy only the data that has changed since the last backup cycle, enabling a full restoration from the combination of the last full backup and the incremental backups following it. This strategy takes less time to accomplish on a daily basis but at the cost of more complex restoration. As restoration is rare, it is a desirable tradeoff.

Testing

During system planning, a test environment is important for system configuration development and testing. Some AIMS may support a test environment that consists of a single workstation with the software components installed in a stand-alone configuration, so that they operate without connecting to a server. Other AIMS may require a more traditional client-server configuration. In either case, the test environment enables the users to refine and test the configuration, including identifying users and setting their permissions, before going live in the production environment. This configuration can then be copied to the production server before going live without having to rebuild the system. The vendor should have access to the test environment so that it can support configuration and transition to production.

All interfaces should be tested, but by definition, they cannot be tested in a stand-alone test environment. Therefore, some coordination with the institution's interface specialist is required. A formal acceptance test may be part of the acquisition contract. Installation and testing of the ADT interface is a logical first choice. If the ADT interface filters patients by some criteria, such as location, it should be confirmed that the patients on the surgical schedule come across the interface. *Transaction latency* should also be determined; this is the time interval between when the ADT transaction is presented to the AIMS side of the interface and when the patient's information is available to an AIMS application. The design should ensure that demographic data for same-day admit patients are available when the patients are first documented in the system, which may be as early as patient entry into preop holding.

The hospital billing interface should be tested to ensure that all of the charges are configured in the system. This function can be tested by creating dummy cases in which all charges are entered as part of the cases. Because the patients are fictitious with fictitious accounts, this test should be conducted in a billing test environment, or reserve accounts for testing purposes should be used. Both credits and debits to patient accounts should be tested to ensure that charge corrections can be handled correctly by the interface.

The laboratory interface should be assessed for the presentation of the desired test results because a patient may have many test results available that have overlapping results (e.g., different lab orders may produce a glucose level). The interval between the time that the results are available from the lab instrument to the time that the results are presented in an AIMS application should be determined. Long latencies in the laboratory interface may limit its usefulness.

Practice cases that utilize all of these interfaces plus the relevant clinical data modules must be tested, and each module will require its own testing procedure. The preoperative module must be tested for usability and completeness. Stakeholders must determine if the right balance has been struck between automatic entries and text entries to optimize efficiency and ensure completeness. The intraoperative module requires similar trials. The monitor capture must function as expected, and the templates must match patient flow. One method of testing involves using real data, but sending them to the test server. This technique allows near-complete testing without prematurely creating a medical record of nonvalid data. Because the data are not real, this method permits testing of features that may be unrelated to the actual case populating the system.

Other strategies can optimize the utility of clinical testing. One is to ensure that different modules are working together properly. For example, preoperative data must display properly in the intraoperative module. In institutions that use medical direction of other anesthesiology providers, some features for faculty will be different from those for CRNAs, Student RNAs, or anesthesiology residents. Including all relevant groups in testing will help to optimize functionality. Finally, system backup and restoration should be tested and practiced within the test environment before switching to the production environment. The worst time to perform the first system restoration is when the system has failed and restoration is required to get the system back on line.

Deployment

Deploying all of the necessary AIMS components to all of the necessary locations for a single go-live date is challenging, if not impossible, for large installations. Even though an AIMS provides the most return on investment when all of the components are used to capture data from preanesthesia evaluation through intraoperative anesthesia care for every anesthetic, large installations may require staging for practical reasons. If an installation is planned for multiple facilities—e.g., a large flagship hospital plus community hospitals and outpatient surgery centers – one staging strategy is to deploy at different facilities at different times. Alternatively, different components might be deployed separately. For example, deploying the intraoperative documentation component before the preanesthesia evaluation component (or vice versa) might be considered. However, some combination of components is required to support the workflow, as in the example mentioned here. Other components may be deployed separately without affecting workflow. Such factors must be considered when planning staged deployments.

End-user training must be undertaken before deployment and must be required of all staff, without exception. Vendors should provide written training materials for users to review. It is usually best to employ in-house trainers or superusers in addition to vendor-provided training resources. These superusers can train the rest of the staff ahead of the go-live date. Just as all groups of users should be involved in testing, trainers should also come from all relevant groups. Allowing users to practice in a test environment before going live is highly recommended. Some form of competency assessment should also be considered, perhaps with staff completing the assessment to acquire privileges to the production system.

For the first few days after deployment, the superusers should be available to help users with their initial records. It is unwise to rely solely on the vendor for this purpose, because the vendor is unlikely to be able to provide a sufficient number of people to adequately cover the users, except perhaps at small installations. Initially, the user might be tempted to keep records manually in parallel with the system. Although such a dual system may be necessary in certain circumstances, it is a substantial burden to provide quality patient care, maintain charts on a new system, and maintain a handwritten record simultaneously. Generally, it is better to limit handwritten records to cases for which the new AIMS is too difficult to use at that particular stage of the learning process.

Failure to use the system must be carefully monitored. Some individuals may need additional training or support. If configuration problems are identified, they must be quickly remedied. Management must determine a date beyond which all records will be generated through the AIMS, except in those locations that are not instrumented, e.g., MRI. One gauge of implementation success is how quickly staff abandon the manually kept record and embrace the electronic record on the AIMS.

Failure is a possibility. During the go-live process, it should be expected that many small flaws will be identified in the system. They should be remedied by the team. If some larger failures occur, it is critical to remedy them as quickly as possible. It may be necessary to rely on manual procedures until the remedy has been implemented. In some cases, failures may even cause a postponement of the go-live process. It is imperative to rapidly determine whether or not a critical failure can easily be compensated for or fixed quickly. A go-live date should not be abandoned lightly, nor should a user persist with an implementation that is not working.

Transition to Maintenance

Once the frenzy of deployment has passed and the core team has recovered, ongoing needs will become apparent. Ideally, after 2–3 weeks, the superusers will no longer be training or troubleshooting common user problems. However, users are still likely to experience occasional problems, unrelated to inexperience, that require some technical support. Relying on the vendor as the sole means of frontline technical support is unlikely to prove sufficient. Therefore, a technical support structure must be planned, managed, and funded.

Building an internal technical support structure can be accomplished in a variety of ways. Regardless of the structure, the goals of technical support are the same (a) rapid resolution of problems affecting clinical documentation and (b) prevention of data loss. Usually, rapid resolution of problems requires some form of support immediately available on site, whether it is from clinical staff (e.g., superusers), a help desk, a dedicated technical support "SWAT" team, or AIMS-savvy Biomedical Engineering support personnel. The type and size of facility will influence the choice for a technical support structure. Some combination of resources will likely be coordinated to provide timely and cost-effective support.

Another maintenance task that will quickly become apparent after deployment is user/personnel maintenance. New users must be added to the system with appropriate permissions assigned, terminated users must be inactivated, and other personnel who are identified in the system but are not users (e.g., surgeons) must be added or inactivated as they are hired or move on. In a large facility, these are weekly, if not daily, tasks. Depending on the frequency of changes, this job may be assigned to someone other than the system administrator who may be in a better position to know when personnel arrive and leave. The vendor will recommend scheduled database and file-server maintenance tasks. Such tasks are required to keep the database server responsive and are the responsibility of the system administrator.

Life-Cycle Issues

The vendor will occasionally offer updated versions of the software. Because the vendor's ability to support older versions of the product may be limited, it is usually recommended that facilities keep their AIMS software current. Unfortunately, deploying AIMS software upgrades requires planning similar to, though somewhat less extensive than, that required for initial deployment. Before proceeding, facilities must carefully evaluate what the new version offers versus the cost of the upgrade, including the cost of the internal resources. In addition to vendor-provided software version updates, workstation operating system updates and patches must be deployed. These can require significant resources as well. For example, the patch to operating systems for Daylight Savings Time in the spring of 2007 was a challenge to many installations.

Facilities should plan to replace their AIMS workstation hardware at appropriate intervals. If the system is large, workstation hardware replacement should be either staggered or budgeted well in advance to avoid unexpected strain on the capital budget. At some point, a facility may contemplate replacing its AIMS with another vendor's system. This decision can be very difficult and demands that many issues be addressed. Foremost is the accessibility of the data housed in the former system. How will they be continued? If the former system's data cannot be converted and loaded into the new system, which may be difficult at best, how long should they be available? Very few current installations of AIMS have faced these difficult questions.

Finally, long-term storage of data must be anticipated. As part of the medical record, the data may need to be preserved for decades. It is possible that the storage media may be at risk of degrading and producing unreliable data. Unlike paper records, the technology for reading unique media may disappear. Because this is an issue shared by all hospital information systems, solutions may be sought through the IT department if and when this situation occurs. One option is to convert the records to images in a common form, such as TIFF or PDF files; although none of the database benefits convey to this mode, the individual patient's record will be preserved.

Conclusion

It is clear that from inception through the life cycle of the product, an AIMS requires careful planning, an ability to deal with detail and the strategic long view, a strong institutional commitment, and, most importantly, adaptability. Implementing an AIMS requires technical knowledge concerning how the hardware and the software function, clinical knowledge concerning how care is delivered, business knowledge concerning how the delivered care translates to hospital and professional billing, and management knowledge concerning the data required to manage anesthesia services effectively. An implementation team that has this collective knowledge is required. Leadership skills are required to focus such a diverse team, to identify the compromises that will be required during implementation, and to acquire the necessary buy-in from the affected staff.

Key Points

- Implementation planning requires the following:

  ○ A project team that represents the various disciplines required to support the system (IT, Biomedical Engineering, Network) and that represents the staff who are affected by the system (anesthetists, anesthesiologists, nursing, management).

- ○ A clear definition of the system scope.
- ○ An understanding of the clinical and business processes that are affected by the AIMS.
- ○ An assessment of the network coverage required for the AIMS.
- ○ A determination of the workstation, server, and interface requirements.
- ○ A plan for the security structure of the system.

- AIMS configuration should map the clinical and business processes, and those familiar with those processes should be consulted as part of the configuration task.
- A test environment should be utilized as part of the AIMS deployment and to support future enhancements:

  - ○ Integrated testing is required for interfaces to other systems such as ADT, billing, and laboratory results.
  - ○ Clinical supervisors must be sufficiently trained to support new users when they go live.

- Deploying a full AIMS as a single event is difficult:

  - ○ Multiple processes, sites, and users are affected, while the size of support infrastructure is generally fixed.
  - ○ Staged release of modules should be considered.
  - ○ Staged geographic implementation should be considered.

- After deployment, a robust and responsive support team must exist to ensure that the system is reliable and available nearly all of the time.

Chapter 5
Ensuring Usability through Human Factors Engineering

Jonathan Kendler and Michael Wiklund

Although the advantages and shortcomings of an AIMS have been debated, in the age of advanced computers, it seems arcane to manually transcribe to a paper form numbers that are displayed on a patient monitor. Potential human errors associated with manual systems include failing to record data due to distraction or forgetfulness, misreading data, and transcribing data incorrectly or illegibly (Fig. 5.1). Entering data into forms is a task that computers perform particularly well, whereas humans are prone to error. In recognition of this reality, the Anesthesia Patient Safety Foundation passed the following motion in 2001: "The APSF endorses and advocates the use of automated record keeping in the perioperative period and the subsequent retrieval and analysis of the data to improve patient safety."[1] Nonetheless, most anesthesia providers continue to document their cases using paper forms more than 20 years after the introduction of the first automated systems.[2] Sometimes, the choice is a matter of economics, with AIMS costs estimated to be $20,000 per OR. Sometimes, clinicians are concerned that automation can decrease their situational awareness during a case. Given how an anesthesia record can factor into medical malpractice proceedings, some clinicians are also concerned about the ease of detecting and accounting for artifacts (e.g., aberrant data) with an AIMS. However, the usability shortcomings of AIMS—many related to design of the software user interface—have historically represented a major obstacle to wider adoption.

Fortunately, the latest generation of AIMS has overcome many of the human factors shortcomings found in earlier systems and includes upgrades such as graphical user interfaces and touchscreens, making them far more usable (Fig. 5.2). Nonetheless, opportunities remain for enhancing their usability. The human factors challenges associated with producing a usable AIMS, as well as broader issues of user acceptance related to AIMS's usefulness, efficiency, and appeal are discussed in this chapter.

About Human Factors Engineering

In the context of user interface design, the term *human factors* describes human characteristics that influence the quality of physical and mental interactions with a given product. Physical characteristics include body size, range of motion, strength, and dexterity. Mental characteristics include information acquisition and processing

J. Stonemetz, K. Ruskin (eds.) *Anesthesia Informatics*,
© Springer Science+Business Media, LLC 2008

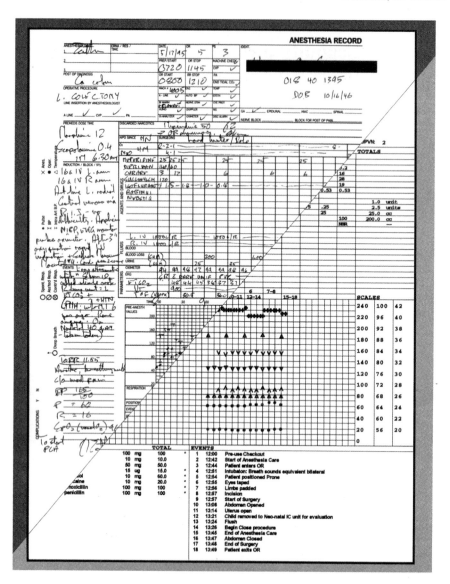

Fig. 5.1 Comparison of handwritten and automated anesthesia record. Cover, ASA Newsletter 59(6), June 1995, reprinted with permission of the ASA

ability, previous knowledge, attentiveness, and learning style. Human factors textbooks contain extensive data and thousands of guidelines on how to design user interfaces that match human capabilities.

The practice of human factors engineering (also called *ergonomics* and *usability engineering*) involves the application of human factors knowledge and guidelines to produce user interfaces that are well suited to the intended users. The discipline

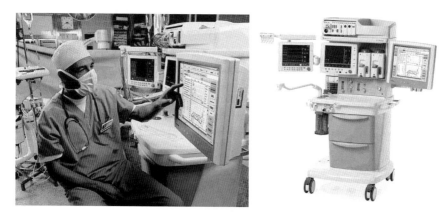

Fig. 5.2 Anesthesiologist reviews data presented on General Electric's Centricity anesthesia system (*left*), which is integrated with the company's anesthesia delivery unit (*right*) (photo courtesy of GE Healthcare)

was formalized in 1950 with the establishment of the Human Factors Society (now called the Human Factors and Ergonomics Society) and is now seeing more widespread application in the medical domain, following the issuance of international regulations and standards that call for its application in the course of a risk management program.[3] Regulator-mandated recalls and embargoes, as well as product liability claims that resulted from use error, have also been strong motivators.

Clearly, AIMS pose extensive human factors challenges and can benefit from the inclusion of human factors engineering in the product development cycle. The following are discussed below:

- Design characteristics known to improve usability
- User feedback regarding the strengths and weaknesses of existing systems and opportunities for innovation
- Benefits and mechanics of usability testing

Usability Considerations

Human factors practitioners utilize established design principles, tempered with professional judgment, to make systems safe, easy, and efficient to use. The principles discussed here are based on the authors' applied design experience, opinions collected from practicing anesthesia providers and AIMS developers, and the human factors literature.

Minimizing Learning Time

While some physicians and nurses will dedicate substantial nonclinical time—perhaps dozens of hours—to learning to use an AIMS, others will not because they have little free time or simply prefer the trial-and-error approach to learning. To accommodate the trial-and-error types, AIMS should enable users to perform at least the most basic tasks without substantial training. They should also minimize the need for supplemental training to master advanced functions, instead enabling users to develop mastery as the natural outcome of extended system use. This type of on-the-job training can be accomplished by user interfaces that enable users to explore new features without concern for causing damage to the system. For example, being able to preview changes to a record before saving them allows users to check for data-entry errors. Similarly, consistently providing "Back" and "Undo" controls enables users to easily correct identified errors.

Ensuring Positive Transfer of Experience

To ease the adjustment from manual anesthesia record keeping to an AIMS, as well as to avoid use errors associated with the presumption of similarity to past approaches, AIMS should carry forward the best characteristics of highly evolved manual records. In that way, users can follow familiar data entry and retrieval routines and avoid cases in which previously learned (i.e., routinized) behaviors cause problems because they do not apply to the new situation—a result termed *negative transfer*. For example, users who are familiar with a horizontal representation of a case's timeline might have difficulty adjusting to an AIMS that presents a vertical timeline, potentially leading them to make documentation or reading errors.

Facilitating Workflow

Anesthesia providers are normally taught to follow definitive medical procedures matched to various clinical conditions and events. Therefore, an AIMS should facilitate established procedures and workflows, rather than force users to adapt their procedures to accommodate a particular system's design. Any procedural changes warranted by using an AIMS should be justified by careful analysis of the associated advantages and disadvantages, with consideration of the human factors principle that technology should adapt to users, not the other way around.

Providing a Sense of Control

Maintaining a sense of control depends on the availability of key information and control options at the time they are required. Especially true of anesthesia workstations that deliver life-supporting therapy, it is also true of an electronic record that requires users to perform tasks, such as documenting medication administration and reviewing preceding events, to determine trends and causes of adverse events. Accordingly, an AIMS's screens should be task-oriented, giving users what they need when they need it, so that they continue to feel in control.

Allowing Flexibility

By virtue of their logic-driven nature, software applications often lock users into specific navigation, information-acquisition, and data-entry patterns. However, human beings, regardless of how logic- and procedure-driven they might be, behave in ways that call for software flexibility. In particular, human beings like to set the pace, rather than having their actions machine paced. They also like to perform tasks in a preferred order, which might vary day to day or case to case, as opposed to a dictated order. Accordingly, AIMS designers should allow for interactive flexibility where possible, rather than requiring users to enter information in a specific order and at a specific pace.

Establishing a Familiar Conceptual Model

The foundation of any software application is its conceptual model—an organizational scheme that ultimately determines the location of content across multiple screens and various pathways to access it. Simple and appropriate conceptual models enable users to "get the big picture" on how to envision and navigate a software application (Fig. 5.3). Complex and inappropriate conceptual models cause users to bog down, making it a struggle to comprehend an application's features and develop a means of using them.

Simple and logical conceptual models beget simple and logical navigation, presuming the consistent placement of necessary controls and continuous feedback regarding one's location in the overall user interface structure (Fig. 5.4).

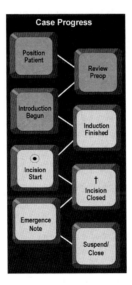

Fig. 5.3 Docusys' organization scheme reflects the case workflow familiar to anesthesiologists (courtesy of Docusys, Inc., Mobile, AL)

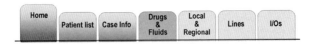

Fig. 5.4 Tabs on General Electric's Centricity anesthesia system enable users to move intuitively and swiftly among information sets (courtesy of GE Healthcare)

Facilitating Situational Awareness

Anesthesia providers must maintain situational awareness of the patient's and the procedure's status, and an AIMS should facilitate this awareness rather than detract from it. Awareness can be enhanced by presenting users with the right information at the right time and providing no more information than necessary. Awareness can be degraded by presenting users with the wrong information, too much information, or information that requires some type of mental conversion before it is useful, as well as demanding the user's attention when it should be directed elsewhere.

Ensuring Legibility

AIMS are bound to present information more legibly than handwritten entries on a paper form. However, software designers can push the legibility limit by using complex-looking fonts, overly small characters, and low-contrast text and background color combinations. Accordingly, designers should gravitate toward sans serif fonts that are sized to be legible from more than an arm's reach and placed on a sharply contrasting background. For example, 14-point, black Arial text on a white background should be quite legible from a distance of 1 meter. Legibility is further improved by adequate spacing between visual elements such as rows of text.

Differentiating Current and Old Data

Because anesthesia providers will make critical decisions based on the AIMS data, they need to know at a glance if they are viewing current or old data. Therefore, information should be coded to clearly differentiate and highlight the most current data. Moreover, intermittently refreshed information should include a time stamp (e.g., 10:54 a.m.) that enables users to note its age.

Highlighting Critical Information

As indicated by eye-tracking devices, a user's eye is likely to jump around an AIMS screen to the most visually conspicuous or distinctive information. Therefore, screen designers should determine which information demands the most attention and then use visual design techniques to make that information stand out. For example, high-priority information can be presented using larger text or numerals, differentiated by color, and placed in screen locations that naturally draw the eye (e.g., the top left corner in Western cultures).

Organizing Data

Large and complex data sets present a myriad of organizational options, but the nature of anesthesia delivery strongly suggests a time-based organization, as reflected in decades of paper anesthesia records. Therefore, many of the current systems appropriately employ a time-based organization system. However, designers can still give users the option of filtering and viewing data in alternative ways.

Visualizing Data

Designers should look for every opportunity to preprocess data and present it in the most naturally meaningful manner (Fig. 5.5). For example, graphs are often superior to data tables as a means to give users the "big picture," but designers can take things further than the kind of graphs produced by applications such as Microsoft Excel. For example, a timeline could be enhanced by graphic labels and status indicators that reduce the amount of information to be read. Data can be color coded to indicate whether they are within or outside the normal range.

Signaling Missing Data and Artifacts

Giving users a sense of control means enabling them to correct the "mistakes" of the AIMS. Because a given system is not a sentient observer of the anesthesia case, it cannot know when special events might lead to artifacts in the data stream.

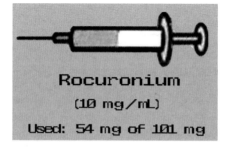

Fig. 5.5 Docusys' main screen, which presents data values in a visual manner to facilitate reading (courtesy of Docusys, Inc., Mobile, AL)

Consequently, such artifacts can appear in the electronic record and require correction. For example, designers can help users to detect artifacts by flagging values that are out of range. They can also speed quality checks by making it easy to make corrections. However, a competing need is the capability to prevent users from falsifying data to hide adverse events.

Using Familiar and Common Terms

It is always important for software applications to "speak" the user's language rather than the developer's. Therefore, recognizing that such users know their own jargon best, designers should be sure to engage representative users to help in selecting terms that are most familiar to them and their facility. In addition to familiar terms, industry-consistent terms must also be used, notably those under development by the Data Dictionary Task Force of the Anesthesia Patient Safety Foundation, which promises to help clinicians shift readily between systems without having to learn a new nomenclature.[4]

Using Acronyms and Abbreviations

Many acronyms and abbreviations (such as NIBP, noninvasive blood pressure) have effectively replaced their long forms, in the same way that "FedEx" replaced "Federal Express" (Fig. 5.6). However, some acronyms and abbreviations have been demonstrated to cause confusion and introduce the potential for error. Therefore, The Joint Commission has published a "do not use" list of abbreviations, acronyms, and symbols, which includes "@," "cc," and most abbreviations of drug names.[5] Accordingly, AIMS must accommodate long text strings, making electronic records larger and requiring an effective means of scrolling or paging.

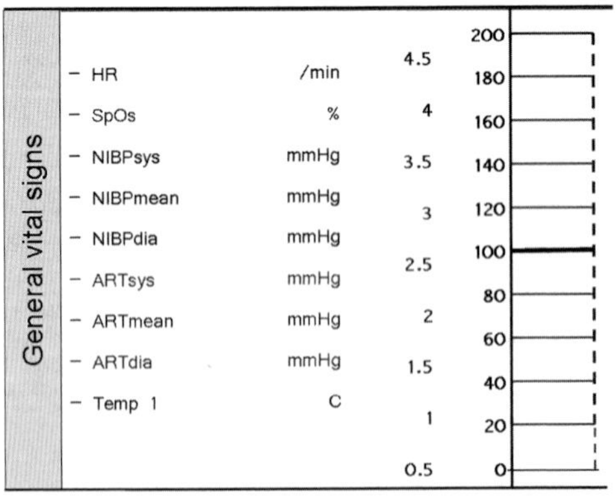

Fig. 5.6 Excerpt from General Electric's Centricity anesthesia machine's main screen uses familiar acronyms and abbreviations (courtesy of GE Healthcare)

Using Symbols

Generally, software application users prefer symbols over text when a symbol can convey information more quickly and reliably. However, symbols should not be used in place of conventional information formats. For example, the term NIBP ultimately functions as a symbol (like FedEx does) and probably should not be replaced with an icon showing an arm and a pressure cuff. Also, the number of symbols should be limited to prevent an interface from looking like a wall of hieroglyphics. As such, symbols are usually best suited for labeling common navigation controls and familiar data sets.

Using Color

While color can play an important role in screen design, excessive use of color is counterproductive. Ideally, developers will use color to draw the user's eye to more important information (as discussed above) and to code information (e.g., distinguishing one class of drugs from another, such as distinguishing blood pressure medications from antibiotics).

Ensuring Visual Appeal

While visual appeal is clearly secondary to an AIMS's functional capabilities, looks still matter. Not only will visually appealing screens increase user satisfaction—after all, they have to look at the screens all day—but they can also enhance usability, given that visual appeal arises from good design practices, such as aligning on-screen information to a grid to facilitate rapid visual acquisition.

Choosing an Interaction Mechanism

Today, the mouse rules as an interaction mechanism used in conjunction with most software. However, the medical environment often makes devices such as touchscreens, trackballs, rotary encoders, and styli the pointing devices of choice. Limited space for a pointing device and cleanability are among the chief factors that drive the final choice(s). Meanwhile, an emerging trend is to provide users with choices, thereby accommodating special needs and preferences and reducing the need for users to become facile with a new device.

Enabling Rapid Data Entry

Strategies by which to accelerate data entry include providing users with lists of common options, such as the names of the months or common drugs, thus limiting the amount of typing and the potential for typing errors. Other strategies include (a) enabling users to manipulate on-screen analog mechanisms, such as moving a pointer on a scale, (b) prefilling data entry fields with default values that may be accepted or readily replaced with alternative values, and (c) giving the user the option to select from lists. Anesthesia providers are not particularly enamored with typing, although as the years pass, an increasing proportion of them should have good typing skills. However, regardless of who is typing, the chance for typos is ever present. In addition, typing is a distraction from direct patient care. Therefore, developers should minimize the typing demands placed upon caregivers.

Correcting Entries

People tend to work faster when they know that it is easy to detect a mistake and quickly correct it. Therefore, AIMS developers should pay particular attention to highlighting potential data entry errors and guiding corrections. Some infusion pumps employ this strategy by alerting users when they program an unusually high dose and indicating the institutionally established limit.

Dealing with Data Loss

Those who depend on electronic data capture systems are usually wary of the potential for data loss. In the business world, electronic files on desktop computers are regularly backed-up onto peripheral devices, and such protection is also the norm among AIMS. However, in addition to ensuring data protection, AIMS users need a fast and convenient means to retrieve "lost" data and continue with their normal clinical activities. Users should be alerted immediately about an AIMS failure that has caused data loss or has somehow reduced the collected data's integrity.

Integration

As discussed in the following section, integrating an AIMS with other anesthesia-related equipment and hospital systems is a cornerstone to overall usefulness. Accordingly, an AIMS should (a) use common terms, symbols, and data visualization schemes; (b) have templates that match with clinical workflows; and (c) communicate fluidly with other equipment and systems. Of course, this goal is obstructed by existing inconsistencies that are independent of a particular AIMS. Therefore, developers can only do their best to follow conventions where they exist and make their systems flexible enough to adapt to a particular institution's conditions and needs.

User Opinions

The authors conducted a survey of 15 anesthesia providers working in more than ten institutions using six different AIMS. The sample included respondents from more than six states in the continental United States. Approximately 75% of the respondents worked at urban teaching hospitals, while the others work at community hospitals. Survey results indicate that anesthesia providers value their AIMS but frequently face usability problems. Moreover, they have many suggestions on how the systems can be improved to be more compatible with their practices. Note that many of the reported views corresponded with the previously discussed design considerations.

General

Overall, survey respondents indicated a positive opinion of AIMS. All participants described AIMS as easier to use than manual systems, primarily due to the minimization or elimination of manual data entry. Most respondents described AIMS as more efficient than manual systems, again because they automatically transfer data from peripheral devices to the system. However, a few respondents noted that even though AIMS are proven to be faster than manual systems, they can be perceived as being slower. New steps, such as navigating through menus or confirming entries, can make AIMS seem as if they are increasing the anesthesiologist's workload.

Approximately half of the participants described AIMS as less prone to use error than manual systems, while the other half described AIMS as more prone to use error. These divergent opinions are probably due to design differences among the systems. For example, systems that incorporate safety-enhancing features, such as dosage checking and cautionary prompts, can help to prevent use errors. Conversely, systems with design shortcomings, such as a complex navigation scheme or an unclear layout, can increase use errors.

Asked to rank-order AIMS design attributes, most respondents named ease of use, user support, and speed of use as most important and named similarity to paper-based documentation, visual appeal, and ease of learning as the least important attributes.

Design Strengths

Multiple Input Methods

Enabling multiple means of interacting with an AIMS helps clinicians to use it efficiently. Survey respondents favored the combination of keyboard-based entry and a touchscreen or rotary encoder (i.e., jog dial). Keyboards facilitate manual data entry, while touchscreens and rotary wheels enable rapid navigation and option/target selection.

Direct Manipulation

Rather than having to navigate through multiple screens and populate numerous data fields, survey respondents noted a preference for directly accessing and modifying data using visual representations (i.e., analog displays) of data values. For example, respondents preferred documenting an event time by clicking on an on-screen timeline rather than typing hours and minutes into a data entry field. Other examples include sliders that allow users to adjust a value with the slide of a mouse and drag-and-drop features. Such interactions save time by minimizing typing. They also facilitate rapid data acquisition in a preprocessed form, thereby reducing mental workload.

Templates

According to survey respondents, case- or unit-specific templates can lower user workload and accelerate documentation tasks. Systems that include case templates allow users to identify the type of case they are documenting and provide them with case-specific features, such as specialized menus and prefilled fields to minimize setup time. Recognizing that different institutions and care units have different needs, respondents lauded systems that featured customizable templates.

Time-based Workflow

Many survey respondents noted a preference for AIMS that are organized to complement real-world anesthesia workflow. In particular, respondents favored systems that present a time-based view of the case, such as a graphical timeline that displays all of the information and associated controls in chronologic order (Fig. 5.7). Such an on-screen representation allows users to document their cases in a manner that matches their mental map of anesthesia delivery.

Memory Aids

Although AIMS automate a significant portion of the documentation process, clinicians are by no means completely rid of manual documentation tasks. Therefore, clinicians remain at risk of forgetting to document certain conditions and events, as well as skipping steps in the documentation process. Many respondents valued AIMS that provide prompts to the user by presenting setup checklists or specific documentation requests that help to ensure a complete anesthesia record.

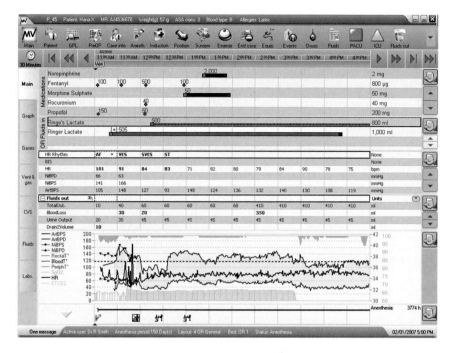

Fig. 5.7 Excerpt from MVOR's (MetaVision for Operating Rooms) main screen presents both data and data visualizations on the same time axis (courtesy of iMDsoft)

User Support

Most anesthesia providers will invest the effort required to master their AIMS. Over time, however, they might forget how to perform certain functions or encounter aspects of the system that they overlooked during their initial studies. Consequently, respondents lauded systems that provided embedded user support, such as instructional prompts and pop-up messages that help to save time and prevent use errors. Importantly, effective embedded support often negates the need to contact customer support, which can be time consuming and expensive for both the hospital and the AIMS manufacturer.

Ergonomics

While most interactions with AIMS occur via the software screen, the system's physical characteristics have a significant effect on usability. For example, respondents favored large computer monitors with clear images, the placement of monitors on adjustable arms that facilitate repositioning during a case, and full-sized keyboards. Moreover, they valued systems that do not place undue constraints on the positioning of other OR equipment.

Similarity to Other Hospital Systems

Just as technical compatibility with other hospital systems is important (e.g., ensuring that power and data communication cables match up with ports), so too is user interface compatibility. Survey respondents noted that AIMS that use terminology, interaction mechanisms, and screen layouts similar to other hospital systems are ultimately easier and more efficient to use. Similarity to other hospital systems allows users to switch among the various systems without having to master new interactions. It also prevents negative transfer of experience from one system to another—a classic cause of use error.

Design Weaknesses

Artifact Notation

Automated data capture is probably electronic record keeping's most valued feature. However, data that enter the electronic record can contain unwanted information—often referred to as *artifact*—such as inadvertent or temporary parameter changes that occur while the anesthesiologist is configuring equipment. When such information gets into the electronic record, the anesthesia provider must detect and flag it or correct it. Unfortunately, many existing AIMS lack a convenient means by which to detect and correct artifacts. For example, respondents described systems in which artifacts can be difficult to detect because they exist in a virtual sea of other data and do not stand out. Also, dealing with artifact can be laborious and distract the caregiver from direct patient care.

Inflexible Workflows

Several respondents described their AIMS as well suited to average cases but poorly suited to more complicated and atypical cases because the systems impose a rigid workflow and data configuration. As an example, respondents described AIMS that require them to complete steps in a predefined order that sometimes conflicts with their clinical approach. Respondents suggested that AIMS should guide clinicians by providing case templates and streamlined workflows, while allowing them to make adjustments with ease.

Lack of Immediate Feedback

Whereas consumer software users have become accustomed to applications that present information in a "what you see is what you get" manner, survey respondents complained about AIMS that present an inaccurate view of case data. As an example, one respondent described a system that "hides" specific data until the user generates a report at the end of the case. He reported that the delayed data presentation had led him to overlook certain conditions and to manually enter certain data several times.

Limited Data Collection

To increase the efficiency of manual data entry and enable verification, most AIMS rely on controlled data entry methods such as drop-down menus, radio buttons, and limited text fields. While such controls facilitate documentation of simple information (e.g., medications used, flow rates, etc.), they can seem limited when used to collect more complicated information (e.g., a patient reaction) for which a more comprehensive or nuanced description would be desired. Several respondents noted that while they appreciated the time-saving benefits of an AIMS, they missed the richer descriptions that they were previously able to quickly jot down on paper.

Poorly Designed Reports

Despite the transition to electronic systems, paper-based documentation continues to play an important role in many clinical environments. Printouts of electronic records allow caretakers to conveniently review, share, and analyze information. However, several respondents criticized their AIMS for producing printouts that are not particularly readable (i.e., they do not ascribe to good document design principles). Respondents noted that despite the benefits of using an AIMS, something as basic as producing poor-quality printed reports can hobble their usefulness.

Impediments to Using Controls

Some respondents described rotary wheels that were difficult to clean and lost their effectiveness after repeated use due to contamination. Also, some complained that it was difficult to type on keyboards with plastic protective covers. Ultimately, respondents stated that physical interfaces should reflect a balance between maintainability (i.e., cleanability) and usability, enabling users to interact with physical components in an effective, comfortable, and reliable manner.

Inadequate Lists and Libraries

Medication and IV infusion libraries have the potential to alleviate significant amounts of manual typing. However, a poorly designed interface to such libraries can increase the anesthesia provider's workload. For example, menus with unconventional organization or navigation schemes can cause the user to spend excessive time searching for a specific medication.

Nuisance Warnings

While respondents lauded safety-enhancing features such as cautionary prompts and messages, they noted that excessive warnings and cautions can hinder the documentation process. In particular, respondents expressed disdain for warning messages related to a technical issue such as entering data in the wrong format.

Overzealous Error Prevention

Many respondents complimented the AIMS for its error-prevention capabilities such as automated dosage checks and entry validation. However, several complained that their AIMS was overzealous with its error-prevention efforts, thereby hindering the documentation process. Respondents suggested that in case of a potential documentation error, an AIMS should seek confirmation from users rather than prevent them from entering particular values. In general, they suggested that the implementation of error prevention means that the system should perform checks and request confirmations, rather than being prohibitive.

Presentation of Nonphysiologic Information

The primary role of an AIMS is to document and present physiologic information. However, some respondents criticized their systems for presenting an excessive amount of nonclinical information. As an example, they described screens littered with technical information related to system connectivity and software status data. Therefore, given the myriad information clinicians have to monitor, both in the AIMS and in other systems, many anesthesia providers will prefer to exclude such nonphysiologic details.

Online Help

Several respondents lauded their AIMS's assistive features, such as instructional prompts and tool tips. However, many respondents complained that their AIMS did not have a comprehensive help system. As such, several stated a preference for complete online help features that include summaries of system features and tutorials that provide step-by-step instructions. They said that such a help system would reduce their dependence on the AIMS manufacturer's customer support services.

Opportunities for Innovation

After identifying the strengths and shortcomings in existing systems, anesthesia providers suggested the following innovations.

Multimodal Interaction

Although respondents cited physical controls, including control wheels and touch-screens, as the most efficient means of interacting with existing AIMS, many indicated an interest in further innovation. Respondents identified voice input as the most promising means of documenting cases, despite the issue of distracting others in the workspace. They also expressed an interest in using biometric authentication (e.g., fingerprint scanners), barcode scanners, and location-aware technologies (e.g., radio-frequency identification tags) in conjunction with the AIMS.

Medication Search

Several respondents noted that poor navigation and search capabilities limit the usefulness of some AIMS drug libraries. Rather than a system that requires navigation through many menus that contain numerous drug categories and types, respondents suggested the addition of intelligent searching features that account for drug synonyms, misspellings, and incomplete entries.

Decision Support

Several respondents suggested that AIMS will reach their full potential once their use transitions from clinicians to assistants. To make this transition, respondents suggested that an AIMS should include reference libraries with dosage suggestions and best-practice descriptions.

Smoother, More Reliable Interaction with Other Systems

Despite technical advances that allow an AIMS to communicate with a variety of other medical devices and information systems, the actual setup and maintenance of such communication remains rather complicated and unreliable. Respondents sought AIMS that "plug-and-play"[6] with the institution's other systems in a simple and reliable manner that prevents the hassle of dealing with a technical problem during a case.

Support for Multiple Users

Most existing AIMS are geared toward single-user interactions; this is an appropriate target, given that anesthesiologists generally hold the primary responsibility for documenting their cases. However, respondents noted that providing access to additional users, including nurses and clinician assistants, could reduce their own workflow.

Better Conceptual Models

Despite the potential innovations associated with new technologies, many respondents noted that an AIMS's overall organization remains a particularly fertile area for innovation. Respondents noted that they still had not used an AIMS that "thought like an anesthesiologist."

Importance of Usability Testing

As with other complex software applications, the quality of the AIMS's user interface will benefit from iterative usability testing with representative users. In lieu of such testing, customers bear the burden of discovering and coping with usability problems that should have been detected and fixed before the application was released to the market. Usability testing involves a representative sample of users performing a representative sample of tasks with a prototype software application. Human factors specialists usually conduct such tests at multiple stages of development, starting with early conceptual designs and finishing with near-final software. Iterative testing ensures the detection of major conceptual design issues early in development, when it is feasible to correct them, and minor problems that might linger as the design reaches maturity. Such testing may be conducted in a usability testing facility, which is similar to focus group facilities that include two rooms separated by a one-way mirror. As an alternative, OR simulators provide a high-fidelity test setting in which various additional inputs and stressors can help to reveal shortcomings in the design of an AIMS's user interface.

Keys to running an effective usability test of an AIMS are:

- A representative sample of prospective users should be recruited, rather than just high-end users (i.e., key opinion leaders). Early tests may involve as few as 8–10 participants, while a later test intended to validate a design should probably involve twice as many participants or more.
- While they use the system, users should be exposed to the normal stresses and distractions encountered in an OR, such as high noise levels, alarming equipment, and demanding personnel.
- In early testing, a "think aloud" testing approach should be employed that calls for test participants to verbalize their decisions and actions, thereby facilitating the detection and analysis of usability problems. During validation testing, "thinking aloud" should be dispensed with to ensure maximum realism.

Early usability testing helps developers to refine conceptual models, user interface structures, overall screen layouts, and information flows (i.e., workflows). Later usability tests tend to identify more discrete opportunities for refinements, such as adding or subtracting content to facilitate tasks and simplifying graphics and wording to improve comprehension. While some developers might feel that usability testing will require too much time and money, evidence suggests that the opposite is true—testing reduces the chance of a time-consuming and costly redesign at the later stages of development.[7]

Conclusion

In another 10 years, it is unlikely that clinicians in technologically advanced nations will use paper records. In many cases, the use of AIMS will be required. Moreover, anesthesia providers who begin their practice using an AIMS will be quite reluctant to switch to a paper-based approach. Therefore, the focus will shift from adoption to optimization, which is where human factors engineering will play an important role, as it already does in some cases.

Ultimately, design refinements in the user interface will help AIMS to blend seamlessly into anesthesia practice. Although some users—particularly older users with manual experience—might miss the control afforded by paper forms, few will miss the tedium and potential for error that accompanied manual systems. Rather, caregivers will be relieved of the added work required to manually maintain components of the anesthesia record, thereby gaining more time to focus on patient care.

Key Points

- Applying human factors engineering to the development of software applications enhances usability; this is particularly important with an AIMS.
- Usability may be enhanced through appropriate use of many guidelines concerning such issues as flexibility, positive learning experiences, and visual appeal.
- AIMS users rank ease of use, speed of use, and support as the most important aspects of usability.
- AIMS users consider multiple entry options, memory aids, and user support as important design strengths.
- Design weaknesses include poor artifact handling, lack of user support, and nuisance warnings.
- Innovation opportunities include new input modalities, decision support, and better integration with existing clinical systems.
- Usability testing provides an opportunity to dramatically improve an AIMS but should be done at the time of development rather than once the application has been deployed to users.

Acknowledgment The authors thank their colleague Eric A. Smith for supporting their writing effort by collecting background technical information and interviewing AIMS developers for this chapter.

References

1. Anesthesia Patient Safety Foundation. APSF Endorses Use of Automated Record Keepers, http://www.apsf.org/resource_center/newsletter/2001/winter/02ARK.htm. Accessed March 12, 2007
2. Anesthesia Patient Safety Foundation. Anesthesia Information Management Systems, http://www.apsf.org/initiatives/infosys.mspx. Accessed March 12, 2007
3. International Electromechanical Commission. IEC 60601-1-6. Medical Electrical Equipment, Part 1–6: General Requirements for Safety—Collateral Standard: Usability. Bruxelles, Belgium, 2006
4. Anesthesia Patient Safety Foundation. Data Dictionary Task Force, http://www.apsf.org/initiatives/ddtf/datams.mspx. Accessed March 12, 2007
5. The Joint Commission. Official "Do Not Use" List, http://www.jointcommission.org/PatientSafety/DoNotUseList/. Accessed February 1, 2007
6. Goldman JM, Schrenker RA, Jackson JL, Whitehead SF. Plug and play in the operating room of the future. Biomed Instrum Technol 2005; 39(3):194–9
7. Wiklund ME. Return on investment in human factors. Med Device Diagn Ind Mag 2005; 8:48

Chapter 6
Data Standards

Martin Hurrell, Andrew Norton, and Terri Monk

The existing and emerging information technology standards that are of relevance to AIMS are discussed in this chapter. The focus is on the use of standards in the AIMS, both in terms of the persistent storage of data and the import of data from and export to other systems. Although the emphasis is on standards that have direct relevance for the storage and communication of anesthetic data, the broader standards "landscape" is also briefly reviewed. Particular attention is given to those standards that provide a supporting infrastructure such as XML (Extensible Markup Language), RDF (Resource Description Framework), OWL (Web Ontology Language), and those that are proposed for the implementation of the EMR/EHR (note that EMR and EHR will be used interchangeably in this chapter to refer to the electronic medical record).

What Data Are "Anesthesia" Data?

The anesthetic episode is embedded in the longitudinal record of patient care; it is therefore natural that the planning and the management of anesthesia are informed and influenced by information from diverse sources, including the EMR. Similarly, information from the AIMS may be used by other systems and caregivers, both in the immediate postoperative phase and in clinical and management audit and research. For these reasons, it is difficult to identify strict boundaries that define "anesthesia" data, but for the purposes of this chapter, they are considered to be mainly those data that comprise the conventional anesthetic record. From a data standards perspective, the technologies and methods that have application to the anesthetic record can be extended without strain to the anesthetic preoperative assessment and to anesthetic outcomes in the immediate postoperative period.

The Uses of Anesthesia Data

Some of the main uses of anesthesia data are:

- Preoperative assessment and planning

J. Stonemetz, K. Ruskin (eds.) *Anesthesia Informatics*,
© Springer Science + Business Media, LLC 2008

- Clinical support in the intraoperative phase
- Medicolegal issues
- Administration and billing
- Clinical audit, research, and epidemiology studies

AIMS create new opportunities:

- Via electronic interfaces to patient monitors and other devices such as ventilators and infusion pumps, AIMS can sample vital signs at much higher rates and with better accuracy and traceability.
- AIMS can facilitate semantic interoperability if observations and events are coded directly at the point of entry.
- AIMS can receive data directly from other IT systems such as the clinical laboratory or patient-administration systems.

Communication and Documentation in the Context of AIMS

The AIMS depicted in Fig. 6.1 may receive information from the EMR and other hospital information systems (scheduling data, patient demographics, labs, images), from patient-connected devices (monitors, ventilators, pumps), and from the anesthesiologist (medications, observations). It stores all of these data in its database and may send data (healthcare providers, procedures performed, events) to the EMR and other systems. Data may be extracted by direct access to the AIMS database, although this demands knowledge of the data model implemented by the AIMS; additionally, if the query is made against the active system database (rather than an archive), (a) the system may be slowed, (b) it is possible that data may be

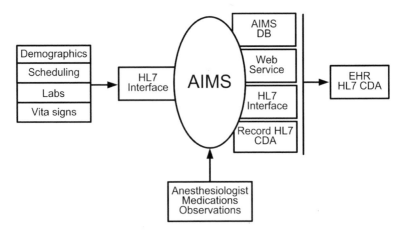

Fig. 6.1 Possible communication with an AIMS

corrupted, and/or (c) the system may crash. Information capture by the AIMS from other systems may be facilitated by utilization of outbound Health Level 7 (HL7)[1] messages or Web services, or by the anesthetic record being available in a form that can be processed by other systems using an appropriate standard such as the HL7 Version 3 (V3) Clinical Document Architecture (CDA).[2]

Storage and communication of data and implementation of AIMS require both a standardized data model and standardized terminology. To these ends, HL7 and the International Standards Organization (ISO) 11073[3] were established with the goal to create robust and modifiable standards. The standards are cornerstones in the initiative, Integrating the Healthcare Enterprise (IHE), which is an international initiative by healthcare professionals and the healthcare industry to improve the way computer systems in healthcare share information. Currently, these standards are supplied by a combination of HL7 and vocabulary standards such as the ISO 11073 nomenclature and Systematized Nomenclature of Medicine–Clinical Terminology (SNOMED CT),[4] both of which have been used by the International Organization for Terminology in Anesthesia (IOTA) to develop a specialized terminology for anesthesia.

The ISO 11073 standards aim to support plug-and-play interoperability between medical devices and other systems. They originated in the 1980s with the Medical Information Bus, which was embodied in the IEEE 11073 standard. The current international standard, ISO 11073, has five parts:

1. 11073–10101 Nomenclature/Terminology
2. 11073–10201 Information Model
3. 11073–20101 Application Profile: Base Standard
4. 11073–30200 Transport Profile: Cabled
5. 11073–30300 Transport Profile: IR wireless

In addition to providing interoperability, the standard can support full traceability of data in terms of the precise source and mode of operation, and it is a core standard in the IHE Patient Care Device Technical Framework. However, adoption by vendors has been slow. Other initiatives, such as CANopen and the Medical Device "Plug-and-Play" Interoperability Program (MD PnP), are also aimed at device communications. This chapter is concerned with the abstract model of medical devices found in ISO 11073 that is linked to a formally structured nomenclature. A detailed description of the use of this standard for device communication is provided in Chap. 7.

The EHR and Its Relationship to the Anesthetic Record

The EHR has many definitions but may be said to comprise a comprehensive, patient-centric electronic record that is ubiquitously available. At a minimum, it includes patient demographics and medical history supported by relevant detailed information about procedures, investigations, and treatments such as laboratory/pathology test results, radiologic images, medications, etc. Some of the standards that are relevant to the EHR are discussed below. The European standard, ENV 13606, defines protocols for the exchange of information between EHRs, including templates that define the context and structure of clinical information. The OpenEHR standard grew out of the Good European Healthcare Record (GEHR) project and embraces both messaging and persistent storage of data.[6] Like ENV 13606, it also defines structures aimed at allowing clinical information to be represented in a standard way.

The HL7 V3 CDA (Release 2)[2] takes a document-centric approach so that case information can be represented as an electronic document, the provenance of which is clearly defined. A CDA-compliant document always contains a human-readable narrative section but may also contain structured information that is machine processessable. These structures are based on the HL7 V3 Reference Information Model (RIM).[1] Thus, the CDA supports the EHR by providing a standard schema for clinical documents. Although not concerned with messaging, it does use the same information model as HL7 V3 messages; in this sense, the structured content of a CDA document and V3 messaging are related.

The Continuity of Care Record (CCR) is a condensed set of the most relevant information about a patient that may be transferred between systems to support the continuity of care. Its formal specification is contained in the American Society for Testing and Materials (ASTM) E2369-05 Standard Specification for CCR.[7] Work has been completed to define a constraint upon the CDA that allows the CCR to be rendered as a CDA-compliant document.[8]

As discussed below, the anesthetic record is a very good example of the CDA definition of a clinical document. If, then, the output of an AIMS were rendered as a CDA-compliant document, how might it fit into the larger EHR picture? One view is represented in Fig. 6.2. In ISO/TR 20514 terms, the model represented is an "extended EHR."

Why Do We Need Data Standards?

The case for the adoption of IT standards in anesthesia is centered on the need to communicate, share, and aggregate information. In addition to receiving information from patient-connected devices and other IT systems, AIMS can also be valuable sources of information. It is quite possible to build custom interfaces to enable information exchanges. In the past, customization was often the norm, especially in the area of patient monitors, for which AIMS vendors developed their own device drivers and parsers to access the data stream and extract salient elements. In principle, communication with other IT systems can be handled similarly. So, why use standards?

The most frequently cited advantage of interfacing standards is that they can reduce complexity and costs in both their development and subsequent maintenance. If each system-to-system connection requires a separate, nonstandard interface, the number of interfaces required to connect n systems is roughly $n^2/2$, $n(n - 1/2)$ to be precise, or approximately 200 if 20 systems are involved.[9] This statistic alone is a powerful case for standardization, although in practice, it must be balanced with other considerations. Standards, by their nature, tend to be complex because they

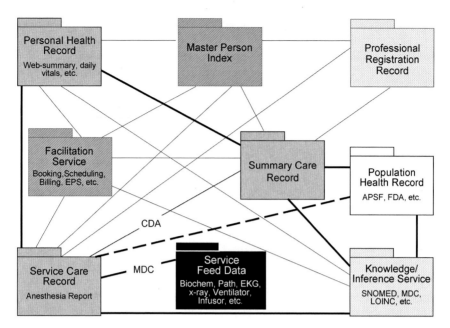

Fig. 6.2 Example of generalized health information infrastructure for anesthesia. Main content flows are represented as *bold lines*. Note that the document itself is populated by information from a variety of sources, including medical devices, where the intermediate actor is the AIMS. In this context, an actor is a person or system who initiates a change

aim to cover a wide spectrum of requirements within an applicable domain. In consequence, substantial time and effort must be invested before realizing the promised benefits. For this reason, proprietary solutions may appear attractive, especially as the immediate stakeholders in any one scenario often have limited requirements. To ease the burden, major standards may be accompanied by metastandards that provide recommended patterns of application for common purposes.

The more compelling case for standards occurs when larger-scale integration and sharing of data are considered. As scale and scope increase, so does the need for standards. While an anesthesiologist may not care what interface is implemented to enter patient demographic data into an AIMS, the IT manager with responsibility for ensuring the interoperability of multiple IT systems will have quite a different perspective. The use of standards-based solutions across the enterprise enhances reliability and reduces costs. Also, limited local interfaces that are based on standards inherit power and potential that may be very helpful as requirements evolve.

Interfaces are only part of the story. True semantic interoperability requires shared ontologies and standard ways to express them. Simple taxonomies are insufficient to allow complex data mining and knowledge discovery. The data that are collected as part of the anesthetic record, when combined with information from other sources, can be a very important resource, especially for studies of surgical outcome. However, as these data travel out from their source, their nature and meaning must remain unambiguous and accessible to a wider domain. Increasingly, data sharing is likely to transcend national borders, so that the chosen standards must have an international perspective as well as a national perspective. HL7 and SNOMED CT are examples that are widely used by the international community.

Underpinning and supporting standards that are specifically related to healthcare are other more general standards that assist in their development and deployment. For example, the HL7 V3 RIM uses the conventions of the Unified Modeling Language[10] (UML) as a means to represent the relationships and properties of its component classes. It uses XML to render message content and persistent artifacts, such as clinical documents, that conform to the HL7 V3 CDA. The IOTA uses OWL, a standard supported by the World Wide Web Consortium (W3C), to represent the conceptual model of domain knowledge that the terminology is used to describe. The specific version used is OWL description logic (DL), which supports reasoning.

A common criticism of standards—that they are too complex—actually serves to highlight why they are so necessary. Very few things are as simple as they first appear; it is not simply because they like to talk that standards committees take as long as they do to arrive at a final version. Major standards are not limited to easy cases; they apply to the really tough cases as well, and they do so using a coherent and embracing model. They also pay strict attention to their compatibility with other relevant standards, taking account of work already accomplished and ensuring that new standards implement lower layers and services in a way that is consistent with how the wider world already works. New interest groups are often seduced into dismissing a major existing standard in their area because they believe that they can create a more elegant solution in half the time. Equally often, the initial optimism fades as the real complexity of the problem becomes apparent and the simple solution must be modified piecemeal to cope with each unforeseen requirement. The inevitable result is either a solution that is not so much simple as simplistic or one that has become very complex but without the intellectual coherence that would make that complexity manageable.

It is often possible to implement lightweight requirements in a way that is compatible with a major standard but that does not involve every feature of that standard. In addition, the implementation of standards-based solutions may be made much easier and more successful by the contribution of metastandards such as IHE, which defines "integration profiles" that recommend specific ways in which other standards should be used to support core processes.

Standards Organizations

A plethora of organizations and standards can claim to bear some relation to the domain of anesthesiology. Some of these are illustrated in Fig. 6.3, although it is by no means an exhaustive list. The sections that follow focus on those standards that

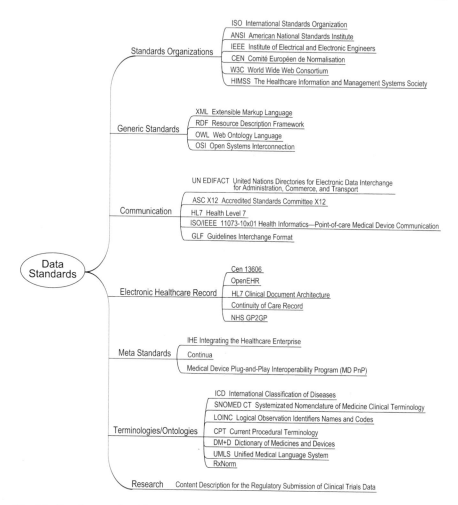

Fig. 6.3 Rough map of healthcare standards

are of direct relevance to the representation and communication of data that are collected by AIMS, such as ISO 11073, HL7 (Messaging and Clinical Document Architecture), and SNOMED CT. Standards are developed, maintained, and made available by standards organizations, the principal single body of which is the ISO, which was founded in 1947. It defines and publishes international standards and consists of approximately 160 representatives from national standards bodies such as the American National Standards Institute (ANSI) and the British Standards Institute (BSI).

Table 6.1 Standards organizations

Acronym	Full name of standard/organization	Web site
ANSI	American National Standards Institute	http://www.ansi.org/
ASTM	American Society for Testing and Materials	http://www.astm.org/
BSI	British Standards Institute	http://www.bsi-global.com/
CEN	European Committee for Standardization (Comité Européen de Normalisation)	http://www.cen.eu/cenorm/homepage.htm
CENELEC	European Committee for Electrotechnical Standardization (Comité Européen de Normalisation Electrotechnique)	http://www.cenelec.org/Cenelec/Homepage.htm
DICOM	Digital Imaging and Communications in Medicine	http://medical.nema.org/
DIN	Deutsches Institut für Normung	http://www.din.de
ETSI	European Telecommunications Standards Institute	http://www.etsi.org
HL7	Health Level 7	http://www.hl7.org/
IEC	International Electrotechnical Commission	http://www.iec.ch/
IEEE	Institute of Electrical and Electronics Engineers	http://www.ieee.org/
IETF	Internet Engineering Task Force	http://www.ietf.org/
ISO	International Organization for Standardization	http://www.iso.org/iso/en/ISOOnline.frontpage
ITU	International Telecommunication Union	http://www.itu.int/net/home/index.aspx
JIS	Japanese Standards Association	http://www.jsa.or.jp/default_english.asp
OASIS	Organization for the Advancement of Structured Information Standards	http://www.oasis-open.org/home/index.php

Standards Development Organizations (SDOs) may be international, national, or regional, e.g., the ISO itself, the ANSI, and the Comité Européen de Normalisation (CEN, European Committee for Standardization), respectively. International and regional standards may reflect different priorities. The 1991 Vienna Agreement allows for standards to be led by either the ISO or the CEN, with the bodies notifying each other of the standards developed to obtain simultaneous approval. Both HL7 and SNOMED are SDOs that are entirely concerned with healthcare issues. Recommendations of specialist SDOs can be presented for review by national and regional organizations. Some of these organizations, their Web addresses, and their relationships, with examples of some healthcare standards, are outlined in Table 6.1 and Fig. 6.4.

Different versions of the same standard may exist at international, national, and regional levels; national and regional versions may incorporate specific variations required by the territory concerned. The ISO includes more than 200 technical

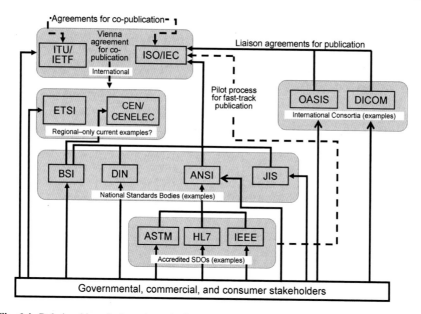

Fig. 6.4 Relationships of selected standards organizations. *ITU* International Telecommunication Union, *IETF* Internet Engineering Task Force, *ISO* International Standards Organization, *IEC* International Electrotechnical Commission, *ETSI* European Telecommunications Standards Institute, *CEN* Comité Européen de Normalisation, *CENELEC* Comité Européen de Normalisation Electrotechnique, *OASIS* Organization for the Advancement of Structured Information Standards, *DICOM* Digital Imaging and Communications in Medicine, *BSI* British Standards Institute, *DIN* Deutsches Institut für Normung, *ANSI* American National Standards Institute, *JIS* Japanese Standards Association, *ASTM* American Society for Testing and Materials, *HL7* Health Level 7, *IEEE* Institute of Electrical and Electronic Engineers

committees (TCs). The TC with responsibility for healthcare-related standards is TC215, which comprises six workgroups, each with a particular focus:

- Electronic health record and modeling
- Messaging
- Healthcare concepts and terminologies
- Privacy and security
- Smart cards
- e-Pharmacy and medicines business

Each of these groups works on standards development within their specific areas. Currently, 24 countries, including the US, are participating in TC215, with another 14 as observer countries.

CEN TC251 is the TC for Health Informatics of the CEN, which is aligned with ISO TC215. Nineteen national standards organizations are members of CEN TC251, which has four working groups that cover topics closely related to those of the ISO working groups presented above:

- Communications: information models, messaging, and smart cards
- Terminology

Table 6.2 Major topics and associated standards

Topic	Standards
Electronic health record and modeling information models	CEN ENV 13606, OpenEHR
Communications and messaging	HL7, ISO 11073
Interoperability	CCOW
Healthcare concepts and terminologies	UMLS, SNOMED CT, LOINC
Privacy and security	HIPAA

CEN ENV Comité Européen de Normalisation, European Prestandards, *HL7* Health Level 7, *ISO* International Organization for Standardization, *CCOW* Clinical Context Object Workgroup, *UMLS* Unified Modeling Language System, *SNOMED CT* Systematized Nomenclature of Medicine–Clinical Terminology, *LOINC* Logical Observation Identifiers Names and Codes, *HIPAA* Health Insurance Portability and Accountability Act

- Security, safety, and quality
- Technology for interoperability (devices)

The subject areas of the ISO and CEN workgroups provide a useful categoric framework. The major topics and some of the standards relevant to each group are summarized in Table 6.2.

Generic Standards

Object-Oriented Analysis and Design and the Unified Modeling Language

Many of the concepts and implementations in the standards world are based on the principles of object-oriented analysis and design (OOAD). This methodology was originally used in software development, but the philosophy is applicable to many systems in the real world. As the name implies, OOAD is concerned with objects. Objects—such as an anesthesiologist, syringe pump, or a drug—bear a close relationship to things that can be classified within a domain. Objects have associated data or *attributes* and are capable of certain operations, behaviors, or *methods* that are bound together. Objects are individual *instances* of a general *class*; for example, both Drs. Smith and Jones are instances of the *anesthesiologist* class. Classes can be organized as a hierarchy, with those at lower levels inheriting the properties of those above. For example, living organisms respire, human beings are living organisms, and anesthesiologists are human beings. The anesthesiologist class inherits the behavior *respiration* from the superclass *living organism*. In the UML, this principle that subclasses inherit properties of the superclasses is also called *generalization*. At the same time, subclasses may define unique attributes and properties that extend or specialize those that are inherited.

The standard way to represent object-oriented designs is via the UML, which enables a number of different views of a model that expose particular aspects of its organization and operation. This functionality is particularly relevant to an understanding of the diagrammatic representation of the HL7 RIM, which uses a UML class diagram. In fact, HL7 has adopted a slightly modified form of the standard UML class diagram; it includes color coding to indicate the nature of the classes that are depicted and is intended to facilitate understanding of HL7. However, the modified form remains completely consistent with the UML.

The Extensible Markup Language

The XML has become ubiquitous in the realization of communication between IT systems. It is used to create structured documents that can be parsed and processed automatically. XML documents are human readable; however, depending upon the nature of the information they contain and the way in which they have been authored, they may not always be easy to understand without supplementary information. A small fragment of an XML document might look like this:

```
<Anesthesiologist>
    <Firstname>John</Firstname>
    <Lastname>Jones</Lastname>
</Anesthesiologist>
```

In this example, "Anesthesiologist," "Firstname," and "Lastname" are tags that identify XML elements. It can be seen that the elements "Firstname" and "Lastname" are nested within the element "Anesthesiologist"; deeper levels of nesting might be used to represent more complex structures.

XML documents can be constrained using XML schema[11] that define, for example, which elements and attributes can appear in a document. XML schemas can include datatype definitions that constrain the form of valid entries. For example, it might be required that contact details be recorded in a particular format; a datatype could be created to define this requirement. Thus, an XML schema can be used to validate an XML document that claims to be compliant. An XML schema has been developed for the anesthetic record.[12]

It is sometimes claimed that XML documents are "self-describing," which implies that their content can be unambiguously interpreted; this is far from the case. In the very simple example shown earlier, most human readers would have little difficulty in understanding that the fragment is intended to convey the identity of an anesthesiologist. This understanding is possible because humans know what anesthesiologists are, that they are people, and that people have first and last names. As a machine is not similarly gifted, an application is not capable of independently interpreting the information. Furthermore, a tag such as "AnesthesiaStartTime" might seem simple enough to interpret, but it might mean different things to different people; therefore, without a common reference, it is ambiguous. XML defines a standard syntax but does not in itself provide meaning.

Healthcare Standards Relevant to Anesthesia

Health Level 7

HL7 is one of the most important standards for anesthesia information management. It defines (a) the ways in which information may be carried by standard messages between systems and (b) a standard for electronic clinical documents. As an organization, HL7 provides a common ground for other standards groups, so that HL7 meetings tend to include groups that are concerned with, among other issues, terminologies, medical device communications, and common authentication schemes, which are also topics for HL7 itself.

HL7 refers to the upper layer of the Open Systems Interconnection (OSI) model, which is the "application layer" concerned with how applications communicate with each other. It impacts directly on the high-level communication issues discussed in this chapter, such as authentication and syntax. The lower layers become progressively more concerned with the nuts and bolts of electronic communication to the point that the lowest layer, "physical," defines the ways in which electronic hardware transmits the basic units of information using wires, optics, or radio waves. HL7 started in the US in 1987 and is now used in more than 20 countries.

HL7 Version 2

In 1988, preliminary work was formalized on HL7 Version 2.0 (HL7 V2), which has been continuously developed until, at the time of this writing, we have Version 2.5.1. Each iteration of Version 2 is backward compatible. New material that is not in the previous standard is simply ignored by systems that support a previous version. However, the *implementation* of standards often lags behind the standards development itself, so that the most widely implemented version of HL7 in 2007 was 2.3.*x*. HL7 V2 in all its variants was designed to facilitate messaging between healthcare IT systems and defines a number of message types that cover most eventualities. Some HL7 communications that are most relevant to AIMS are detailed in Table 6.3.

HL7 V2 messages have a clear structure that allows them to be parsed in a standard way by a receiving application. Each message comprises one or more

Table 6.3 Messages relevant to AIMS

Message type	Uses
ADT	Patient demographic data from the Hospital Information System
Scheduling	Information about operating schedules (sessions and associated cases) to be accessed by the AIMS
Results and observations	Import of lab results and export of information about intraoperative events, vital-sign data, etc.

ADT admission/discharge/transfer

segments, each of which has a segment identifier (segment ID) that identifies the kind of information with which it is concerned. For example, the message header (MSH) segment describes how to parse the information that follows. It also includes the version of HL7 that is being used. Before the advent of XML, elements of information in HL7 message segments were demarcated by special characters, a method that is still supported. These characters allow an application to identify where each segment starts and ends, where the fields that it contains start and end, and how to identify the components and subcomponents in the message content. In other words, the message can be considered as a nested structure and the separators allow the levels of nesting to be unwrapped correctly so as to extract the information. The form of elements of HL7 messages is constrained by datatype definitions that are part of the standard, e.g., dates and times. Usually, the transmission of a message is associated with one or more events, *trigger events*, which are also indicated in the message header and may be human or machine generated.

Messages may be broadcast with or without an indication of the targeted system(s) for which they are intended. This occurrence can involve significant overheads for the receiving system, in that relevant messages may have to be intercepted and identified. Also, because the period of availability of broadcast messages may not be known, it may be necessary to make local copies for later analysis. An alternative is to request the information as and when required. For example, patient demographic information linked to a hospital identification number can be requested by using an HL7 query. This method is arguably more efficient and more secure, but the method is not always supported by systems that could supply the information.

A particular issue with HL7 V2 has been the so-called optionality—in particular the use of locally defined message segments known as *Z-segments*. Z-segments are locally agreed upon extensions to the standard that can only be interpreted with special knowledge of the local contract. Also, although newer versions are backward compatible, systems that use an older version of the standard may not be able to understand some content in messages that are compliant with a newer version. HL7 V2 does not define a standard data model, and it is quite possible for different messages to be used to convey the same information.

HL7 Version 3

Whereas the different iterations of HL7 V2 were developed using the same general philosophy of bottom-up message design, V3 adopted a completely new approach. It was developed using the principles of object-oriented design and was founded on a formal RIM. All valid HL7 V3 artifacts, such as messages, are based on the V3 RIM. The RIM is described using the conventions of the UML. The six core classes that constitute the so-called HL7 V3 backbone are shown in Table 6.4.

The RIM comprises approximately 70 classes, which are specializations of the six core classes. In that not all of the classes that are in the RIM are likely to be needed to fulfill the requirements of a particular domain, a natural step is to define

Table 6.4 Core classes in the HL7 Reference Information Model

RIM class	Examples
Act	Referral
	Supply
	Procedure
	Observation
	Medication
	Financial act
Entity	Living subject
	Person
	Organization
	Place
	Health chart
	Material
Role	Employee
	Patient
	Scheduled resource
	Certified practitioner
	Assigned practitioner
	Specimen
Participation	Performer
	Author
	Witness
	Subject
	Destination
Act relationship	Compositional
	Reference
	Succeeds
Role link	Direct authority
	Indirect Authority
	Replaces
	Part
	Backup

a subset of those that are required. The result of this process is referred to as a *Domain Message Implementation Model* (D-MIM), which can be further specialized to produce *Refined Message Implementation Models* (R-MIMs) that reflect the more specific needs of subdomains. Finally, to produce a practical specification for a given message, it is necessary to produce a serialized version that defines the sequence in which the units of the message are processed—called a *Hierarchical Message Description* (HMD). These stages represent a progression from very generalized expressions to those that can be used in the real world. The HL7 organization has produced a number of tools that facilitate this process and perform validation. HL7 uses a modified form of the UML to make class diagrams more readable and easy to understand. It introduces color coding of classes to facilitate discerning from which of the RIM core classes each subclass is descended: green for *entity*, yellow for *role*, blue for *participation*, and pink for *act*.

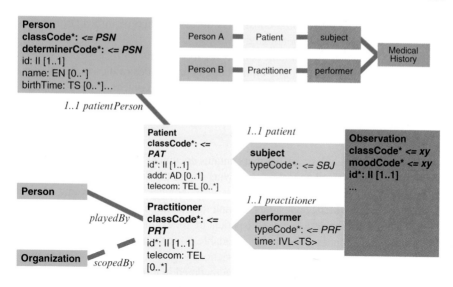

Fig. 6.5 Example of HL7 R-MIM (figure courtesy of Dr. Kai Heitmann)

In the example shown in Fig. 6.5, two people, a patient and a practitioner, are involved in a clinical observation that contributes to the patient's medical history, depicted by the linked boxes at the top right of the figure. The green box at the top left depicts an *entity* "Person," who is playing a *role*; "Patient," who participates in an *act*; "Observation," as the "subject." A second person plays the *role* "Practitioner" and is scoped by (belongs to) an "Organization" (which might be specifically identified). This person *participates* in the observation *act* as the performer of the act. Other attributes can be defined for each class to add more information and specificity to the model.

HL7 Clinical Document Architecture

The HL7 CDA is an XML-based document markup standard that specifies the structure and semantics of clinical documents for the purpose of exchange. It is developed and maintained by the Structured Documents TC within HL7. By leveraging the use of XML, the HL7 RIM, and coded vocabularies, the CDA makes documents both machine readable (so that they are easily parsed and processed electronically) and human readable (so that they can be easily retrieved and used by the people who need them). A CDA document is a defined and complete information object that can include text, images, sounds, and other multimedia content.

The HL7 CDA clinical document contains observations and services and has the following characteristics:

- *Persistence*—continues to exist in an unaltered state for a time period defined by local and regulatory requirements.
- *Stewardship*—maintained by an organization entrusted with its care.

- *Potential for authentication*—constitutes an assemblage of information that is intended to be legally authenticated.
- *Context*—establishes the default context for its contents.
- *Wholeness*—authentication of a clinical document applies to the whole and does not apply to portions of the document without the full context of the document.
- *Human readability*—human readable, guarantees that a receiver of a CDA document can algorithmically display the clinical content of the note on a standard Web browser.

A CDA document includes a header that contains document metadata and information that assists in tracking authentication and ownership of the document and in document management, including version control. It also includes data concerning clinical encounters, care providers, and patients. Using information in the header, it is possible to link documents that relate to the same patient to, for example, the EHR. The content of the document is contained in a human-readable component that may include images as well as text and that can be divided into sections to give structure and enhance readability. Finally, the same information can be rendered in a form that is machine processessable, so that the content of a CDA document can be analyzed or extracted for other purposes, such as research. CDA documents can be included in HL7 messages.

HL7 Special Interest Group for the Generation of Anesthesia Standards

In 2005, a Special Interest Group for the Generation of Standards in Anesthesia (SIGGAS) was established within HL7, sponsored by the Patient Care TC. The aims of SIGGAS are to:

- Identify critical data standards specific to anesthesiology that are necessary for standardized quality and outcomes reporting and measuring.
- Identify and promote required terminology to support reporting and measurement.
- Identify and promote requirements for a standardized anesthesia record to facilitate exchange and aggregation of perioperative data.
- Coordinate and cooperate with other groups interested in using anesthesia data standards.
- Enable and promote use of these standards nationally and internationally.
- Identify appropriate anesthesia constraints against existing HL7 artifacts.

SIGGAS includes representation from the IOTA and the Anesthetic Patient Safety Foundation (APSF) Data Dictionary Task Force (DDTF) and works with other groups interested in anesthesia and perioperative data standards and performance measurement.

Clinical Terminologies for Anesthesia

Anesthesiologists are familiar with structured information in clinical records. Conventional paper anesthetic records contain multiple elements where data are recorded in lists, checkboxes, or fields that have actual or potentially constrained

Table 6.5 Scope of clinical terminologies: international, national, and local

Type	Examples
International	• ICD-9, ICD-9CM, and ICD-10 • SNOMED CT • LOINC • MEDCIN
National	• Nation-specific procedural classifications ° OPCS 4.x (UK) ° CPT (US) • National datasets (e.g., cancer) • National formularies and drug dictionaries (e.g., RxNORM)
Local	• Local datasets for record keeping, audit, and research • Local data dictionaries for AIMS

ICD International Disease Classifications, *SNOMED CT* Systematized Nomenclature of Medicine–Clinical Terminology, *LOINC* Logical Observation Identifiers Names and Codes, *MEDCIN* a medical terminology engine, *OPCS* Office of Population Censuses and Surveys, *CPT* Current Procedural Terminology

values for data entry. Despite the efforts of AIMS proponents, the market infiltration of these systems remains relatively low. Although many reasons could be cited, it is clear that several events must occur to improve AIMS market penetration, including creation of a data dictionary and development of a qualitative method by which to report and compare data between AIMS and other IT systems.

The purposes of clinical terminologies are many and varied and include encoding of clinical data, audit functions, research, epidemiology, statutory reporting requirements, statistical analysis, and financial reimbursement. Consequently, terminologies have been developed to meet these requirements, but it is inevitable that a specific terminology will not adequately support all of them. The difficulties encountered in developing clinical terminologies are not always immediately apparent.[13] A number of clinical terminologies, with an indication of their scope—international, national, and local—are listed in Table 6.5.

Systems such as SNOMED CT often include terminology and mapping for a number of national or international controlled vocabularies or classifications. ICD, OPCS 4, Laboratory LOINC, and some nursing terminologies are all incorporated into SNOMED CT. MEDCIN is another extensive clinical terminology, with over 250,000 concepts and the capability of crossmapping to coding systems such as SNOMED CT, CPT, ICD, and LOINC. Beyond this level of integration are systems such as the National Library of Medicine Unified Medical Language System, a metathesaurus of over 1 million biomedical concepts and 5 million terms derived from 143 international, national, and local vocabularies (including language variants). This system comprises a metathesaurus organized by concept and meaning, and a semantic network of nodes (concepts or objects) and links (relationships between nodes). The specialist lexicon contains tools to enable searching of medical records by examining syntax, morphologic form, and orthographic information.

Controlled clinical terminology for anesthesia has been developed, with some anesthesia-relevant terms having existed for many years in epidemiologic classifications. One of the first initiatives to develop a systematic, comprehensive, clinically rich language was the development of Clinical Terms Version 3 (Read Codes V3) in the UK in the clinical terms project (1992–1996). Earlier versions of the Read Codes [V1 (1984)—4-byte, 10,000 codes, and V2 (1988)—5-byte, 30,000 codes] were developed to support computerized primary care systems in the UK. They are still extensively used in UK primary care computer systems, often allowing additional free text information to be recorded against a coded entry. The Read Codes will be gradually superseded by SNOMED CT in these systems. The clinical terms project aimed to expand the scope of the Read Codes to meet the needs of the secondary and tertiary care sectors. Over 50 specialty working groups were established, including Anesthesia, Pain Management, and Intensive Care. By 1999, Clinical Terms Version 3 (CTV3) contained over 250,000 clinical terms and concepts.

In 1965, the College of American Pathologists developed the Systematized Nomenclature of Pathology (SNOP), which was extended into the first release of SNOMED in 1974. By 1979, SNOMED II contained 44,500 concepts, and it contained 130,500 by the release of SNOMED III in 1993. By 1999, SNOMED Reference Terminology (RT) had been developed in collaboration with Kaiser Permanente and provided a unified clinical terminology for health states, diseases, pathophysiology, treatments, and outcomes. In March 1999, agreement was reached between the College of American Pathologists and the UK National Health Service (NHS) to unify SNOMED RT and CTV3. This work was completed by January 2002 and contained 325,000 concepts, 800,000 synonyms, and more than 950,000 links (semantic relationships). It included extensive crossmaps to other classifications and vocabularies. The SNOMED CT structure was voted as an ANSI standard in August 2002.

SNOMED CT was adopted as the clinical terminology standard for the UK NHS Programme for IT in 2003. In May 2004, SNOMED CT was made available free of charge to US healthcare providers through the Unified Medical Language System metathesaurus. In 2007, the International Healthcare Terminology Standards Development Organization (IHTSDO) was established as a not-for-profit association chartered in Denmark. The founding charter members included the US, the UK, Australia, New Zealand, the Netherlands, Canada, Sweden, Denmark, and Lithuania. IHTSDO now owns the intellectual and commercial rights to SNOMED CT and is charged with its continued development.

In 2002, the APSF established a group, the DDTF, to develop a standardized anesthesia terminology for use in AIMS. An agreement between APSF and SNOMED International to enhance the anesthesia content of SNOMED CT was signed in 2003. The DDTF work has assumed an international aspect, with partners in the UK, Canada, Australia, and the Netherlands, and is now known as the IOTA. This group collaborates with other relevant standards bodies, including standards groups within HL7 and in the medical devices domain.

As SNOMED CT is a massive terminology, consideration must be given to implementation that enables efficient use by the clinician without his being overwhelmed with excessive or inappropriate terminology choices. This scenario can be realized by the development of subsets, which can be flagged and identified within the terminology. Subsets can vary enormously in size and scope, depending on the clinical requirements.

NHS Connecting for Health is making use of the OpenEHR standards in the development of archetypes and templates based on the reference model in CEN ENV 13606. An *archetype* is a reusable model of a domain concept (e.g., blood pressure). Archetypes are written using an Archetype Description Language (ADL) to describe the information needed to fully represent a concept, and they may be populated with clinical terminology. A *template* is a specification of archetypes to form a screen design (or message specification) that removes optional parts of archetypes not needed in the context of use, and it selects terminology from that available within the archetypes. An extensive archetype and template library is in development for use in applications by NHS Connecting for Health EHR. Anesthetically relevant examples currently include templates for obstetric anesthetic assessments and procedures.

Clinical Ontologies for Anesthesia

The role of reference ontologies is to define classes and their relationships in a way that allows their meaning to be understood and that forms a basis for inference. An ontology represents domain knowledge by defining relevant concepts and their relationships to each other in a formal way.

Various languages have been developed over time to describe ontologies; the latest of these languages is OWL, which is a standard of the W3C and is intended to underpin the so-called Semantic Web.[14] It is based on another W3C standard, the RDF. Three versions of OWL exist—Lite, DL, and Full. OWL DL supports logical inference, so that the domain knowledge contained in an ontology that is defined using OWL DL can potentially be used to drive decision support. OWL files are rendered using XML but would rarely be accessed in their native form by a human reader. Fortunately, certain tools make it possible to create and edit ontologies that are rendered in OWL without having to look at OWL itself. Probably the most widely used is Protégé with the OWL plug-in that can be freely downloaded. Protégé-OWL has been developed jointly by Stanford University in California and the University of Manchester in the UK. OWL is widely used to represent biomedical ontologies, including those for oncology, proteomics, and genomics. An OWL ontology can reference one or more other OWL ontologies, so that existing work can be used as a foundation or contribution to new work. An excellent introduction to the use of Protégé-OWL can be found at http://www.co-ode.org/resources/tutorials/protege-owl-tutorial.php.[15]

Conclusion

The introduction of an AIMS to a facility presents both a challenge and an opportunity. The opportunity is to leverage data contained in the electronic record to enhance patient safety through analyses of data from many different hospitals and even different countries. These data may be expressed with an accuracy and granularity that is simply unattainable using conventional manual records. The challenge is to ensure that various systems record data in a standard way, so that they may meaningfully be exchanged and compared. The anesthetic record is first and foremost a clinical document, and the HL7 V3 CDA represents a basis for a standard anesthetic record specification. While the CDA can support the overall structure of the record, a standard terminology is also essential. The IOTA has identified more than 3500 terms, most of which are included in SNOMED CT. The IOTA term set is also aligned with the ISO 11073 nomenclature, so that unambiguous and complete terms for data obtained from patient-connected devices are available. Finally, work is underway to supplement the anesthesia terminology with an ontology expressed in OWL that enriches the definition of the terms and may in the future provide a basis for decision support within AIMS.

Key Points

- The APSF has formally recommended the adoption of AIMS in the US.
- Implementation of AIMS, which has been static at below 5% for many years, is likely to increase significantly.
- In the context of wider use of AIMS and the EHR, the anesthetic record becomes an important source of information that can be leveraged to drive improvements in quality of care and outcomes.
- To ensure that data from AIMS can be accessed in a way that is cost effective, efficient, reliable, and secure, it is necessary to use standards as the foundation for storage and communication.
- The major initiatives with immediate relevance to using standards in information storage and communication are ISO 11073 (for communications with patient-connected devices), HL7 (for communication between systems and for the representation of the anesthetic record as a clinical document), IHE (as a framework), and SNOMED CT, including the IOTA terms (as a reference terminology).
- Other standards (e.g., OWL) will become of increasing importance with the development of domain ontologies.

References

1. Health Level 7 Standards. http://www.hl7.org. Accessed January 22, 2008
2. Dolin RH, Alschuler L, Boyer S, Beebe C. HL7 Clinical Document Architecture, Release 2.0. http://xml.coverpages.org/CDA-20040830v3.pdf. Accessed January 22, 2008
3. ISO/IEEE 11073. http://www.iso.org/iso/iso_catalogue.htm. Accessed January 22, 2008

4. International Health Terminology Standards Development Organization. http://www.ihtsdo. org. Accessed January 22, 2008
5. Integrating the Healthcare Enterprise. http://www.ihe.net. Accessed January 22, 2008
6. OpenEHR. http://www.openehr.org. Accessed January 22, 2008
7. ASTM International. http://www.astm.org. Accessed January 22, 2008
8. HL7 Implementation Guide: CDA Release 2—Continuity of Care Document (CCD). A CDA implementation of ASTM E2369-05 Standard Specification for Continuity of Care Record (CCR), which may be used in lieu of ASTM ADJE2369, 2006. http://www.hl7.org. Accessed January 22, 2008
9. Mead CN. Data interchange standards in healthcare IT—computable semantic interoperability: Now possible but still difficult, do we really need a better mousetrap? J Healthc Inf Manag 2006; 20(1):72
10. Unified Modeling Language. http://www.uml.org. Accessed January 22, 2008
11. van der Vlist E. *XML Schema: The W3C's Object-Oriented Descriptions for XML*. Sebastopol, CA: O'Reilly Media, 2002
12. Gardner M, Peachey T. A standard XML schema for computerised anaesthetic records. Anaesthesia 2002; 57:1174–82
13. Rector A. Clinical terminology: Why is it so hard? Meth Inf Med 1999; 38(4):239–52
14. Daconta MC, Obrst LJ, Smith KB. *The Semantic Web: A Guide to the Future of XML, Web Services, and Knowledge Management*. Indianapolis: Wiley, 2003
15. Horridge M, Knublauch H, RectorA, *A Practical Guide to Building OWL Ontologies Using the Protégé-OWL Plugin and CO-ODE Tools*, ed. 1.0. Manchester: University of Manchester, 2004

Chapter 7
Device Interfaces

Melvin I. Reynolds

The focus of this chapter is medical device interfaces in the context of anesthesia service delivery, including a discussion of some of the business, clinical, and technical issues and constraints that have applied in the past and are likely to continue to impose themselves in the future. Device data interfaces designed and used exclusively for single-vendor communications are not discussed because many such interfaces are closed and proprietary, and to use them, a customer must access a proprietary black box.

Background, Motivation, and Application

Device interfaces are required when one system must communicate with another system or with a user. Until very recently, it had been difficult to identify practical communication *use cases*; "use case" is a specific term that defines how a given piece of software will be used.

Memory

Medical devices used in the OR in the 1960s and 1970s almost entirely employed analog circuitry that had effectively no memory. The only method of outputting any of the signals was to produce a printed recording, which was usually the default interface. It was not until oscilloscopes became more compact and lower in cost that electronic displays became an integral part of measurement systems. The outputs from these early systems were therefore either the prime recorder output or a replica of that output used to drive an integral recorder. These analog outputs were most often presented as an array of plugs and jacks. Output signals usually consisted of the amplified signal (for vital signs, a waveform of some sort), and later, they consisted of a DC voltage proportional to the desired derivative of the raw signal (e.g., heart rate from an EKG).

In the 1970s, medical devices began to incorporate first solid-state, then integrated circuit, and soon after, microprocessor electronics. Their ability to use digital signal processing led to significant improvement in the stability and usefulness of their output

J. Stonemetz, K. Ruskin (eds.) *Anesthesia Informatics*,
© Springer Science + Business Media, LLC 2008

data. However, for the development of AIMS, the more significant detrimental impact was the innovation of on-device memory in medical devices, which enabled trending of intraoperative data. The ability to print these trends may have undermined the development of integrated data management and more comprehensive—and commercial—information systems.

Event Logging and Decision Support

Simply charting derived vital-sign information is only one reason to implement an AIMS. An ideal system should appropriately annotate the record and use specific combinations of information to provide clinical decision support. Such support was thought to be capable of delivering, in the short term, artifact suppression, smart-alarm management, and population of decision-support "information blackboards," or repositories of data, that would enable various algorithms to make useful inferences to guide clinical management. In some instances, the target of such advice included crisis and incident management—the beneficiaries often stated to be "junior staff"; in other instances, the advice was intended to enable work simplification by routine control of "single" functions, such as depth of anesthesia. Although reports of the experience of such decision-support systems are many, the systems have only rarely been integrated into AIMS.

Managing Complex Situations

The conjunction of some of these various aspirations led, not surprisingly, to analogies being made to airplane flight-deck control "cockpits," where the patient vital signs are likened to external flight information (location, altitude, airspeed, etc.), while the data associated with the anesthesia process itself are likened to the aircraft setting and status readouts. While the analogy is helpful in some respects, it is misleading in two significant respects: (a) the complexity of the combined technical systems of an airplane is far less than that of human physiology, which has more disparate but interrelated (and poorly understood) functional entities, and (b) the set of technical subsystems that comprise an airplane is not subject to intentional physical reconfiguration while it is in flight. New measurement and therapeutic modalities are often incorporated "midflight" into anesthesia systems in response to changes in both patient status and surgical procedure.

An AIMS in the Enterprise

As the 1980s progressed, the growing capability of computer technology encouraged thoughts that the availability of information from individual anesthetic encounters would enable better clinical and administrative management within anesthetic departments and in ORs with which they were associated, as well as more effective integration throughout the entire hospital enterprise. These thoughts mirrored the sort of functional integration that was then well underway in industry, where production-floor devices were being integrated with production management and control, which in turn, were being integrated into stock and financial systems. This analogy is worth recalling throughout this chapter.

Successful Management of Interfaces

The contextual background provided is noteworthy because expectations place direct and sometimes difficult-to-reconcile requirements upon a device-communications interface. In 1989, Gardner and coworkers succinctly expressed the requirements for successful management of device interfaces, including:

- Representation of real-time signals (noting that the relevant time base may typically be in the range of milliseconds to minutes)
- Representation of derived (vital-sign) data signals (typically the relevant time base may be in the range of seconds to hours)
- Indications and descriptions of physiologic-status alarms
- Device-setting representation and bidirectional device-control communication
- Support of "on-the-fly" connection/disconnection and establishment/pull-down of communication as devices are added and removed from the patient-care environment
- Retention of electrical and data safety in medical devices and communication equipment, particularly as the data are used for purposes other than clinical care
- Support of data consistency and transparency from the interdevice network, to the AIMS, into enterprise systems—and even beyond into regional, national, and international secondary-use systems[1]

Uses of Interfaces

The data communication requirements encountered by manufacturers and biomedical engineers who perform maintenance and troubleshooting of medical devices, either in the field or in workshops, bear noting. The early analog outputs from medical devices lent themselves to the simple diagnostic instruments that were available at the time; subsequently, digital outputs made it possible for devices to present data, often in very cryptic formats that varied from model to model.[2] In the case of simple, low-cost devices, external communication is sometimes a relatively low design priority that is shoehorned into spare processor capacity after the needs of signal processing and user-interface support are fulfilled. As long as the system diagnostic needs of the device engineer are fulfilled, the designer may regard his task as complete. Unfortunately, the cryptic and variable nature of the interfaces continues to today. Fortunately, many of these simple interfaces generally use plain (ASCII) text and numerics to communicate.[3] However, data formats remain highly variable despite advances in communication technology,[4] and little or no consistency exists between devices, even when they have been developed by the same manufacturer.

Interoperability

Definition of Interoperability

In 1990, the Standard Computer Dictionary of the Institute of Electrical and Electronic Engineers (IEEE) defined *interoperability* as "the ability of two or more systems or components to exchange information and to use the information that has been exchanged."[5] This remains an accurate definition but perhaps falls short of more recent expectations that information exchange will happen without the user having to undertake any special task. A more recent publication therefore proposed a more complete definition: "The capability to communicate, execute programs, or transfer data among various functional units in a manner that requires the user to have little or no knowledge of the unique characteristics of those units."[6] In either case, the implied need is first for *functional interoperability* (i.e., shared architectures, methods and frameworks, and technologies) and, second, for *semantic interoperability* (shared data types, terminologies, and coding systems), which relates well to a concept that is now somewhat out of fashion—that of Open Systems Interconnection (OSI).[7] In this approach, the entire gamut of communication technology is broken into seven separate layers, the so-called OSI 7-layer model of the International Standards Organization (ISO) (Fig. 7.1).[8] Retaining the concept of layered services, however, remains important for reasons that become clear later.

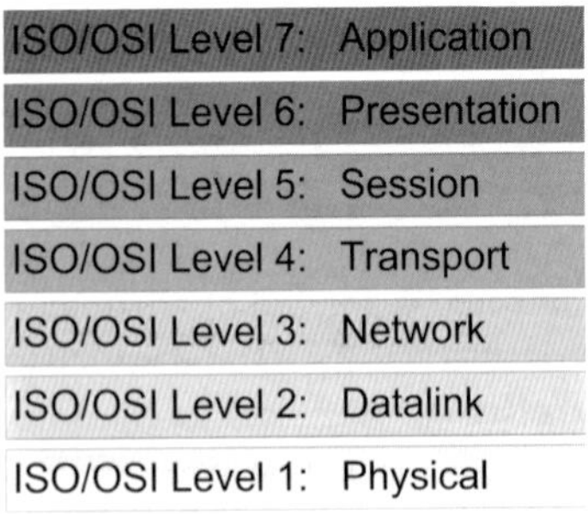

| ISO/OSI Level 7: Application |
| ISO/OSI Level 6: Presentation |
| ISO/OSI Level 5: Session |
| ISO/OSI Level 4: Transport |
| ISO/OSI Level 3: Network |
| ISO/OSI Level 2: Datalink |
| ISO/OSI Level 1: Physical |

Fig. 7.1 The ISO OSI 7-layer model of communication—conceptual layers of elements used in all communication in information systems. It should be noted that such a cleanly differentiated approach is seldom possible in real implementations, but attention to maintenance of clean break points assists in enabling work to be reused in combination with newer technologies as they emerge

Legislation

No discussion of medical device data communication would be complete without reference to the legislative framework in which devices are placed on the market, used, and maintained. The European Union (EU) Medical Devices Directive (MDD) governs the manufacture and use of medical devices placed on the market in the EU. The Food and Drug Administration (FDA) has regulatory responsibilities for this area in the US.

Historically, conformance to the provisions of the MDD has been assessed by compliance to mandated standards that were produced in support of the "new approach." In practice, this means that a number of ISO and International Electrotechnical Commission (IEC) standards are mirrored (sometimes with additional provisions) in European equivalent standards bodies [European Committee for Standardization (CEN) and European Committee for Electrotechnical Standardization (CENELEC)] and cited by the *Official Journal of the EU* in support of the MDD.[9-11] The European versions of standards mentioned in the section on Device Safety are those that are currently most commonly used in support of the MDD. In March 2007, the EU Parliament adopted a revised form of the MDD, which includes "stand-alone software" placed on the market for diagnostic or therapeutic purposes. At present, the precise interpretation of adoption of this revision remains unclear, but the time frame for its introduction was set at 2010. A possible interpretation is that the Directive now covers all software designed for healthcare use, though informal communications with the UK Medicines and Healthcare Devices Regulatory Agency indicate that they will continue to interpret "stand-alone software" only as being applicable to control and interpretation of other Active Medical Devices.

Standards

As in other areas of standardization, a rambling array of standards impacts the area of device interfacing. After examining some underpinning principles, we will briefly consider the standards with the least immediate impact before examining the most extensive body of work on the topic in more detail.

Device Safety

Depending on interpretation, the standards in this section could be applicable, in part or in whole, to health informatics software in general (see "Legislation" section). These standards refer to requirements for electrical devices that communicate directly with patients. The two major groups working in this area are IEC TC62, "Electrical equipment in medical practice," and ISO TC210, "Quality management and corresponding general aspects for medical devices." In addition to the two main groups working on device safety, ISO technical committees (TCs) work on specific types of devices, and other committees in both the ISO and IEC work on more generic aspects of safety; however, a full discussion all of the committees is beyond the scope of this chapter. The three primary committees are the IEC TC62—electrical equipment in medical practice, the ISO TC210—quality management and corresponding general aspects for medical devices, and the ISO TC121—anesthetic and respiratory equipment. None of these committees has a specific focus on device-communication standards, but all of them have produced documents that directly impact aspects of these standards, as discussed below.

Logistics and Tracking

A number of European and International standards are concerned with identification of material objects. In the past, these were in conflict, but GS1 was established to coordinate the former European and US standards on a global basis.[12] GS1 states that it is dedicated to the design and implementation of global standards and solutions to improve the efficiency and visibility of supply and demand chains globally, with the goal of simplifying global commerce by connecting the flow of information with the flow of goods. The GS1 "system" of standards is the most widely used supply-chain standards system in the world.

GS1 Healthcare User Group

The mission of the GS1 Healthcare User Group (GS1 HUG) is "to lead the healthcare industry to the effective utilization and development of global standards with the primary focus on automatic identification to improve patient safety."[13] Its vision is "to become the single source for regulatory agencies and trade organizations (manufacturer, wholesaler, hospital, and pharmacy) to seek input and direction for global (identification and logistics) standards in the healthcare industry" (a not atypical interest-centric view of the healthcare domain).[13] The four focus areas for the HUG are prevention of medical errors, product authentication, tracking and tracing, and increasing total supply-chain efficiency.

Although it is possible to implement fully interoperable aspects of logistics and tracking systems without resorting to GS1 (i.e., via careful application of the ISO and IEC standards to which GS1 contributes), by driving adoption of increasingly coherent international standards in the supply and demand chains, GS1 has considerable power to enable safe and efficient deployment of products to patients. The medical device-communication (MDC) field has considerable interest in enabling traceability and real-time tracking, though some technical and cultural challenges must be overcome at the semantic representation level. An allied group of technologies, real-time location services (RTLS), are fast being deployed to enable devices with radio-tag, WiFi, or mobile phone identifiers to be located in three dimensions in real time. Potential applications would allow continuous remote monitoring during movement of preoperative and postoperative patients.

Communication Technology Protocols

Although the topic of communication technology protocols has enormous impact, we will here only highlight the current and emerging technologies because the continual evolution of communications dictates that it is the principles that emerge from such an overview that are important rather than the specifics, which can be examined on a case-by-case basis.

RS232 Protocol

Medical devices currently use a range of communication technologies to carry information content. Most common is a variant on the RS232 Electronic Industries Alliance (EIA) protocol (actually EIA-232).[2] Common problems were, and remain, nonstandard pin assignment of circuits on connectors and incorrect or missing control signals. This lack of adherence to the published standards has resulted in the proliferation of breakout boxes, patch boxes, test equipment, books, and other aids for the connection of disparate equipment, all of which have served to add complexity to the use of RS232 for many applications.

RS485 Protocol

RS485 (actually EIA-485) is an OSI electrical specification for a physical layer of a two-wire, half-duplex, multipoint, serial connection using differential signaling.[14] Like EIA-232, EIA-485 only specifies electrical characteristics of the driver and the receiver and does not specify or recommend any data protocol. However, it enables the configuration of inexpensive local networks and multidrop communications links at transmission speeds of 35 Mbit/s at up to 10 m and 100 kbit/s at 1200 m, and can relatively span distances of over 1200 m. In the early 1990s, implementations of this technology, though commercially unsuccessful because the problem of semantics was not addressed, demonstrated the viability of plug-and-play medical device networks for interfacing to acute care information systems.[15]

Ethernet-Based Protocols

The second most widely used communications technology employed by medical devices is Ethernet,[4] most commonly using IEEE 802.10, so-called 10BASE-T, but with the higher speeds and wireless (IEEE 802.11) becoming increasingly common. Wired connections use the RJ45 connector (actually 8P8C), but confusingly, this is also sometimes used for RS232. The international MDC standards groups are working with industry leaders to define appropriate profiles of IEEE 802 standards for use in point-of-care device communications.

Radio-Frequency Wireless Protocols

The number of radio-frequency wireless protocols has proliferated in the last 5 years. For most information communications purposes, the Ethernet-based IEEE 802.11 "WiFi" (or its faster derivatives) are used; this is true for medical devices as well. However, for shorter-range communications, the Bluetooth (now IEEE 802.15.1:2002) system has some attractions, particularly now that some of the interference issues involved when it coexists with WiFi (802.11) have been mitigated. Though it appears that entities within the very short-range wireless ("body area network") community are competing to make recommendations, the MDC standards community is working with the Bluetooth SIG Medical Devices Working Group[16] to profile the 802.15.1 standard for use in point-of-care device communications. Other standards that cover sensor-area networks to wide-area networks are also being adapted for medical device use.

Infrared Protocol

A few devices (generally those used for point-of-care blood tests) use infrared communications because they can be used to collect a series of measurements and take them to a base station, where the data are transferred for inclusion in the permanent medical record. The technology used is known as *IrDA*, named after The Infrared Data Association (http://www.irda.org).[17] This protocol is a simple and efficient way to connect devices. The MDC standards group assisted the Point-of-Care Communications Industry Consortium (POC-CIC) to profile the IrDA standards for use in point-of-care test communications specifications. The resulting Clinical and Laboratory Standards Institute (CLSI) standard[18] and two transport technology standards are listed in the section on International Medical Device Communication standards (CEN ISO/IEEE 11073).

Fieldbus Protocols

Fieldbus is a network system for industrial, real-time, distributed control over different topologies. Although the technology has been available since 1988, completion of the international standard took many years and resulted in the current IEC 61158 standard ("Industrial communication networks—fieldbus specifications..."), which comprises 66 parts and relates to eight different protocol groups called "Types." At least 16 competing fieldbus standards are in widespread use, and it is this fragmentation that makes it difficult to select a front-runner in the healthcare area. At the present, Controller Area Network (CAN)[19] and CANopen[20] are the most high-profile standards in terms of interdevice control being used by a few manufacturers of OR, X-ray, and lighting system equipment.

CAN was considered as the basis of the original CEN work on vital-sign representation but was rejected because it did not support a plug-and-play situation well, the assumption being that the network in which plug-and-play devices operated would be shutdown before any configuration changes occurred. This situation has changed somewhat, and one of the fieldbuses (CAN) is now used for some device-control purposes by some major manufacturers.[20] It is being actively promoted for "plug-and-play" MDC and has some semantic primitives associated with the low-level protocols, though apparently it is still not designed for midflight plug and play. The "Operating Room of the Future" project at the Center for Integration of Medicine and Innovative Technology (CIMIT) in Boston has been, since 2004, working with some equipment vendors to use CAN technology in support of intelligent control of equipment.[21]

The Uncertainty Dilemma

From an interoperability perspective in the context of healthcare, the field has two conflicting requirements for the technologic (as opposed to the semantic) aspects of communication. The first requirement is for a simple "connect (as and when we want) and it will do the rest" operation for users, especially as the move to provide more home/personal-based care proceeds. The second requirement is for communication of medical device data to be conducted in a fully safe, secure, and reliable manner. No off-the-shelf technology available at present can deliver both of these requirements without some compromise or addition of costly safeguards.[22] In what Kennelly called "The RS-232 Uncertainty Dilemma," he observed, "...hospitals think they have purchased a useful option on their devices. RS-232 is simply a cable, connector, and voltage specification." He went on to state:

> RS-232-based approaches to electronic data capture from patient-connected bedside devices have a more fundamental flaw. The software drivers for most devices change with different internal firmware revisions. This means that two identical looking devices need

entirely different device drivers. This precludes the successful larger scale use of any nurse-based device driver-loading scheme. At one hospital, an internal survey showed that they had ventilators from four different manufacturers in their acute care settings. From these manufacturers, they had a total of ten different model numbers. These ten models had a total of forty different device drivers, caused by different revisions of internal firmware. This represents a complicated matrix of required drivers and actions that cannot be managed by clinicians who rightly prioritize patient care actions over data communications. Finally, since the vast majority of device RS-232 ports are never used by hospitals, many of them simply do not work.[23]

Nearly 10 years later, it is still difficult to fault Kennelly's analysis—and it could as well have been applied to any communication transport technology.

New technologies such as WiFi, radio-frequency identification tags (RFID), and RTLS can be incorporated in a single device.[24] These combinations are now becoming commonplace, and while individually each has a valid part to play, the utility of such combinations for medical devices has yet to be demonstrated.

Information Representation

Although the diversity of communications transport technologies used by device manufacturers is a barrier to interoperability, it is nevertheless a much more tractable problem than the diversity of approaches to *representation of information*. In most cases, either a hardware adaptor can be bought or made, or a new protocol driver can be written to solve a communications transport problem. However, interpreting the data produced by devices often requires deep knowledge of each software revision of each model of each device. This is because the communication aspect of devices is, in priority of function, relatively unimportant and therefore is often left to occupy (or be cut to fit) spare processing and bus capacity. Thus, as models evolve, the information made available can be reduced or expanded by company engineers to fit the demands of more immediate design criteria.

It is important at this point to be clear about the nature of device data, in particular with respect to communication of clinical information in the context of the healthcare enterprise, be that an individual OR or a group of hospitals. Plug and play, as in point-of-care devices, requires a highly detailed and structured nomenclature for safe communication, whereas clinical reporting can generally rely on the training and interpretative ability of the healthcare professional to interpret a variety of terms that may be used to convey the same basic concept. For this reason, a clinical terminology such as Logical Observation Identifiers Names and Codes (LOINC)[25] displays a level of granularity between approximately one-fifth and one-twentieth of that required to permit safe device data communication, as summarized from the conclusions of a detailed study by Kraemer and colleagues.[26]

Analysis of LOINC and CEN ISO/IEEE 11073 Nomenclature

The LOINC nomenclature is oriented to the requirements of clinical reports and the healthcare record, whereas the ISO/IEEE 11073-10101 MDC nomenclature is focused on the requirements of medical device communication, monitoring of vital signs, and charting of critical care medicine.

The overlap between the LOINC and MDC nomenclature is rather small for most fields that are covered by both terminologies, such as anesthesia, cardiology, and neurology. Although a relatively large overlap has been found for terms used in EKG description and classification, LOINC does not cover many nomenclature items useful for describing EKG or EEG patterns, a consequence of the fact that these patterns are recognized and described during vital-sign monitoring but are less often reflected in the summarizing reports finally provided for the healthcare record.

LOINC does not cover the nomenclature needed for waveforms. Matching and, hence, translating to LOINC is possible for only a small number of items from the MDC nomenclature. For hemodynamic measurement terms, 26 out of 147 items (17.7%) have equivalents, and for respiration/ventilation terms, 12 out of 202 items (7.9%) have equivalents. This discrepancy is the consequence of the limitations of a multiaxial mapping of two nomenclatures from different environments. LOINC, therefore, is not a useful alternative nomenclature in the device-communication environment, and MDC nomenclature is no substitute for clinical terminology in an information-system application such as an AIMS.

Other Terminologies

The Anesthesia Patient Safety Foundation working group on terminology, the International Organization for Terminology in Anesthesia (IOTA)[27] (see Chap. 6), has presented preliminary studies that indicate that the relationship between Systematized Nomenclature of Medicine–Clinical Terms (SNOMED CT)[28] and MDC is similar to that seen between LOINC and MDC and that the description of devices within SNOMED CT is rather inconsistent at present. IOTA is undertaking work to define the optimal linkage of MDC into SNOMED CT for consistent reporting of device-derived information into clinical documents and databases.[29]

The Global Medical Devices Nomenclature (GMDN), a coding structure for describing adverse events related to medical devices, is designed for and used by regulators as the basis for globally harmonized data exchange.[30,31] It therefore has insufficient specificity to enable it to operate as an on-the-wire terminology for device communication; its designed use is more analogous to that of LOINC or SNOMED CT. Similarly, the nomenclature used for traceability by GS1 is designed for item-, pack-, or pallet-level description of items and is not detailed enough for device communication.[31]

In summary, both SNOMED CT and LOINC are suitable for the purposes of human communication at the clinical level but not for plug-and-play interoperability to, from, and between devices. Nor are their terms related to devices sufficiently crisp that they could be safely used to draw any sort of inference when data are aggregated from different patients or episodes (regardless of how effective they might be at the clinical descriptive level). Similarly, the various terminologies designed in ISO TC121 and TC210 to track problems, trace use, and provide glossaries of terms are insufficiently structured to enable unambiguous communication to, from, and between medical devices. Recognizing the need to permit clean operation of these terms for their legitimate purposes, the MDC standards enable the manufacturer to add a variety of these more general descriptors to medical device communication, but always in association with the unambiguous MDC term.

International Medical Device-Communication Standards

A single set of standards has emerged to enable language-independent communication between medical devices and related computer systems; these, for reasons that are explained later, are commonly called the CEN ISO/IEEE 11073, MDC or, most commonly, $x73$ standards.

Background

In the mid-1980s, a group of anesthetists, intensivists, clinical engineers, and medical device vendors began to define the Medical Information Bus (MIB) within the standards organization of the IEEE under the project identifier P1073.[32] Their goal was to overcome the problems of dealing with proliferating communications protocols as they tried to develop clinical information systems. At the time, they anticipated using the bus-like capabilities of RS485 as the main transport; hence, the familiar designation of MIB. By 1989, reasonably stable transport proposals had been developed and some preliminary work had been accomplished on allocation of codes to a set of common terms—the Medical Device Data Language (MDDL). These drafts resulted in a number of prototype implementations in the US and Europe by the early 1990s,[1,15,33] but progress on the standards stalled. At about that time, the CEN[10] initiated work in a similar field, and the responsible committee started work on standards for Vital Signs Representation (VITAL) and interoperability of patient-connected medical devices.[34,35] This work engaged some of the IEEE P1073 workers, and a high degree of commonality of approach emerged. When, in 1999, the ISO agreed to establish a committee for health informatics, one of the most active working groups was that for medical device communications, and it was quickly agreed that all of the IEEE and CEN work should be shared and coordinated into a single set of coherent standards for MDC. The group agreed that IEEE would be the primary publisher, with identical texts being made available internationally under the same identification number (11073) through the ISO and from CEN through European national standards bodies. By this time, the RS485-based bus approach had been abandoned as the main transport (the decision being to use common commercial and, where possible, mass-marketed technologies). Therefore, MIB was discouraged as a moniker, and $x73$, or sometimes MDC, was born. In 2006, the powerful industries behind the Continua Alliance,[36] after extensively researching the other possibilities, decided that $x73$ provided the most promising basis for implementing their plans for an ecosystem of personal health devices.

The CEN ISO/IEEE 11073 standards are, therefore, the only coherent standards addressing MDC, resulting in a single set of internationally harmonized standards that have been developed and adopted by ISO and CEN member countries. CEN ISO/IEEE 11073 standards enable communication between medical devices and related computer systems. They provide automatic and detailed electronic data capture of patient vital-sign information and device operational data. According to the charter of the joint group working to develop these standards, the primary goals are to provide real-time, plug-and-play interoperability for patient-connected medical devices and to facilitate efficient exchange of vital-sign and medical device data that are acquired at the point of care in all healthcare environments. In this context, *real time* means that data from multiple devices can be retrieved, time correlated, and displayed or processed in fractions of a second; *plug and play* means that all the clinician or patient has to do is make the connection, without stopping and restarting devices—the systems automatically detect, configure, and communicate without any other human interaction. *Efficient exchange of medical device data* means that information that is captured at the point of care (e.g., patient vital-sign data) can be archived, retrieved, and processed by many different types of applications without extensive software and equipment support and without needless loss of information.

The standards now cover the full spectrum of health-related devices from critical and acute care use (patient monitors, dialysis machines, ventilators, infusion pumps, etc.) to over-the-counter personal well-being monitors (exercise, heart rate, weight, etc.). They comprise a family of standards that can be combined to provide connectivity optimized for the specific devices being interfaced. The standards have four main sections:

- *Data services* (a) are described by an object-oriented data model that forms the basis for all messages, (b) are described by a nomenclature that has been optimized for vital-sign data representation, and (c) enable device-specific standards (specializations).
- *Application profile services* provide data-encoding specifications and service models to support both event-driven and polled communication architectures, as well as additional services such as remote control.

- *Transport services* provide reliable connections using off-the-shelf technologies that are commonly used in the industry (e.g., RJ45 connectors, CAT-5 cables, IrDA protocols, TCP/IP, RS232, Ethernet, WiFi, etc.).
- *Application gateways* define interactions between 11073-enabled systems and other application-level protocols and services, including Health Level 7 (HL7)-enabled applications.

Component standards from these areas may be layered together to provide a full ISO OSI 7-layer communications stack that supports plug-and-play interoperability from the cable connector (if wireless is not used) through to the application. The clinician need only make the connection (in the case of wireless, the user must acknowledge that the correct device is "connected"). In addition to these clear sections, one loose grouping of documents (the 11073-*xyyzz* series) provides more general information about the series, and another loose grouping (the 11073-9*yyzz* series) shares some aspects of the "stack" series but is not guaranteed to interoperate cleanly within the stack (usually because these documents accommodate legacy terminology).

Overview of the CEN ISO/IEEE 11073 Series

In most instances, the *x*73 documents are jointly published by CEN member organizations (the European national standards bodies), ISO member organizations (national standards bodies globally), and IEEE in various formats. In a few instances, groups other than IEEE have initially published *x*73 documents. In most instances, the full titles of the published documents are "ISO/IEEE 11073-*xyyzz*, Health informatics—Point-of-care medical device communication—..." if published by ISO or IEEE and "EN ISO 11073-*xyyzz*, Health informatics – Point-of-care medical device communication—..." if published through CEN (note that these also have a national prefix, e.g., BS for British Standard). The work plan, project contacts, and background materials are available from http://www.11073.org. The standards and related guidance documents that are or will be in production (search for "11073" at IEEE—http://tinyurl.com/yr2nmw, ISO—http://tinyurl.com/7ato5 , or CEN—http://tinyurl.com/29byc8) are shown in full in Table 7.1.

CEN ISO/IEEE 11073 Specialization Standards

These modality-oriented standards are all derived from the underpinning semantics described in the -1*yyzz* series. The -103*zz* Health informatics—Point-of-care medical device communication—Specialization series are, at this writing, not being progressed to publication because of higher perceived priorities within the workgroup; but a number are mature and form the basis of the -104*zz* series.

Table 7.1 CEN ISO/IEEE 11073 standards

CEN ISO/IEEE 11073 overview and related guidance documents	
11073-series #	**Document title: "Health informatics—Point-of-care medical device communication—…" (unless shown in full)**
-00000	Framework and overview (under revision in 2008—to replace obsolete IEEE 11073)
-00101	Guidelines for the use of RF wireless technology—Technical report (IEEE publication only)
-00103	Personal Health Device Communication—Technical report—Overview
-00201	Recommended practice—profile template
CEN ISO/IEEE 11073 semantics standards	
11073-series #	**Document title: "Health informatics—Point-of-care medical device communication—…" (unless shown in full)**
-10101	Nomenclature (terminology)
-10102	Nomenclature—annotated ECG (used in support of FDA clinical trials dossiers)
-10103	Nomenclature—implantable device cardiac (IDC)
-10104	Nomenclature—virtual attributes
-10201	Domain Information Model
-10202	Domain Information Model—XML schema format
CEN ISO/IEEE 11073 specialization standards	
11073-series #	**Document title: "Health informatics—Point-of-care medical device communication—…" (unless shown in full)**
-103zz	…Device Specializations (-10301, …—infusion device; -10302, …—vital-signs monitor; -10303, …—ventilator; -10304, …—pulse oximeter; -10305, …—defibrillator; -10306, …—ECG monitor; -10307, …—blood pressure; -10308, …—temperature; -10309, …—airway meter; -10310, …—cardiac output; -10311, …—airway gas analyzer; -10312, …—hemodynamic calculator; -10313, …—pulmonary calculator; -10315, …—weighing scale; -10316, …—dialysis device)
-10400	Personal Health Device Communication—device specialization—common framework
-10404	Personal Health Device Communication—device specialization—pulse oximeter
-10406	Personal Health Device Communication—device specialization—heart rate monitor
-10407	Personal Health Device Communication—device specialization—blood pressure monitor
-10408	Personal Health Device Communication—device specialization—thermometer
-10415	Personal Health Device Communication—device specialization—weighing scale
-10417	Personal Health Device Communication—device specialization—glucose meter
-10441	Personal Health Device Communication—device specialization—cardiovascular fitness and activity monitor
-10442	Personal Health Device Communication—device specialization—strength fitness equipment

(continued)

Table 7.1 (continued)

-10471	Personal Health Device Communication—device specialization— … independent living activity hub
-10472	Personal Health Device Communication—device specialization— medication monitor

CEN ISO/IEEE 11073 application profile standards	
11073-series #	**Document title: "Health informatics—Point-of-care medical device communication—…" (unless shown in full)**
-20000	Application profile—framework and overview
-20101	Application profile—base standard
-20103	Application profile—clinical context management (CCoM)
-20200	Application profile—association control function
-20201	Application profile—polling mode
-20202	Application profile—baseline asynchronous mode
-20301	Application profile—optional package, remote control
-20401	Application profile—common networking infrastructure
-20601	Health informatics—personal health device communication— application profile—optimized exchange protocol

CEN ISO/IEEE 11073 transport standards	
11073-series #	**Document title: "Health informatics—Point-of-care medical device communication—…" (unless shown in full)**
-30000	Transport profile—framework and overview
-30200	Transport profile—cable connected
-30300	Transport profile—infrared wireless
-30400	Interface profile—cabled Ethernet
-30503	Transport profile—RF wireless—local area network (wLAN)
-30505	Transport profile—RF wireless—wide-area (mobile phone) network (wWAN)

CEN ISO/IEEE 11073 gateway standards	
11073-series #	**Document title: "Health informatics—Point-of-care medical device communication—…"**
-60101	HL7 (V2.x) observation reporting interface (ORI)

CEN ISO 11073 miscellaneous standards	
11073-series #	**Document title: "Health informatics—Point-of-care medical device communication—…" (unless shown in full)**
-90101	Health informatics—analytical instruments—point-of-care test (CLSI POCT1-A2)
-91064	Standard communication protocol—computer-assisted electrocardiography (EN1064 SCP-ECG)
-92001	Medical waveform format—encoding rules (JIS MFER)

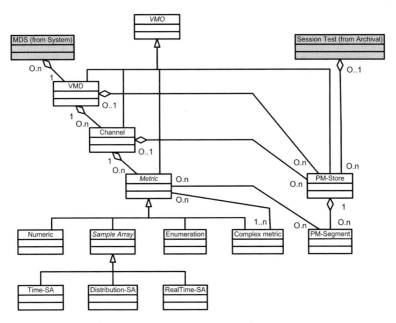

Fig. 7.2 The Domain Information Model (DIM) for the medical subject of the *x*73 standards (from ISO/IEEE 11072-10201). This UML diagram (see Chap. 6) shows a hierarchical aggregation of device elements, with the metrics being the data measured or calculated by devices. *MDS* medical device system (abstraction for system comprising one or more medical functions), *VMO* virtual medical object (an abstract representation of an object in the Medical Package of the DIM), *VMD* virtual medical device (an abstract representation of a medical-related subsystem of an MDS), *PM* persistent metric, *SA* sample array (for real-time/waveform, time/trend, distribution)

Medical Device Semantics

The underpinnings of the CEN ISO/IEEE 11073 series lie in just two standards: the Domain Information Model (Fig. 7.2) and the Nomenclature. Between them, they provide a robust and unambiguous means of describing how devices and their subsystems, together with the associated measurements, are related. They also provide the language-independent syntax for defining terms (systematic name) associated with different aspects of the MDC domain. This syntax can then be used to ensure that the required on-the-wire or database term (and its shorthand code) is globally unique. All *x*73 standards are identified in electronic communications by a globally unique object identifier; when the context-free code (an even smaller one is used "on the wire" once communication is established) is combined with this object identifier, the resulting information is guaranteed to be globally unique in any electronic communication. If allied with the unique address of the device and a time stamp, any item *x*73 data can be traced to its source device from whatever database in which the information is deposited. A selection of common terms, the *x*73 Ref_ ID (the unique abstract and in-message term), and the full context-free (32-bit) code are listed in Table 7.2. The systematic names, common abbreviations, and short (16-bit) codes are omitted.

Table 7.2 Example from ISO/IEEE 11073-10101 showing common terms, *x*73 Ref_ID, and full code

Common term	*x*73 Ref_ID	*x*73 full code
Noninvasive blood pressure (systolic)	MDC_PRESS_BLD_NONINV_SYS	150021
Noninvasive blood pressure (diastolic)	MDC_PRESS_BLD_NONINV_DIA	150022
Noninvasive blood pressure (mean)	MDC_PRESS_BLD_NONINV_MEAN	150023
ART (systolic)	MDC_PRESS_BLD_ART_SYS	150033
ART (diastolic)	MDC_PRESS_BLD_ART_DIA	150034
ART (mean)	MDC_PRESS_BLD_ART_MEAN	150035
PAP (systolic)	MDC_PRESS_BLD_ART_PULM_SYS	150045
PAP (diastolic)	MDC_PRESS_BLD_ART_PULM_DIA	150046
PAP (mean)	MDC_PRESS_BLD_ART_PULM_MEAN	150047
Pulmonary artery wedge pressure	MDC_PRESS_BLD_ART_PULM_WEDGE	150052
Central venous pressure	MDC_PRESS_BLD_VEN_CENT	150084
Unspecific temperature	MDC_TEMP	150344
SpO_2 parameter label	MDC_PULS_OXIM_SAT_O2	150456
Respiration rate	MDC_RESP_RATE	151562
End-tidal CO_2 concentration	MDC_AWAY_CO2_ET	151728
Inspired minimum CO_2	MDC_AWAY_CO2_INSP_MIN	151738
Transcutaneous CO_2 partial pressure	MDC_CO2_TCUT	151756
Inspired halothane concentration	MDC_CONC_AWAY_HALOTH_INSP	152176
Inspired sevoflurane concentration	MDC_CONC_AWAY_SEVOFL_INSP	152180
Inspired isoflurane concentration	MDC_CONC_AWAY_ISOFL_INSP	152184
Inspired oxygen concentration	MDC_CONC_AWAY_N2O_INSP	152192
End-tidal oxygen concentration	MDC_CONC_AWAY_O2_INSP	152196

ART arterial, *PAP* pulmonary artery pressure

Although the *x*73 working group has concentrated on common, off-the-shelf technologies for transport, it has been important to ensure that these can actually deliver plug-and-play functionality during "in-flight" use. Therefore, it has been necessary to define how sending devices and related data recipients behave during connection and disconnection in order to ensure that all data can be handled as quickly and safely as is technically possible. A schematic representation of how this is achieved is shown in Fig. 7.3. A state machine diagram showing the high-level transitions required to achieve connection by a device is provided in Fig. 7.4; each high-level state is actually achieved by many more detailed transactions. Such detailed device-communication arrangements are, of course, necessary. However, in routine use, they should all be entirely hidden from clinical users, who, if the requirement is simply to populate a chart, need only know that the communications gateway from a device is delivering appropriate, timely information in a manner

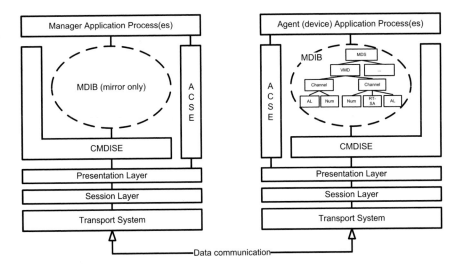

Fig. 7.3 The logical interface between two *x*73-connected systems. This schematic shows how sending devices and related data recipients relate through a mirrored set of logical entities and services. This figure can be compared with Fig. 7.1. to see how the layers of the ISO OSI model act in practice. *MDIB* Medical Device Information Base (provides standardized representation of device information elements), *ACSE* Association Control Service Element (provides methods to establish logical connections between systems), *CMDISE* Common Medical Device Information Service Element (provides generalized object access services), *MDS* medical device system, *VMD* virtual medical device (an abstract representation of a medical-related subsystem of an MDS)

that the receiving AIMS "understands." For this reason, the MDC group started to work with HL7[37] to ensure that the device semantics could be safely carried in HL7 enterprise-level messages. The result was the *x*73 HL7 V2.*x* observation reporting interface standard, which has now become the basis of profiles and demonstrations of the Integrating the Healthcare Enterprise (IHE)[38] (see below).

Are the CEN ISO/IEEE 11073 Standards Needed?

The CEN ISO/IEEE 11073 standards are the only coherent standards that address medical device interconnectivity and have resulted in a single set of internationally harmonized standards that (a) have been developed and adopted via clinical and technical contributions from within ISO and CEN member countries and (b) include contributions from the most significant manufacturers. That they have taken far longer to develop than their early protagonists could have imagined is due in large part to the emerging complexity of the task, in large part to the relative lack of drive from the user sector, in some part to the desire by industry to retain competitive distinctions, in small part to the rapid evolution of technology, and in some part to the emergence of the interface technology market. Nevertheless, they now at least provide complete profiled solutions for medical device connectivity, starting at the physical cable or wireless

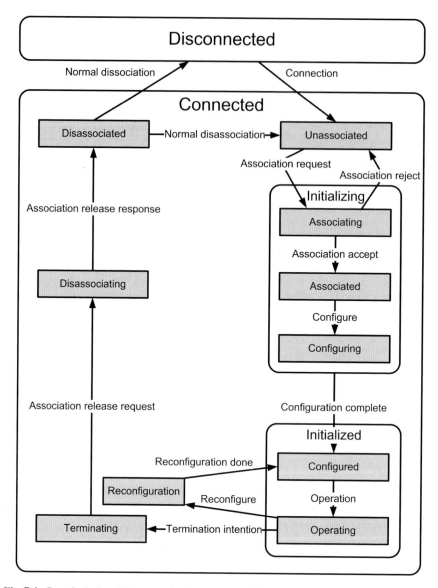

Fig. 7.4 Generic device *x*73 communications-state machine, which shows the different high-level states that a plug-and-play medical device must negotiate to behave well when connected or disconnected on the fly within a patient-centric information communication environment

connection and continuing through to the abstract representation of information and the services used for its management and exchange; in other words, they provide all seven layers of the ISO OSI 7-layer communications model (Fig. 7.1).

The CEN ISO/IEEE 11073 standards enable full disclosure of device-mediated information[33,39] so that measurement modalities are declared in detail and the associated metrics and alerts are communicated, together with any user-configured changes to settings. In addition, the device can communicate its manufacturer, model number, serial number, configuration, operating status, and network location—all in real time. These CEN ISO/IEEE standards have been developed in close coordination with other standards development organizations, including IEEE 802, IrDA, HL7, DICOM (Digital Imaging and Communications in Medicine), and CLSI. More recently, a related IEC/ISO Joint Working Group and an IHE group have been formed to assist still wider integration. The adoption by the Continua Alliance of the $x73$ standards as the vehicle for personal health data communication from consumer-purchased and consumer-managed devices has, since 2007, propelled the CEN ISO/IEEE 11073 standards into very large and fast-growing global markets and is driving adoption among the world's largest corporations, some of which are embedding support of $x73$ functions in their equipment.

A liaison between the IEEE 11073 standards group and the Center for Devices and Radiological Health (CDRH) of the US FDA helps to ensure that patient safety and efficacy concerns are addressed in the standards. Use of the standards is required for device communication by the National Programme for Information Technology (NPfIT) of the UK National Health Service. They were also included in the recommendations related to patient medical record information message formats that support HIPAA-compliant implementations; these recommendations were presented by the US National Committee on Vital and Health Statistics to the Department of Health and Human Services.

Vendor Standards Interpretations

As a cynic is said to have once observed, "the good thing about standards is that there are so many to choose from." This truism is only slightly less accurate in the area of health informatics than it is in most industries; however, for medical device communication, there is only one set of standards, deliberately harmonized with other areas of health informatics, that can deliver integrated functionality from the wire (or air) to the data representation in the clinical application—for the purposes of this book, the AIMS. These standards are the evolving set of ISO/IEEE 11073 standards. However, it must be said that, until 2007, very few major vendors of medical devices were advertising the availability of ISO/IEEE 11073-compliant communications, although some had been implementing them for a number of years. It is possible that marketing departments neglected to mention this compliance because they wished to lock customers into ongoing procurements by ensuring that change would be technically difficult. This apparent reluctance has done much to increase the timidity of purchasers in asking for open standard communications from medical devices, resulting in tentative requests in outline specifications being withdrawn in the face of statements from the manufacturer that, "there is no demand for that." In the relatively closed world of a regulated device market, only the robust insistence of clinical professionals, backed by their procurement staffs, is likely to ensure that the vision annunciated by Gardner et al. in 1989[1] is likely to persuade vendors to make their devices communicate in an open and interoperable manner. In the wider world of over-the-counter personal health devices, industry adoption of the ISO/IEEE 11073 standards is already well underway, and only time will tell how the cultural and commercial collision impacts both sectors.

Medical Device Communications in the Enterprise

Standards evolve to address business needs of the affected constituents. The gradual introduction of information technology into healthcare has caused providers and vendors to cooperate on standards for healthcare data communications. Three major standards efforts are ongoing for the healthcare clinical setting: CEN ISO/IEEE 11073, HL7, and DICOM. CEN ISO/IEEE 11073 addresses the needs of patient-connected bedside medical devices. HL7 addresses the needs of batch-based processes such as orders, results, and admission/discharge/transfer. DICOM addresses the needs of radiology and medical imaging. The major difference between ISO/IEEE 11073 and HL7 is the wide disparity in use cases; these are highlighted below. IHE is tasked with bringing together the various complementary standards that are identified as best able to address particular clinical scenarios. It has used ISO/IEEE 11073, HL7, and DICOM standards, together with others from the larger IT industry, to deliver tested specifications for application profiles of use in the enterprise. We examine the role of IHE for medical device communications at the end of this section.

Relationship Between CEN ISO/IEEE 11073 and HL7

This section briefly addresses the relationship between, and the different business requirements for CEN ISO/IEEE 11073 and HL7, the major worldwide standard used for communication between information systems in healthcare (see Chap. 6). The major difference between the two standards is the computing models for which they are designed. HL7 is designed for use by PC- and workstation-type machines that have significant computing power available for communications, whereas the $x73$ standards are designed for use by devices that are run by microcontrollers and microprocessors and therefore have very limited processing bandwidth available for communications.

HL7 messaging assumes point-to-point transmission of an (event-triggered) initial message from a sender to a receiver, followed by a (sometimes optional) response or acknowledgment message from the receiver back to the sender. The $x73$ service model provides "real-time" access to object instances using a data communication link between a manager system and an agent system. CEN ISO/IEEE 11073 standards define two separate messaging paradigms: one for dynamic exchange of information structures and another for mostly context-free, polling-mode access to medical data.

Human Client versus Machine Client

HL7 has a basic assumption that the end user of the information is a screen (or print) read by people; thus, its messaging method is ASCII based. ISO/IEEE 11073 is highly optimized for use by processor-based devices, with the assumption that the immediate user is also a computer. This choice in communications models has caused some higher level of complexity in the design and adoption of this standard, but it also results in significantly simpler processing for computer software writers. HL7 assumes that most transactions are completed by providers and are not performed in real time. Even machine-to-machine transactions, such as a report to a clinical data repository, assume an eventual human use without further computer processing.

The net result all of these business differences between HL7-based information-system applications and medical devices has been a mutual recognition that a common standard could not be achieved. Both groups, however, agreed that compatibility between the two standards was highly desirable and could be best achieved at the level of application layer messages. Such work has been undertaken for several years. The first effort at achieving compatibility between the two standards was made in 1995, when the IEEE 11073 meetings were moved to become part of the HL7 meeting schedule and agenda. This effort continues today and has been consolidated into a dedicated Working Group for Devices in HL7, enabling the HL7, ISO, and IEEE 11073 groups to hold joint meetings three times each year. On occasion, these meetings take place outside of the US and have enabled participation by other regional standards organizations (such as CEN in Europe), which have displayed a strong desire to work toward global compatibility with device messages.

Integrating the Healthcare Enterprise

IHE is an initiative by healthcare professionals and industry to improve the way computer systems in healthcare share information. IHE promotes the coordinated use of established standards such as DICOM and HL7 to address specific clinical needs in support of optimal patient care. Systems developed in accordance with IHE communicate better with one another, are easier to implement, and enable care providers to use information more effectively. Physicians, medical specialists, nurses, administrators, and other care providers envision a day when vital information can be passed seamlessly from system to system within and across departments and made readily available at the point of care. IHE is designed to make their vision a reality by improving the state of systems integration and removing barriers to optimal patient care.

The IHE was conceived by the Healthcare Information and Management Systems Society and the Radiological Society of North America. The American College of Cardiology has joined them as a major sponsor in recent years. The IHE brings together a wide range of stakeholders to develop the framework and process for industry to achieve new levels of systems integration. IHE enables vendors to cooperate in implementing standards for communication among information systems, while giving users—medical practitioners and information technology professionals—an important advisory role in that process.

The American College of Clinical Engineers was awarded sponsorship for patient care devices (PCD) under IHE. The PCD domain includes point-of-care devices used at the bedside and in the ED, OR, ICU, and other acute care settings. It deals with a wide variety of work flows throughout the healthcare system—perhaps most notably, those associated with the integration of the patient-centric, device-derived data with the wider, enterprise-level, communication of clinical information. The PCD technical Framework Profiles that are available at this writing are:

- *Device to enterprise*—maps ISO/IEEE 11073 semantics to an HL7 V2 ORU^R01 message
- *Device observation filter*—profiles an HL7 publish/subscribe mechanism for specifying what information should be communicated
- *Patient device ID binding*—profiles how patient and device identifiers are bound and unbound

The PCD technical Framework Profiles that are in production at this writing are:

- *Simple medical device plug and play*—profiles ISO/IEEE 11073 standards for plug-and-play connectivity
- *Alarm communication management*—profiles device alarm communication between the point of care and the enterprise
- *Infusion pump integration*—profiles a device-to-enterprise-based exchange for ensuring the Five Rights of medication administration, as defined by The Joint Commission (see Chap. 11)
- *HL7 V3/CDA device information representation*—profiles HL7 V3 model constructs for *x*73 information and defines a consistent representation in CDA documents

Implementation

Although in writing about the topic of implementation, one risks stating the obvious, it is worth reviewing a few general principles, even for those readers who are content that they all have been addressed in their planning. We have observed that although a good deal of effort has been invested in support of the CEN ISO/IEEE 11073 MDC standards, they had, as of the beginning of 2008, made relatively little impact upon the regulated medical device market. As a result, a number of opportunistic strategies have been adopted to fill the gap left by the lack of full interoperability. It is worth examining the strategies that have been used and considering their advantages and shortcomings. However, we will first review how most devices currently behave.

Device Communication

Almost all vendors of medical devices that enable their products to communicate electronically do so (at least in 2008) using proprietary formats—of connectors, as we have already seen—and in the representation of the information, which can be much more problematic. The challenges lie in having to elicit not only the documented aspects of the device communication (often, obtaining this documentation takes persistence and depends on personal relationships), but also those undocumented aspects, such as whether the device simply sends new data as it generates them, how and when it refreshes discontinuous data such as noninvasive blood pressures, how out-of-range signals are handled or suppressed, etc. The device will typically provide quasi-English language-derived data (heart rate, respiration rate, etc.) but typically will not give real-time waveform signals (such as EKG) in an easily accessible form, although for most regular AIMS-charting activities, this is not a significant problem.

In general, most devices deliver unsolicited results messages from the interface and, as the data become available, from the medical device. Some interfaces then pause to wait for an application-level (AIMS or its proxy) acknowledgment. Sometimes, messages are sent at user-configured time intervals, and some device interfaces do not wait for acknowledgments. If a device sends data only in response to a request (either a one-time query, or one of a series of polling requests), then it must be determined if the device will send all of the data accumulated since the last request or only the most recent (ignoring all intermediate data). The major patient-monitoring vendors all market intermediary systems than can convert data used on their proprietary networks to HL7 messages, and those messages have a high degree of commonality. However, in the context of an AIMS, the case for networking like devices between ORs is not as clear as in an ICU, where it may make operational sense; the cost of the intermediate gateway device may be prohibitive if it cannot cope with third-party devices.

The biggest problem comes last, however. Even if the temporal performance of the device interface were to be clearly articulated such that it would be one of a set of options (standardized), it would still leave the problem of *information representation*. This concept is illustrated most simply by a sample set of actual device parameters to real representations that are currently used by various vendors (Table 7.3). This short set of common examples illustrates what a formidable task it is to ensure that receiving applications can accurately and safely interpret this sort of communicated data into charted or recorded form; only one label term (out of 22) is consistent across all vendors. Note, too, that in some instances, the label is combined with the units of measurement, making on-the-fly computation very difficult. Another point worth noting is that in modular medical devices in which the measurement/therapy subsystems can be hot swapped, the behavior of the systems varies; some always report physical locations (i.e., bus locations), whereas others dynamically reconfigure so that labels shown to the communications interface are altered. This added complexity means that great care must be exercised when reading and controlling such modular systems, particularly if they are delivering therapy.

It is important to mention that to deliver peer-to-peer interoperability, the devices must not just exchange data. They must also exchange their shared understanding of that data (the "Initializing" stage in Fig. 7.4). For example, connecting a pulse oximeter to an infusion pump does nothing unless the pump "knows" that it is connected

Table 7.3 Comparison of actual communicated terms from three vendors' devices with $x73$ common term

Common term	Vendor 1	Vendor 2	Vendor 3	X73 Ref_ID
Noninvasive blood pressure (systolic)	NBP S	NBP-S	NBP[a]1	MDC_PRESS_BLD_NONINV_SYS
Noninvasive blood pressure (diastolic)	NBP D	NBP-D	NBP[a]2	MDC_PRESS_BLD_NONINV_DIA
Noninvasive blood pressure (mean)	NBP M	NBP-M	NBP[a]3	MDC_PRESS_BLD_NONINV_MEAN
ART (systolic)	ART D	AR[b]-S	ART[a]1	MDC_PRESS_BLD_ART_SYS
ART (diastolic)	ART S	AR[b]-D	ART[a]2	MDC_PRESS_BLD_ART_DIA
ART (mean)	ART M	AR[b]-M	ART[a]3	MDC_PRESS_BLD_ART_MEAN
PAP (systolic)	PA S	PA[b]-S	PAP[a]1	MDC_PRESS_BLD_ART_PULM_SYS
PAP (diastolic)	PA D	PA[b]-D	PAP[a]2	MDC_PRESS_BLD_ART_PULM_DIA
PAP (mean)	PA M	PA[b]-M	PAP[a]3	MDC_PRESS_BLD_ART_PULM_MEAN
Pulmonary artery wedge pressure	PWP	PAW	PAWP	MDC_PRESS_BLD_ART_PULM_WEDGE
Central venous pressure	CVP	CVP[b]	CVP	MDC_PRESS_BLD_VEN_CENT
Unspecific temperature	T	TMP-[b]	T[b]	MDC_TEMP
SpO_2 parameter label	SpO2	SPO2-%	SpO2	MDC_PULS_OXIM_SAT_O2
Respiration rate	RRc	RR	RESP	MDC_RESP_RATE
End-tidal CO_2 concentration	etCO2	CO2-EX	ETCO2	MDC_AWAY_CO2_ET
Inspired minimum CO_2	iCO2	CO2-IN	IMCO2	MDC_AWAY_CO2_INSP_MIN
Transcutaneous CO_2 partial pressure	tpCO2	TC CO2	tcpCO2	MDC_CO2_TCUT
Inspired halothane concentration	iHAL	HAL-IN	inHAL	MDC_CONC_AWAY_HALOTH_INSP
Inspired sevoflurane concentration	iSEV	SEV-IN	inSEV	MDC_CONC_AWAY_SEVOFL_INSP
Inspired isoflurane concentration	iISO	ISO-IN	inISO	MDC_CONC_AWAY_ISOFL_INSP
Inspired oxygen concentration	iO2	O2-IN	inO2	MDC_CONC_AWAY_N2O_INSP
End-tidal oxygen concentration	etO2	O2-EX	etO2	MDC_CONC_AWAY_O2_INSP

[a]Provides an indication that this measure is an instance in a triplet (three-part variable), which is identified in the coded expression by an offset numeric

[b]Provides an instance identifier related to the number of recurrences of that type of measurement from the device

ART arterial, *PAP* pulmonary artery pressure

to a pulse oximeter and shuts off if the saturation drops below a certain value. The Medical Device Information Base is shown in Fig. 7.3; all shared understanding is dependent on this being a clear mirror of the minimum information needed to achieve true interoperability (see earlier section). Most devices will establish only limited sets of "understanding" based on their capability with respect to their peer; most AIMS will "know" about a very wide range of device types.

Current Device-Communication Architectures

Two basic models of device-communication architecture have been, or are being, used for device communication with other devices and computers such as AIMS; the third architecture is the "emergent" standards-based approach:

- Customized device-to-recipient communication
- Converters to common semantics for communication to recipient
- Inherently open standard communication between devices and over network(s)

Customized Device-to-Recipient Communication

Customized device-to-recipient communication (Fig. 7.5) is the oldest and still widely used strategy for getting a medical device (usually a patient monitor) with a proprietary communications interface to provide an information system with data. Because the interface is intended only to be applicable to one instance of a device and one instance of a computer program, the communications, parsing, and database code can all be handcrafted to fulfill the specific needs. It is difficult to accurately estimate the time that this "handcrafting" takes, but it is not unusual for a highly skilled software engineer to take more than a week to get a relatively simple device such as a pulse oximeter to reliably place data (e.g., saturation and pulse) into a database. Accessing event data or devices of greater complexity presents a much greater challenge.

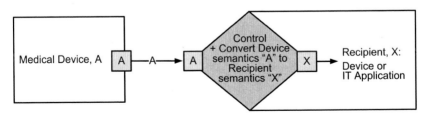

Fig. 7.5 Customized device–database communication. Schematic showing the semantic transition that must be made when a closely coupled interface is implemented using customized software in the receiving device or system

Custom-developed software works on an individual basis but may fail if other software, such as medical device firmware or the receiving application, has been updated. Custom software is costly to execute but could provide as much transfer of information as the communication technologies permit. The oldest variant of this implementation architecture enables a group of devices (typically up to 4, 8, or 16) to be hardwired for database communication that covers each patient-centric area. The difficulties of software coding for data handling are similar to those for customized 1:1 communication, except that the task is multiplied by the number of device types to be used. The additional complexity arises from having to recognize which data are being presented and having to establish suitable data flow control. The approach is therefore most often used where relatively standard RS232 protocols are observed by the devices. Each connector (port) on the device-clustering equipment (usually a "terminal server") must be assigned to a particular device type, and if the clinical user connects the wrong piece of equipment, erroneous data communication or a total failure of communication may result.

Converters to Common Semantics for Communication to Recipient

The architecture of converters to common semantics for communication to the recipient is similar to the previous "many devices" implementation, except that the terminal server function is up-rated to that of a data server, as it has enough computing power to translate all of the recognized device-specific communications to a common set of semantics (Fig. 7.6). The difficulties of device semantics and data flow control are therefore separated from the recipient application, which generally

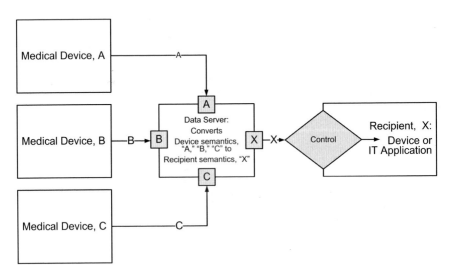

Fig. 7.6 Converter to common semantics for communication to recipient. A "converter" architecture implementation with a data-server function translates all of the recognized device-specific communications to a common set of semantics

determines whether to accept a constant flow of data or to poll the data server for information when required. Usually, each port on the data server still has to be assigned to a particular device type, though a few more powerful—and costly—variants are said to be able to interpret the communications from any device regardless of the connection port (this presupposes that the device type being connected is known to the data server).

The increased costs implied by this more user-friendly architecture mean that it is usually deployed downstream of a patient-centered group of devices, which may often use a terminal server as a means to put their serial (RS232)-carried data onto an Ethernet backbone. The data server is then shared by more than one set of patient data but can route its data to the associated application (which, because of the device data architecture, is often then a centrally served system, with each workstation in communication with the single server). All devices still have to be "known" to the data server, and many converters ignore all but the most commonly charted data.

A major variant of the "converter" architecture involves conversion of semantics at the MDC's port (or somewhere along a cable from that port) by use of a converter box (dongle). In some cases, these dongles can convert RS232-based communication to Ethernet. This approach means that the user can plug a new device into any available communications port in the patient area and have it communicate with the recipient application. From a user perspective, the use of dongles for data conversion purposes is an attractive option so long as they can be powered from the host device (not always the case). Their bulk is not too great compared to the host device, and they cannot be accidentally detached from the intended host. The disadvantages remain the relatively high cost of developing the conversion software. One now-defunct European system from the mid-1990s made a virtue out of necessity by including an LCD display in such a converter. This then enabled the information-system users to be sure that they had the correct device recognized by the information system, which would also show information about any therapy that the device was supposed to be delivering and seek an "is this correct?" confirmation to the information system.

Inherently Open Standard Communication between Devices and over Networks

Although the architecture used in the previous example could be adapted to convert networked systems to the ISO/IEEE 11073 semantics, it is less likely that devices could deliver the same level of plug and play with full disclosure (i.e., the intermediate conversion to common semantics is not a matter of only converting the most commonly used data and ignoring the rest). Similarly, $x73$-enabled devices and any of the systems using shared semantics could use those semantics in more than one information system. However, in reality, because such different systems would only exist if they served different uses, it is likely that they would require the less commonly converted semantics and would be poorly served by such lowest-common-denominator approaches. The use of standardized ISO/IEEE 11073 communications

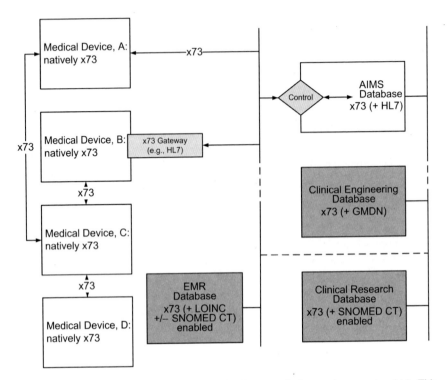

Fig. 7.7 Inherently open standard communication between devices and over network(s). This schematic shows how use of standardized communications not only delivers unified semantic interoperability but also enables delivery of real-time data and enables midprocedure plug and play of devices without the user having to search for additional hardware or the correct port on a data concentrator

not only delivers unified semantic interoperability, but also enables delivery of real-time data and enables midprocedure plug and play of devices without recourse to additional hardware or searching for the correct port on a data concentrator (Fig. 7.7). It remains to be seen whether the signs of widespread vendor adoption that were visible at the IHE demonstrations in 2007 and 2008 will be converted into market demand.

Marketing and Availability of x73 Standards

As of this date, few devices are actively marketed as having ISO/IEEE 11073 standards capability, although a number have this capability but do not advertise it. Although many interface-system vendors exist, only one is strongly active in both the North American and European markets. Most others are geographically localized

from the vendor. An alternative is threefold (a) identifying an interface vendor that has, or will develop, test, and debug interfaces that meet the customer's specifications; (b) asking about migration to using open $x73$ standards; and then (c) introducing a time-to-deploy clause.

The use of custom-developed solutions written by the institutional IT staff is discouraged. Those that start such tasks as willing experimenters rapidly become bored with the tedium of fighting to achieve interface specifications that are meaningful and then endlessly debugging software that works correctly *most* of the time (and then fails for no apparent reason). Detecting which devices are connected, where, and with what intended system interaction is a complex problem well beyond the capability of most hospital IT departments. Unless a very simple, hardwired connection between one or two devices and a single AIMS dataflow is what is required, it is advised that a preexisting product be purchased.

Aspirations for the Future

Unfortunately, the time that it has taken to develop and publish universal standards for management of device interfaces has tended to set aspirations at a fairly low level. To review the desiderata listed at the beginning of this chapter:

- Representation of real-time signals
- Representation of derived (vital-sign) data signals
- Indications and descriptions of physiologic-status alarms
- Device-setting representation and bidirectional device-control communication
- Support of "on-the-fly" plug and play
- Retention of electrical and data safety
- Support of data consistency to the AIMS and enterprise, regional, national, and international secondary-use systems

From the intervening material, we can see that these requirements can all be delivered by the $x73$ standards—if only it were possible to buy a product that supports those standards. So, this must be Aspiration #1. Aspiration #2 must be using the accurate, rich data that could be acquired with $x73$-enabled systems to accomplish some simple artifact removal, with the immediate impact that this could have on reduction in false alarm rates.[1,33] Aspiration #3 would be the use of artifact-free data to build useful, smart, physiologic warnings. A great deal was written on this idea in the late 1980s and into the 1990s, but interest dwindled because of the chore of writing device drivers and eliminating disruptive artifacts. This same approach could, when allied to physician-entered (or therapeutic-device-contributed) data, be used to warn about iatrogenic effects in real time.[41] Aspiration #4 is a progression from #3. It would see treatment protocols designed on the basis of rich data and implemented using real-time feeds of that data.[39] Repositories of complete and comparable data should enable routine variance, effectiveness, and utilization analysis.

Conclusion

In the absence of standards for MDC, data are captured manually or with custom equipment (both at considerable expense), or not at all. Capturing data manually is labor intensive, recorded infrequently (particularly when it matters most), and is prone to human error.[1,23,33] Use of expensive, custom connectivity equipment increases the cost of healthcare delivery and tends to lock healthcare providers into single companies or partnerships that provide "complete" information-system solutions, making it difficult to choose best-of-breed technologies or the most cost-effective systems.

Without standards, even when similar devices do provide communications, consistency is lacking in the information and services that are provided, thus inhibiting the development of advanced care delivery systems or even comprehensive patient health records. For example, because of lack of shared semantics throughout the point-of-care environment, it is the rare system (if it exists at all) that collects real-time data from multiple devices and potentially uses the information to detect patient safety problems (e.g., adverse drug events) or to quickly determine a patient's condition and, with minimal clinician involvement, optimally adjusts a device's operation.

As Robinson pointed out in an article in *IEEE Micro* in 1999:

> The problem in healthcare is not one of a lack of standards. What is needed is a demand for the level of service that is achievable only with standards. Once that demand is there, the standards will be broadly implemented and then rapidly improved. Perhaps then, healthcare can make strong use of information technology to rapidly and professionally care for patients.[42]

In short, appropriate use of MDC standards could help patients achieve better health more quickly and at a lower healthcare cost. However, until use of standard interfaces becomes widespread, use of appropriate technology for medical device interface engines represents the lowest-risk option.

Key Points

- Insistence on the use of CEN ISO/IEEE 11073 standards would provide in-system and intersystem comparability of data.
- Comprehensive integration of data from clinical and environmental systems can prevent errors and inefficiencies across the continuum of care.[43]
- Medical system interoperability can create healthcare provider empowerment by providing an infrastructure for innovation (see Chap. 6).[43]
- The customer should clearly articulate the primary goals of institutional medical device communication.
- What data are needed, when, where, and by whom are essential items that must be defined in the process of designing a network. Readers are encouraged to think outside the box.
- The customer must ensure that supply contracts include wording about ensuring interoperability, both at purchase and in the future.

Acknowledgments The completion of this chapter would not have been possible without the prior work and contributions of many international coworkers from the field of medical device communication, notably Todd Cooper, Kai Hassing, Michael Krämer, Thomas Norgall, Paul Schluter, and Jan Wittenber, as well as others too numerous to mention individually.

References

1. Gardner RM, Tariq H, Hawley WL, et al. Medical information bus: The key to future. J Clin Monit Comput 1989; 6:205–9
2. Electronics Industries Association. *EIA Standard RS-232-C Interface Between Data Terminal Equipment and Data Communication Equipment Employing Serial Data Interchange.* August 1969. Reprinted in *Data Communication Library*, Greenlawn, NY: Telebyte Technology, 1985
3. *Information Systems—Coded Character Sets—7-Bit American National Standard Code for Information Interchange (7-Bit ASCII), ANSI INCITS 4-1986 (R2007).* New York: American National Standards Institute, 2007. http://webstore.ansi.org/RecordDetail.aspx?sku=ANSI+INCITS+4-1986+(R2007). Accessed February 7, 2008
4. *IEEE Standard for Local and Metropolitan Area Networks: Overview and Architecture, IEEE 802-2001 (R2007).* New York: Institute of Electrical and Electronics Engineers, 2001. http://standards.ieee.org/getieee802/802.html. Accessed February 7, 2008
5. *IEEE Standard Computer Dictionary: A Compilation of IEEE Standard Computer Glossaries.* New York: Institute of Electrical and Electronics Engineers, 1990
6. *Information Technology—Vocabulary, Fundamental Terms: ISO/IEC 2382-01:1993.* Geneva: International Organization for Standardization, 1993
7. *Information Technology—Open Systems Interconnection—Basic Reference Model: The Basic Model, ISO/IEC 7498-1:1994.* Geneva: International Organization for Standardization, 1994
8. International Organization for Standardization, 1 ch. de la Voie-Creuse, Case postale 56, CH-1211 Geneva 20, Switzerland. http://www.iso.org/iso/home.htm. Accessed February 7, 2008
9. International Electrotechnical Commission (IEC), 3 rue de Varembé, P.O. Box 131, CH-1211 Geneva 20, Switzerland. http://www.iec.ch. Accessed February 7, 2008
10. European Committee for Standardization (Comité Européen de Normalisation, CEN), 36 rue de Stassart, B-1050 Brussels, Belgium
11. European Committee for Electrotechnical Standardization (CENELEC), 35 rue de Stassart, B-1050 Brussels, Belgium
12. GS1, Blue Tower, Avenue Louise, 326, BE 1050 Brussels, Belgium. http://www.gs1.org. Accessed February 7, 2008
13. http://www.gs1.org/hug/. Accessed February 11, 2008
14. *TIA-485-A, Electrical Characteristics of Generators and Receivers for Use in Balanced Digital Multipoint Systems (ANSI/TIA/EIA-485-A-98) (R2003).* Arlington, VA: Telecommunications Industry Association, 2003
15. Kampmann J, Lau G, Kropp S, et al. Connection of electronic medical devices in ICU according to the standard "MIB." Int J Clin Monit Comput 1991; 8:163–6
16. BlueTooth SIG Medical Devices Working Group. http://bluetooth.com/bluetooth/press/sig/bluetooth_sig_aims_to_improve_healthcare_experience_through_interoperability.htm. Accessed February 7, 2008
17. The Infrared Data Association. http://irda.org. Accessed February 7, 2008
18. *Point-of-Care Connectivity; Approved Standard—Second Edition. CLSI Document POCT1-A2:2006.* Wayne, PA: Clinical and Laboratory Standards Institute, 2006

19. *ISO 11898-1:2003, Road Vehicles—Controller Area Network (CAN). Part 1: Data Link Layer and Physical Signaling*. Geneva: International Organization for Standardization, 2003
20. CAN in Automation (CiA) e. V., Am Weichselgarten 26, DE-91058 Erlangen, Germany. http://www.can-cia.org/. Accessed February 7, 2008
21. Center for Integration of Medicine and Innovative Technology (CIMIT), 165 Cambridge Street, Suite 702, Boston, MA, USA
22. *ISO TR 21730:2007, Health informatics—Use Of Mobile Wireless Communication and Computing Technology in Healthcare Facilities—Recommendations for Electromagnetic Compatibility (Management Of Unintentional Electromagnetic Interference) with Medical Devices*. Geneva: International Organization for Standardization, 2007
23. Kennelly RJ. Improving acute care through use of medical device data. Int J Med Inform 1998; 48:145–9
24. *IEEE 11073-00101:2008, Health informatics—Point-of-Care Medical Device Communication. Guidelines for the Use of RF Wireless Technology—Technical Report*. New York: Institute of Electrical and Electronics Engineers, 2008
25. *Logical Observation Identifiers Names and Codes (LOINC)*. Indianapolis: Regenstrief Institute. http://www.regenstrief.org/medinformatics/loinc. Accessed February 7, 2008
26. Krämer M, Norgall T, Penzel T. Short Strategic Study: Strategies for Harmonisation and Integration of Device-Level and Enterprise-Wide Methodologies for Communication as Applied to HL7, LOINC, and ENV 13734, CEN/TC 251/N01-033rev2. Brussels: European Committee for Standardization, 2001
27. International Organization for Terminology in Anesthesia (IOTA). http://www.apsf.org/initiatives/ddtf/iota_contact.mspx. Accessed February 7, 2008
28. Systematized Nomenclature of Medicine–Clinical Terms (SNOMED CT). International Health Terminology Standards Development Organisation (IHTSDO). http://www.ihtsdo.org/. Accessed February 7, 2008
29. Monk T, Sanderson I. The development of an anesthesia lexicon. Semin Anesth Perioperat Med Pain 2004; 23:93–8
30. *ISO/TS 20225:2001, Global Medical Device Nomenclature for the Purpose of Regulatory Data Exchange*. Geneva: International Organization for Standardization, 2003
31. The Global Medical Device Nomenclature (GMDN) Agency. http://www.gmdnagency.com. Accessed February 7, 2008
32. Institute of Electrical and Electronics Engineers, Standards Association, 3 Park Avenue, 17th Floor, New York. http://www.ieee.org/web/standards/home/index.html. Accessed February 7, 2008
33. Vawdrey DK, Gardner RM, Evans RS, et al. Assessing data quality in manual entry of ventilator settings. J Assoc 2007; 14:295–303
34. *ENV 13734:2000, Health informatics—Vital Signs Information Representation*. Brussels: European Committee for Standardization, 2000
35. *ENV 13735:2000, Health informatics—Interoperability of Patient Connected Medical Devices*. Brussels: European Committee for Standardization, 2000
36. Continua Health Alliance, c/o VTM, Inc., 3855 SW 153rd Drive, Beaverton, OR 97006, USA. http://www.continuaalliance.org. Accessed February 7, 2008
37. HL7 International. Health Level Seven, Inc., 3300 Washtenaw Avenue, Suite 227, Ann Arbor, MI 48104, USA. http://www.hl7.org/. Accessed February 7, 2008
38. IHE International. Integrating the Healthcare Enterprise, c/o Healthcare Information and Management Systems Society (HIMSS), 230 East Ohio Street, Suite 500, Chicago, IL 60611-3269. http://www.ihe.net/. Accessed February 7, 2008
39. Morris AH. Developing and implementing computerized protocols for standardization of clinical decisions. Ann Intern Med 2000; 132:373–83
40. National Institute of Standards and Technology (NIST) validation tools. National Institute of Standards and Technology, Information Testing Laboratory, Software Diagnostics and Conformance Testing Division, Medical Device Communication Testing, 100 Bureau Drive,

Stop 8900, Gaithersburg, MD 20899-8900, USA. http://xw2k.nist.gov/medicaldevices/index.
html. Accessed February 7, 2008

41. *The Report of the Expert Working Group on Alarms on Clinical Monitors in Response to Recommendation 11 of the Clothier Report: The Allitt Inquiry.* London: Medical Devices Agency, 1995

42. Robinson GS. Healthcare needs standards. *IEEE Micro* 1999; 19(3):5, 87

43. Goldman JM. Update on the Medical Device Interoperability Program. Presented to the Massachusetts Health Data Consortium Clinical Networking Forum, November 6, 2007. http://mdpnp.org/uploads/Clinical_Networking_Forum_6Nov2007.pdf. Accessed February 7, 2008

Chapter 8
Architecture

Sachin Kheterpal

As described in previous chapters, AIMS have evolved from stand-alone physiologic parameter recorders to complex, cross-departmental information management systems.[1-4] As the role of the AIMS has changed, so too has the technical architecture. Clearly, users' demands for increasingly comprehensive functionality have driven technical innovation, but technical advancement has undoubtedly allowed for functional innovation and maturation of AIMS.

The original anesthesia record keepers performed a local function. Data from anesthesia and monitoring equipment were downloaded to a nearby computer and stored there. A paper printout served as the lasting output of these systems; local data were purged.[3] Early AIMS development reflected the functional requirements and technical opportunities of that time. The original systems had localized architecture with minimal networking to centralized servers and little interfacing with other information systems. In contrast, more recent models reflect a technical and functional environment that requires reliable uptime networking, stringent medical record keeping, and integration with other perioperative information management systems (OR management systems, inventory systems, etc.) and hospital information systems (admission/discharge/transfer systems, laboratory information systems, etc.). The newer AIMS offer distributed storage systems, data redundancy options, and interfaces. However, they come with a concomitant complexity that may require robust IT support and management tools.

A constant throughout this functional and technical evolution has been the rapidly changing definition of the term *current*. As a result, the technical architecture discussion that follows must be interpreted in the context of this ever-changing state of the art. More importantly, technical architecture has no "right" or "wrong." The functional requirements, IT infrastructure, and budgetary limitations of a given perioperative environment will dictate the optimal AIMS and technical architecture for a given institution. For example, although a network-dependent distributed environment might be optimal for a large tertiary care center with many anesthetizing locations and extensive preoperative and postoperative needs, a stand-alone, anesthesia machine-based AIMS might be appropriate for a community hospital with ten ORs.

J. Stonemetz, K. Ruskin (eds.) *Anesthesia Informatics*,
© Springer Science + Business Media, LLC 2008

Architectural Elements of an AIMS

Data Storage

One of the most fundamental characteristics of any software is the data-storage location. Some applications, such as word processors and presentation software, typically store data locally on the hard drive of the computer running the software. Although network drives can be used, the software interacts transparently with these drives as if they were local hard drives. Other distributed software, such as a Web-based electronic mail application, is fundamentally designed to operate in a networked environment and store its data in centralized servers. The computer running the software does not store the data locally. Rather, it reads and writes all data to the centralized servers and acts solely as a presentation and computational device. Similarly, an AIMS can store data locally or centrally. The choice of one strategy over another allows the use of certain desirable features and results in specific limitations.

Local storage of data allows the AIMS to function independent of a local area network that connects computing devices. An advantage of this setup is that network failures do not impact AIMS usage. Given the mission-critical nature of point-of-care (POC) clinical software, local data storage is a vital feature. In addition, the overall acquisition and maintenance costs are much lower than those of a networked model because of the limited number of components involved. Additionally, a skilled IT team is not required to support a complex network infrastructure. However, clinical data stored only on the computer (or device) are not available for review or editing at other locations; all interaction with the data must occur at the initial computing location. Consequently, as the patient moves from the OR to the PACU, the data cannot move with her. Information must then be transferred in a mobile medium—usually in the form of a paper printout. In addition, local-storage space is limited, necessitating that the data eventually be deleted or archived, which, as well, limits the method of future access to a patient's anesthetic records to a paper printout.

Centralized data-storage architecture separates the data-storage location from the POC computing location. Although the computing device at the POC is used to display the application user interface, data are stored remotely and accessed via a network, with no permanent data stored locally. Clearly, this centralized data-storage architecture requires a robust and reliable network, but it enables many capabilities. First, a patient's data can be accessed at many locations, possibly concurrently. For example, data entered in the OR can be reviewed by PACU or ICU staff awaiting the patient's arrival. Second, data can be aggregated into the centralized data storage from multiple information system sources, allowing the development of interfaces (see Chap. 7) that merge laboratory, demographic, OR management, pharmacy, and other hospital information system data. Thus, the application can serve as a holistic clinical information resource for the user. Third, a centralized data-storage architecture typically allows for expansion of data storage over time. Although not limitless, centralized data storage can enable long-term storage of patient records for retrieval at a later date. Unless hospital or regulatory policies require it, a paper printout need not serve as the official medical record copy. If the patient requires anesthesia in the future, an AIMS with centralized data storage could easily retrieve prior intraoperative records.

Centralized data-storage architecture is also associated with some disadvantages. A pure centralized architecture creates a critical dependency on network uptime. If the network fails for any reason, the POC application is unable to function, even in a read-only mode. Because no data are stored locally, a constant, reliable network connection between the application and the central server is necessary to store or retrieve patient information. This dependency can be a serious shortcoming given the life-critical nature of the OR environment. Substantial costs are associated with centralized data-storage architecture. Whereas an AIMS with local storage requires only the POC workstation to be functioning, with centralized architecture, the network and servers must be maintained in constant uptime.

To reap the benefits of both local and centralized architectures, some AIMS offer a centralized architecture with an emergency failover, or redundant capability, to local storage in situations of network or server downtime. In such systems, a subset of system functionality is available even when the network or server fails, enabling a user to continue reviewing or entering data into the patient's anesthetic record, even though networked functions such as retrieval of laboratory values or previous anesthetic administration are unavailable. More importantly, functions dependent upon centralized data access, such as retrieval of dynamic clinical or administrative content, are possible during a network or server failure period. This functionally elegant hybrid requires complex technical underpinnings, and because local and centralized data must be maintained in synchrony, some performance limitations may occur. Fortunately, the need for a local failover is becoming more infrequent as network and server unscheduled downtime becomes more and more rare. Advancements in network management tools and server tuning and diagnostics are allowing system administrators to make downtime a truly rare event.

Database Management Systems

A database management system (DBMS), which can run either locally or centrally, must be used to store the AIMS data. Independent of the location, several types of DBMS exist and can be grouped into four major categories: flat file, healthcare specific, relational, and object oriented.[5]

Flat-file data management systems were used primarily in the 1980s before the rapid expansion of enterprise relational DBMS. Flat-file systems are based on simple file storage technology, and proprietary software is generally required to access the data. Unfortunately, because this custom software is specific to each vendor, industry-standard tools cannot be used to access the data for reporting, backup, or development. The vendor's development pace can be slowed by the need to train developers on this proprietary software.

Healthcare-specific DBMS are also offered in the marketplace. The most common is known as MUMPS (*M*assachusetts General Hospital *U*tility *M*ulti-Programming *S*ystem)—a data management system designed for the storage of healthcare data and related concepts. Based upon hierarchical databases, MUMPS systems have limited crosspatient analysis abilities and a limited ability to expand clinical concepts. Furthermore, challenges can be associated with integrating these healthcare-specific DBMS with other clinical information systems that may have valuable data. Finally, because this type of DBMS is healthcare specific, it cannot utilize the software advances made in other industries.

Relational DBMS (RDBMS) are the most commonly used management systems in the general software industry and are the current "standard of care." RDBMS allow software developers to create and manage the complex relationships between concepts. Microsoft and Oracle offer two prominent RDBMS. Lesser-used systems include DB2, Informix, and Sybase. These models leverage general advances in DBMS software because they are used across all industries. In addition, many off-the-shelf tools can enable access to the data, and the large pool of talented RDBMS developers is an excellent resource. Unfortunately, a substantial licensing cost is associated with most commercial RDBMS. The AIMS vendor must pass the price on to the customer unless the hospital already has an enterprise license. Newer shareware RDBMS are being developed to minimize this cost.

Object-oriented DBMS, such as Cache (http://www.intersystems.com), are the most recently developed and most advanced data management software. They were developed in the mid-1990s to enable improved response times and simplified programming, as compared with those of RDBMS. Object-oriented databases allow the storage of data to better represent conceptual relationships. However, as processing power has increased, hardware costs have decreased, and RDBMS tools have improved, much of the promise of object-oriented DBMS has been rendered unnecessary. Given the training and migration costs of switching to object-oriented databases, most vendors have remained with RDBMS.

Point-of-Care Software

In general, AIMS software can be grouped into three broad categories: medical device, traditional client/server, and Web based. Each type of software implementation demands a unique IT infrastructure. A medical-device AIMS resides on the device itself—most commonly on an anesthesia machine or a physiologic monitor. The software-user interface is incorporated into the device itself. As monitoring and device interfaces have advanced, so too have the AIMS housed on them. The integration of the device and software into one physical entity reduces the potential possible points of failure. In addition, the user interface is familiar to the clinician because it is the foundation for their interaction with the device. As a result, training is often limited to workflow and business logic. However, because of the rigorous CE-Mark and FDA 510K processes essential to medical devices, the software is also subjected to a more rigorous development, validation, and marketing process. Though this may improve the robustness of the product, the speed of development may lag behind other nonmedical-device software platforms. In addition, the software development tool set might not be able to take advantage of operating system and development language advances across industries.

Before the advent of Web browsers, most modern software required a variety of files to be installed on the local workstation. These files provided the instructions for how the software should perform, display information, and interact with the user. The primary interaction between the workstation (known as the client) and the location of the patient data (known as the server) was the exchange of data. A balance of duties exists between the client and server computers; hence, the term *client–server application*. Unfortunately, this type of software provides distribution and maintenance challenges for a hospital's IT staff. Because most of the instructions for the application's behavior are stored locally in files on the workstation, the files must be updated on all workstations by the IT staff. The applications invariably depend not only on the AIMS vendor's files, but also on files shared across vendors and applications that are distributed by the operating system vendor. As clinical IT offerings expand, client–server applications may become victim to unintentional interactions between two applications that share a common file. Updates to the file by one vendor could have a disastrous impact on another vendor's application. However, new management and automation tools allow upgrades to be sent to the client workstations through the network and enable careful version checking for the files shared across vendors. Most important, the development tools for client–server software are extremely mature and allow advanced user interface development. They have progressed through multiple generations of improvement and offer a very robust development environment with very detailed control over the workstation itself.

Web-based software uses Web browsers to perform the display function and stores the application instructions in a more centralized location known as a Web or application *server*. Rather than distributing instruction files to every POC workstation, most of the AIMS business logic is stored on the Web server. Ubiquitous Web browsers that are already installed on the POC workstation then interpret these instructions from a specific Web server. The workstation interacts with the Web server not only for data, but also for display instructions, validation rules, and business logic. When a vendor offers software upgrades, files can be updated on only a limited number of centralized Web servers. Web software is especially advantageous when the workstations that access the system are extremely large in number or in unpredictable locations. For example, access to an OR schedule from hundreds of surgeons' offices is enabled by Web software. Because the development tools available for Web-based software are not as mature as those for client–server development, user interfaces and robustness are less advanced. This drawback is rapidly being mitigated through extensive efforts by the software industry. A more challenging drawback can be inconsistency between the Web-browser software and the instructions on the Web server. Although the instructions can be based on a crossvendor industry standard known as *hypertext transfer protocol* (HTTP), some advanced capabilities and instructions might require a specific browser version or vendor. In addition, easier access to the application is associated with increased security risk; therefore, security concerns may be heightened.

The latest software tools blur the lines between client–server and Web-based applications. Using technologies that maintain a centralized store for the instructions, they also copy software that interprets the instructions to individual workstations—eliminating dependency on the browser vendor and version. Decreased dependency on the browser also enables more advanced user interfaces and complex business logic to be run efficiently. Microsoft's .NET and its rival's JavaBeans technology are examples of this emerging software model.

Finally, some software is designed specifically to run on mobile, handheld devices that have unique requirements for ergonomics, speed, and screen size. The widely variant user interfaces of a desktop computer and handheld Palm or PocketPC demand that software be designed specifically for the mobile device, even though it might be similar to that run on a desktop.

A combination of all three types of software is possible and may actually optimize the speed, usability, and cost of the system.

Point-of-Care Hardware

Most potential customers recognize the importance of choosing the right software model and vendor, and they recognize the difficulty of this task. However, choosing the correct POC hardware remains a very challenging decision that is often overlooked by customers. The workstation bears a number of POC demands. Given the potential for nosocomial infections, the institution's infection control leadership must review the potential POC hardware. Stationary, mounted hardware must be capable of being cleaned as part of the routine housekeeping process during patient turnover. Typical cleaning agents could harm hardware not designed for the POC environment. Hence, water-resistant keyboards that lack crevices capable of housing infectious materials are often chosen. One should also confirm that the hardware is reliable in difficult environments. Certain clinical situations (burn units and NICUs) warrant a room temperature outside the typical operating range of a standard off-the-shelf workstation. Also, although they are mounted, stationary workstations are routinely moved by maintenance and housekeeping staff. Exposure of the equipment to this level of maneuvering should be considered when evaluating the necessary durability. In addition, a small footprint is helpful to minimize the space consumed by the information system in already-cramped patient care areas. Finally, regardless of which hardware is chosen, it must be mounted or secured in an economical and effective manner. Although the price of workstations continues to plummet due to the commoditization of computer hardware, simple mounting arms and carts remain relatively expensive items that often can exceed the cost of the workstation itself.

Despite these healthcare-specific POC hardware demands, most current AIMS can be deployed on any standard, modern personal computer. However, this flexibility brings with it an overabundance of options. In addition, each POC—advanced testing clinic, preoperative holding room, OR, offsite procedure site, imaging suite, PACU, ICU, or general care floor—presents its own challenges and opportunities for the IT department. Potential customers may wish to work with the healthcare-specific division of a general computer hardware manufacturer. Furthermore, vendors' user groups are invaluable sources of advice and experience that can substantially reduce frustration, cost, and project delay. Unfortunately, access to this resource typically occurs only after installation. Though the highly competitive computer hardware industry offers many pricing options, the initial capital costs must be balanced with the long-term operating maintenance expenses associated with each hardware option.

Some vendors offer unique functionality that requires vendor-specific hardware. Proprietary hardware such as special keyboards, entry keypads, or syringe pumps can be specialized for the AIMS feature set. Even if proprietary hardware is not required, some advanced functionality could require hardware such as barcode readers or radio-frequency sensors, and a typical IT department is not familiar with this equipment or comfortable supporting it.[6] The value of the advanced functionality must be assessed in terms of the potentially high initial cost, ongoing maintenance effort, and IT training requirements. Optimistically, these issues will wane as AIMS and other POC information systems increase their market penetration.

Physiologic Device Interfaces

Clearly, integrating the physiologic and device-setting data from POC devices is a critical element of a perioperative clinical information system.[7,8] The frequent vital signs and device settings collected in the OR, PACU, and surgical ICU demand a more efficient means of transferring digital data from these devices to the computerized clinical record. Commonly interfaced devices include physiologic monitors, anesthesia machines, ventilators, gas analysis monitors, and ancillary monitors such as those for bispectral index (BIS) and continuous cardiac output. Less commonly interfaced devices include heart–lung bypass machines, infusions pumps, and digital urimeters.

To enable the remote viewing of waveforms, many physiologic monitoring implementations from the leading vendors have included a "monitoring network," which carries vital-sign information to central viewing stations. These networks can be leveraged to interface device data into the AIMS. Via a centralized interface server, information is copied from the monitoring network to the AIMS database server—the source of the anesthesia record data (Fig. 8.1). Because each vendor's monitoring network uses a slightly different language to transmit the device data, it is critical to ensure that the interface server is capable of interpreting a given monitoring vendor's language, or protocol. If the physiologic monitors already display data from other devices, such as the anesthesia machine, ventilator, gas analyzer, or ancillary monitors, the monitoring network will probably also contain information from these additional devices. Connecting these ancillary devices generally requires

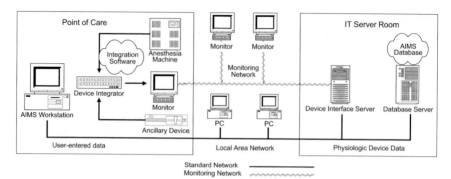

Fig. 8.1 Device connectivity option 1—monitoring network plus device integration using monitor

some type of integration device in each OR. In this situation, the interface server may fulfill all of the device integration requirements. Some common brand names for these devices include UnityID from GE Medical Systems and VueLink from Philips Medical Systems.[2]

If the ancillary devices (anesthesia machine, ventilator, etc.) cannot be integrated into the monitoring network, a distributed strategy may be necessary. Most devices offer an outbound data port in the rear of the device; specifically, an RS232 port can be used to connect the medical device to another processing device. This processing device can be a local PC that is running device integration software or dedicated device integration equipment. In either case, the device's information is temporarily stored locally and then forwarded to the centralized database storage server. If the local PC is used to perform the device integration work, it can also serve as the AIMS workstation used by the anesthesia provider—the device integration software can run silently in the background (Fig. 8.2). This local mechanism of device integration can be used for nearly any device that is not capable of connecting directly to a network—heart–lung bypass machines, infusion pumps, and even bench lab testing equipment. In addition, if a monitoring network cannot be implemented for either cost or technical reasons, the primary physiologic monitor can be integrated locally (Fig. 8.3).

The AIMS vendor is responsible for developing device-integration software that can translate between the device's unique communication protocol and the vendor's data-storage mechanism. Maintaining an expansive and up-to-date library of supported devices can prove challenging. In fact, many vendors have chosen to outsource the development of these specialized software libraries to companies that exclusively focus on device interfaces, such as Capsule Technologies (Andover, MA).

Networking Considerations

As discussed previously, different AIMS implementations require different types of data storage (centralized or local) and network infrastructure. An honest assessment

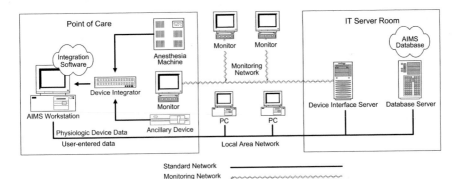

Fig. 8.2 Device connectivity option 2—monitoring network plus device integration using the AIMS workstation

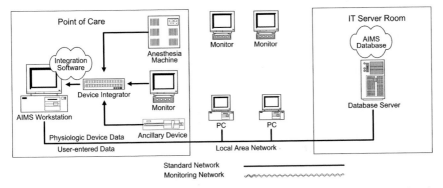

Fig. 8.3 Device connectivity option 3—no monitoring network, with all integration using the AIMS workstation

of the institution's network infrastructure, reliability, and expandability must occur prior to project planning or vendor selection. Networks with poor reliability or those lacking constant support staff might require a redundant local-storage model. The absence of a wireless network might preclude implementation of software that affects mobile ICU or acute pain service teams. In any case, each vendor must be asked for their minimum and recommended network requirements to minimize the number of surprises during the implementation. An important point of distinction involves how the AIMS and medical-device data streams will be separated from routine administrative applications on the network. Some customers and vendors will not require any separation. Others may prefer physical (i.e., different physical cables and routers) or logical (i.e., virtual private networks with specific encryption) separation to improve reliability or guarantee performance.

Interfacing Considerations

A complete discussion of hospital information systems interfaces is beyond the scope of this chapter. They are discussed at length in previous chapters. However, a brief discussion regarding outbound notification options is appropriate.

Increasingly, AIMS have moved beyond solely the medical record to a workflow-management role. Rather than simply storing and retrieving clinical data, AIMS offer rules-based logic and decision-support capabilities. These topics are discussed at length in following chapters. However, implementing these capabilities has an architectural impact. A mechanism for outbound notification is essential. In some cases, a distinct application run on the POC workstation serves as a decision-support module. This application constantly polls for clinical conditions that warrant an alert. The creation of a distinct application separates the development process for the decision-support module from the application itself. This separation may have some benefits in improved application stability and parallel development tracks. However, it may also add to the maintenance workload of the IT staff.

In other cases, an AIMS can be used to send notifications via alphanumeric paging or email. A growing body of anesthesia literature indicates that both notification methods improve compliance with institutional goals. Email can be used for non-urgent issues such as documentation compliance, billing reminders, or quality assurance notification.[9] An abnormal postoperative lab value or event could trigger the delivery of an email to the anesthesia providers involved in the case. For more urgent issues, the providers can be sent an alphanumeric page.[10,11] For either mode of contact, an outbound notification server must be established. First, the institution's IT staff should be contacted to establish what communication protocol can be used to send an automated alphanumeric page or email. Next, the AIMS must be configured to associate a unique identifier with each person who may be the target of the notification. An alphanumeric paging identifier may be completely distinct from any other identifiers for that user. In some cases, alphanumeric pagers can be accessed by sending an email to a specific address. The body or subject of that email serves as the pager message itself.

Data Modeling Concepts and Their Impact

Normalized versus Denormalized Data

Just as the location of data storage profoundly impacts the functionality of an AIMS, the data modeling strategy affects the functionality of an application.[5] A "denormalized" data model stores a given concept in multiple tables to enable simpler queries, improved processing, and easier reporting. For example, a denormalized data model would store the patient name in both the patient information table and in the operative schedule table. By storing the data in both tables, a query to identify which patients were scheduled for an operation on a given day would have to retrieve information only from the operative schedule table, making data retrieval—be it for transactional or reporting purposes—easier. However, the trade-offs are extensive. First, if the patient's name is updated, it must be propagated across many tables, a task that impacts performance. Second, storing the data redundantly in multiple tables results in wasted storage space. Finally, if all tables that contain a particular data concept are not accurately updated, inconsistencies could result.

In a perfectly normalized data model, a given data concept is stored only in a single table. In the example, only the patient information table would have the patient's name, thereby decreasing data-storage requirements, eliminating the need to update multiple tables, and eliminating the possibility of data inconsistency. However, this, too, is associated with a drawback; normalized data models necessitate complicated queries joining several tables together to gather even the simplest information, such as an operative schedule. In addition, the data retrieval process exacts a high processing load because of the need to access multiple tables. Finally, this complicated data retrieval process creates challenges for future soft-ware developers and those attempting to extract data for reporting purposes.

In reality, no AIMS can be described as perfectly normalized or completely denormalized. Each vendor and data architect blends the two strategies to balance the tradeoffs of each. However, the choice of one model over another often is dictated by and reflected in the feature set of the AIMS. It can be a good idea to ask an IT professional to perform a basic review of the data model as part of the vendor-selection process. Such a review will provide a glimpse of the future challenges and opportunities that the user can expect.

One possible solution to the choice of data models is a combination of both a normalized database that is referred to as an *online transactional processing* and an *online analytical processing* database that is used to archive data and provide report-ing functionality. Certainly, products that use this functionality have gained popular-ity in the healthcare field, as is evidenced by Microsoft's acquisition of Azyxxi, a healthcare-specific application framework.

Configurability

The constant changes in clinical standards, medical technology, and regulatory requirements demand that an AIMS be easily configured after the system is imple-mented. Changing pressure from groups such as The Joint Commission requires that the information system be able to adapt its screens, questions, and process flow. Some aspects integral to the information system might require specific application logic updates from the vendor. The instructions for certain behavior may be stored in executable files, dynamic linked libraries, or control files, as opposed to the database configuration. In this case, the vendor must provide an upgrade to the institution to implement the change. These upgrades must be carefully coordinated with the institution's IT department. Other behavior changes may simply be content or configuration settings that are stored in the database or other content-defining files. These settings can be more easily changed than the programming code written for the application. In either case, it is important to understand how content and basic configuration changes are managed. Some vendors require that only vendor-supplied staff be able to make the changes. Although this policy may improve the robustness of the changes and free the department from such worries, it also makes the department dependent on the vendor's timelines and cost demands. If the vendor offers configuration tools that can be used by the institution's staff, it is essential that the tools be easy to use and that the staff be adequately trained. Such internal training allows the institution to make changes without waiting for the vendor but does consume some internal staff resources. During the vendor selection process, it may be prudent to specifically identify which aspects of application behavior and content the vendor must change and which are configurable by the institution, as these issues will have a significant impact on the system's utilization and user satisfaction soon after go-live.

Security, Privacy, and Access Considerations

A full review of security, privacy, and access considerations is beyond the scope of this chapter (the topic is discussed in detail in Chap. 23). However, a brief discussion of the architectural decisions that have a major impact on the security and access profile of an AIMS is warranted.

Preventing Inappropriate Access to Data

A typical hospital in America lacks even basic safeguards against unauthorized access to a paper medical record. Any person wearing appropriate medical attire and carrying a confident attitude could likely walk up to the chart rack and begin perusing the record for sensitive information. An AIMS is held to a much higher standard than a paper medical chart because systematic safeguards are possible when implementing a mature AIMS. Many of the necessary requirements are explicitly detailed in HIPAA. Though HIPAA applies to both paper and electronic medical records, many of its most stringent requirements affect EMRs. Despite the length of the HIPAA text itself, many areas still require interpretation by each vendor and customer. As a result, the legal and medical records departments of each institution affected by an AIMS should be consulted for their interpretation of HIPAA. The spirit of the complicated act is to ensure that only users with a need to know have access to specific patients and elements of the record. Additionally, a user's access must be logged and auditable. Many sites also implement hardware-based safeguards to complement software-based safeguards against inappropriate access to clinical data. These may include workstation inactivity time-outs, workstation passwords distinct from application authentication, and rolling security code remote access.

Ensuring Access

Although HIPAA typically is referred to when defining ways to limit access, it also contains language that establishes the clinical importance of being able to gain access when needed. It specifically guides institutions to ensure that clinicians have the data necessary to make sound clinical decisions. Leaders of projects to ensure remote, wireless, or mobile access should consider referring to HIPAA when seeking justification for their cause.

Access History

One key provision of HIPAA requires a healthcare provider to be able to furnish a comprehensive list of all those who access a given patient's record; this requirement has a major architectural impact on an AIMS. First, it requires that all accesses be authenticated and based on a specific user ID. Group authentication or anonymous authentication is no longer an option. Second, each time a patient record is opened and closed, the event must be logged for possible future retrieval. Each screen of an AIMS that displays patient information must have its own logging-in place so that as a user moves from the preoperative H&P of one patient to the postoperative note of another, the process is logged. Finally, this audit trail of access must be available in perpetuity. Although HIPAA does not specifically state how long the data must be stored, one can assume it must be available much longer than the patient's stay itself. The period of archive has architectural impact on data-storage requirements, archiving strategies, and reporting tools. AIMS must offer a reporting mechanism to extract this access history data easily and promptly.

Impact on AIMS

These complex legal and regulatory concepts may seem to be beyond the scope of a clinical information system. However, the architecture and functionality of an AIMS can compromise security, privacy, and access requirements. The seasoned AIMS customer must establish a detailed security, privacy, and access requirement list that measures each potential vendor and application. For example, software that stores identifiable patient data locally for reliability purposes would create significant liability if it did not use encryption. In addition, exciting AIMS features such as an electronic OR schedule whiteboard would be in violation of HIPAA if protected health information such as patient name, address, or date of birth were accessible without specific user authentication.

Disaster Preparedness

As increasing volumes of critical clinical data are stored online, a sound data redundancy and disaster preparedness strategy is essential to AIMS architecture. Historically the purview of medical records departments, ensuring timely access to clinical data is now also the responsibility of the clinical staff most affected by a data outage.

Disaster preparedness is broadly defined as the policies, infrastructure, and people necessary to provide access to information system data in the case of online data access failure. A comprehensive strategy details the following:

- Possible failure points
- The impact of each failure point
- Trigger points for enacting the disaster preparedness failover
- The actions to be taken by each member of the disaster preparedness team

For example, a network outage in one part of a hospital might cripple clinical work-stations in that area, leaving the remainder of the information system intact. A strategy designed to address this specific challenge should be in place. A larger outage that includes the center housing the data and application servers would have a distinct impact and response. In concert with the institution's IT staff and medical records department, the leadership of an AIMS deployment should establish the disaster preparedness strategy. Some institutions create an official response, called a "code white," that indicates the need to begin paper documentation. A single POC failure may be addressed by the information system itself. As discussed previously, some AIMS offer a redundant data-storage strategy that allows a workstation to continue functioning even if the network or central data storage is compromised. A typical disaster preparedness strategy includes redundancy and automatic failover at crucial architectural points: network switches and routers, database servers, storage area network, and data-storage center.

Database servers are often "clustered," enabling two identical servers to serve as backup for each other. A primary processing server is used during most periods. A second server is inextricably linked to the primary server and is constantly poll-ing the server to ensure that it is accessible and responsive. If any critical failure is detected, the secondary server automatically redirects all network traffic to it and alarms the appropriate server support staff. End users would only perceive a delayed response time. This failover mechanism is available in a variety of operat-ing systems and is enabled via off-the-shelf, crossindustry software. A less expen-sive failover mechanism involves the manual creation of a second server. If the IT staff detects a primary server failure via user feedback, it can bring the backup server online and direct network traffic to it. This mechanism is less robust and will involve a short application downtime.

Failure at the data-storage level can be handled similarly. A redundant array of independent drives (RAID) storage system ensures data accuracy by storing a given piece of data in multiple disk drives. A group of disk drives is managed by a RAID controller, which distributes data elements across the drives. The failure of a single drive does not result in any data loss because data stored on a given drive are already replicated on another drive. Different levels of RAID redundancy correlate with variant failure tolerance. When a drive fails, a technician can replace it in real time without any application downtime. In addition, RAID systems are housed in parallel in storage area networks that can possess their own redundancy mechanisms.

These RAID, or storage area network, systems are backed up onto mobile storage media (e.g., tape or DVD). In a robust disaster preparedness strategy, these data media are housed offsite in a physically separate location. In the case of a severe physical disaster, such as a fire or a flood, these media can be used to restore the information system data. As expected, extensive user downtime would occur while the server and the data are configured.

It is clear that a comprehensive disaster preparedness strategy is not only essential but also very resource intensive. The replication of computing environments or installation of complicated redundancy mechanisms is an expensive proposition. However, this cost could be miniscule compared to the potential clinical and political challenges faced if the data cannot be recovered in a timely fashion.

Reporting Infrastructure and Considerations

Although operational efficiency is a primary driver for the implementation of an AIMS, robust reporting is also an important element. Many justifications for the return on investment are based on the clinical, operational, and financial improvements offered by analysis across patients. The ability to quickly and easily retrieve key metrics about a perioperative process allows for data-based change initiatives. However, the technical complexity of reporting requires foresight and planning.

Reports can be categorized into *standardized* and *ad hoc*. *Standardized reports* are usually built into the AIMS and are based on industry-wide indicators: case volume, cases by anesthesia type, cases per provider, billable units. These reports are easily created on a regular basis without substantial effort. Perioperative process reports and indicators are more prevalent than clinical indicators because surgery scheduling and management systems are much more widespread than AIMS. As a result, years of iterative improvement have resulted in industry-standard reports. To prevent wasted effort, project planning must ensure that the reports sought from the AIMS are not already offered by another existing information system. *Ad hoc reports* are unique reports that answer specific clinical, operational, or quality improvement questions at a given institution. They may require considerable technical expertise or simply an understanding of the clinical data and its accuracy.

During the vendor and application selection process, the customer must clearly understand the limitations of the ad hoc reporting tools available. In many situations, the flexibility and ease of ad hoc reporting is improved by the implementation of a separate denormalized reporting database. Although the transactional database may be optimized for application functionality, reliability, and performance, it may not be the optimal data structure for reporting. As discussed previously regarding an online analytical processing database, a separate reporting database, housed on a distinct physical server, may be a necessary luxury for certain customers. Off-the-shelf reporting tools such as Crystal reports, GQL, or SAS can be directed against denormalized reporting databases. These robust tools increase an institution's flexibility by creating independence from the AIMS vendor's limited offerings.

It is important that customers not assume that collected data can be the source of easy crosspatient reports. For example, although the system may document the type of endotracheal tube type and size, it might be difficult to create a report on the type of endotracheal tube only. It may be necessary to decompose an overall data element into more discrete reportable elements. Tradeoffs may be necessary between reporting flexibility and ease of use by the end user. Discrete content often requires more selections by end users. During the planning and implementation of the clinical content, the vendor and institution must discuss the type of reports envisioned. However, many institutions cannot predict their future reporting needs because of the dynamic research environment, ultimately defining a content-development philosophy that balances reporting and ease of use.

Finally, the configurability of the system can impact the ease of reporting. To make content customizable and configurable while maintaining fast response times, one might need to abstract the clinical concepts and data so that certain data describe what data are stored in other tables. These content-describing data are known as *metadata*. Conversely, systems with very robust reporting may limit the configurability because the reporting tools assume specific content and concepts. The configurability–reporting tradeoff must be considered carefully and should factor in the decision of which AIMS to purchase.

Interoperability Considerations

A complete discussion of interoperability architecture is beyond the scope of this chapter. It is discussed at length in Chap. 6.

Typical Vendor Challenges

The relationship between vendor and customer is a partnership in all cases. Whether this partnership remains a positive one beyond the contracting phase often depends on mutual respect, honesty, and accurate expectations. Several challenges are often experienced when working with external vendors.

Mixed Architectural Environments

Many customers choose a particular vendor because of the comprehensive application feature set. However, AIMS feature requirements evolve as the anesthesiologist's role evolves. Consequently, the vendor community attempts to satisfy this ever-changing requirement list. The result is a mixed architectural environment that reflects either an acquisition-based heritage or the evolutionary nature of software development.

Significant consolidation in the vendor community continues. As a result, a given vendor's AIMS may actually be a packaged offering of multiple architectures housed under one corporate identity, brand, and marketing team. Underneath the integrated packaging or user interface could lie completely disparate architectural philosophies, limitations, and opportunities. The purchasing process should include a detailed discussion regarding the heritage of each product and its underlying component technologies. This interaction may reveal additional costs, valuable functionality, or features that are lacking. A discussion regarding data flow between the product components offers a concrete starting point that may reveal the architectural variations.

A mixed technical architecture can also occur through the natural evolution of products. As user needs change, a vendor may choose to incrementally expand existing functionality or undertake a wholesale rewrite of certain components because of limitations in the previous iteration of the software. These advances often are accompanied by newer technologies and philosophies that may result in varying database or POC software architectures.

Minimum versus Necessary System Requirements

It is impossible to predict accurately the exact architectural requirements of an AIMS during the planning phases. Given the rapidly changing cost and performance profile of computer hardware, initial bids and plans are often outdated by the time a project is actually initiated. However, this challenge does not free the vendor or the customer from attempting to predict what the role of the AIMS will be several years after implementation. The customer should be able to establish the care areas affected, number of expected users, and response time expectations. In return, the vendor must offer a bid based on these customer expectations. However, the recommended system requirements may actually reflect a lower response time expectation or a previous customer's needs. Given the prevalence of fixed budgets in AIMS implementations, it may be impossible to revisit the hardware estimates made early in the process. The vendor should be asked to commit to a performance level based on a specific hardware profile and customer functionality. If the AIMS does not meet the performance goals, the vendor is held responsible for the unanticipated hardware upgrades.

Conclusion

Any treatise regarding technology architecture is hampered by the rapid advance of capabilities. As such, the issues addressed in this chapter were kept to a general level. The issues will remain independent of the specific vendors or technologies available at the time this text is being reviewed. Several major themes have emerged:

- Awareness of the tradeoffs of each technologic option is essential.
- Accurate expectation management early in the planning stages will create a more accurate project plan.
- Frank discussions with the vendor regarding customer needs and vendor options will decrease conflict.
- The evolution of technology and vendor consolidation will create heterogeneous architectural environments.

As discussed in other chapters, emerging data and interoperability standards offer the exciting opportunity to merge data from an AIMS into other information systems. Effective use of these standards will enable research, reporting, and communication. Furthermore, it could enable the componentization of information systems. Customers would no longer be required to choose a single AIMS, full of tradeoffs. A given vendor's intraoperative record keeper could be combined with the preoperative module of a second, while the reporting infrastructure of a third could be the foundation for it all. This "brave new world" is based not on the creation of standards but on the adherence to standards by vendors and customers alike. The widespread use of standards-based content, communication, and software would allow an entirely new architectural model and interoperability.

Key Points

- Data storage is the primary consideration of AIMS architecture. Successful management of central versus local data storage is pivotal to efficacious utilization of these systems.
- Data stored in an AIMS are typically managed with a DBMS, which is generally one of four types (flat file, healthcare specific, relational, and object oriented).
- When selecting an AIMS, it is important to consider POC hardware, network configurations, and interfacing capabilities.
- Normalized data, configurability, and security of access are important data-modeling concepts that must be understood by the customer.
- Because an AIMS is a mission-critical application, disaster preparedness plans regarding the system must be evaluated.
- Reporting functionality is essential to yield value from the use of an AIMS.
- The relationship between vendor and customer must be a partnership, and the parties must have a mutual understanding concerning the mixed-system environment and system requirements.

References

1. Bashein G, Barna CR. A comprehensive computer system for anesthetic record retrieval. Anesth Analg 1985; 64(4):425–31
2. Strauss PL, Turndorf H. A computerized anesthesia database. Anesth Analg 1989; 68:340–3
3. Edsall DW, Deshane P, Giles C, et al. Computerized patient anesthesia records: Less time and better quality than manually produced anesthesia records. J Clin Anesth 1993; 5(4):275–83
4. O'Reilly M, Talsma A, VanRiper S, et al. An anesthesia information system designed to provide physician-specific feedback improves timely administration of prophylactic antibiotics. Anesth Analg 2006; 103:908–12
5. Elmasri R, Navathe SB. *Fundamentals of Database Systems, 4th ed.* Boston: Addison Wesley, 2003:340–3
6. Egan MT, Sandberg WS. Auto identification technology and its impact on patient safety in the operating room of the future. Surg Innov 2007; 14(1):41–50; discussion 51
7. Reich DL, Wood RK, Jr, Mattar R, et al. Arterial blood pressure and heart rate discrepancies between handwritten and computerized anesthesia records. Anesth Analg 2000; 91:612–6
8. Vigoda MM, Lubarsky DA. Failure to recognize loss of incoming data in an anesthesia record-keeping system may have increased medical liability. Anesth Analg 2006; 102(6):1798–802
9. Blum JM, Kheterpal S, Tremper KK. A comparison of anesthesiology resident and faculty electronic evaluations before and after implementation of automated electronic reminders. J Clin Anesth 2006; 18:264–7
10. Kheterpal S, Gupta R, Blum JM, et al. Electronic reminders improve procedure documentation compliance and professional fee reimbursement. Anesth Analg 2007; 104(3):592–7
11. Spring SF, Sandberg WS, Anupama S, et al. Automated documentation error detection and notification improves anesthesia billing performance. Anesthesiology 2007; 106(1):157–63

Chapter 9
Preoperative Systems

David Young and Gordon Gibby

The preoperative period is the time during which critical patient data are gathered, processed, and disseminated. This information is used to plan for and schedule personnel, equipment, and a myriad of subtasks to ensure a smooth day in the OR. The level and the thoroughness of planning determine the efficient utilization of personnel and facilities, which impacts actual costs and, equally important, "frustration costs" to patients and staff. A proper preoperative process contributes significantly to patient safety, decreases institutional costs, and ultimately determines a large portion of the cost of national surgical healthcare. Preoperative patient care is an area of medical specialization that lends itself very readily to the application of the technologic tools of information management. A wise hospital administration will ensure that access to and use of the preoperative informatics system is not restricted to the anesthesiologists but is made available to surgeons, schedulers, equipment technicians, preoperative and postoperative nurses, and supply specialists, so that it provides a finely crafted tool for communication between all of these personnel. In practice, the method of preoperative patient management varies greatly from one institution to another and is determined by budgets, space, available personnel, and historic factors. The four most prevalent preoperative patient evaluation models utilized today are discussed in this chapter.

Preoperative Evaluation Models

Surgeon's Office Evaluation and Triage

While the surgeon's office evaluation is currently used, it was essentially the only process used for preoperative evaluation until the 1980s. The process proceeds as follows: the patient's H&P examination is performed in the surgeon's office, diagnostic procedures and consultations are ordered based on hospital guidelines, and OR equipment needs are determined from the limited surgical posting. In this self-contained system, the patient's health information and test results are often not available to the hospital or anesthesiologist until the morning of surgery.

J. Stonemetz, K. Ruskin (eds.) *Anesthesia Informatics*,
© Springer Science + Business Media, LLC 2008

Preoperative Phone Triage

Hospital nurses telephone patients to gather health history information. They then work with the anesthesia care team to direct patients for medical consultation when appropriate. Surgical planning operates independently. This process is still in common use today. However, it is costly due to the nursing hours involved; in addition, if the call center uses an open-entry data system, patient information may be incomplete.

Nurse-Run Preoperative Clinic

Patients visit a hospital-based site where a health history is taken in person. Using guidelines provided by the anesthesia care team, nurses direct the patients to primary care providers or specialty consultants for further medical workup and to designated laboratories for diagnostic testing. This process is also in common use today. It can be costly for the hospital and time consuming for the patient.

Physician-Run Preoperative Clinic

In this model, the patient visits a hospital-based clinic staffed by nurses and physicians (anesthesiologists, internists, and/or hospitalists) or nurse practitioners. After an initial health history is obtained, the patient is seen by the physician for a full preoperative assessment if indicated. In this model, laboratory, electrocardiogram, and x-ray facilities are also on site, reducing patient inconvenience and improving interdisciplinary communication. Although this model is the most comprehensive, cost restraints limit this type of clinic predominately to large academic settings. According to published studies, costs for the physician-run preoperative clinic range from approximately $26.00 per patient at The Cleveland Clinic to $145.00 at other centers.[1] Fisher published a landmark study that demonstrated the overall benefits, including reduced cancellations.[2] Despite the increased cost, a recently published study highlighted the multiple benefits realized from employing this model, including a 17% increase in diagnosis of previously unrecognized comorbid disease processes.[3] Another study found that a computerized preoperative evaluation resulted in increased hospital coder recognition of comorbidities over a handwritten system (resulting in a financial benefit to hospitals), primarily because the coders would read the laser-printed preanesthetic evaluation and ignore the handwritten evaluations.[4,5] Further positive financial impact of these additional comorbid conditions has been studied, and the results are currently being prepared for submission for publication.[6]

It is clear that the full-service preoperative physician-run clinic is the best model for a complete preoperative evaluation of patients. Most European countries are required by law to provide this type of preoperative center. However, in the US, resource-constrained hospitals must often choose another, less costly path for preoperative evaluation.

The implementation of an integrated information system is one solution to the high costs associated with preoperative evaluation. This solution also improves patient outcomes, as it provides an ability to triage the preoperative patient to the appropriate evaluation pathway. Not all surgical patients need to be seen in a preoperative clinic; however, depending upon the surgeon to make this determination is not the optimal solution.

Preoperative Evaluation Module

AIMS must include a robust preoperative evaluation module that creates, at a minimum, the requisite anesthesia H&P, which must contain a thorough review of systems and a physical exam, as well as specific information tailored to an anesthesia assessment.

Patients in the US often receive their care from several facilities that do not readily share medical information. A static EMR contained within a single system cannot provide caregivers with all relevant information on a patient because it only provides the information that is stored within. Furthermore, most health information contains very little data regarding a patient's prior experiences with anesthesia or confirmation of family history reaction to anesthetics. Such disjointed communication, even though electronic, necessitates a complete reassessment of the patient's current health history at the time of surgery that includes information on the proposed surgery, along with history of the medical condition that led to the surgery. A review of systems provides additional details on other medical conditions. A list of medications (ideally with dosages) and allergies (with detailed descriptions of reactions) is also needed. Past anesthetics used for previous surgeries and any difficulties should be noted, and documentation of current vital signs and an anesthetic-oriented physical exam, with particular attention to the dentition, airway, cardiovascular, and pulmonary systems, is paramount. In the presence of neurologic abnormalities, a carefully completed exam will prove extremely valuable should questions arise later. Current laboratory results and major diagnostic tests such as an exercise stress test, cardiac catheterization, CT studies, etc., should be available to the practitioner and either included or linked. The possibilities for anesthesia and the choices, risks, and consents discussed with the patient should also be documented. A list of specific data elements that should be included in any comprehensive preoperative module of an AIMS is provided in Table 9.1. This module will only cover the essentials of the preanesthesia evaluation and will not include functions required for consult documentation or other evaluation scenarios.

Historically, institutions that have adopted an AIMS typically completed the implementation and go-live effort of the intraoperative product prior to introducing the preoperative module. However, the consensus of several physicians who have

Table 9.1 Data elements required for preoperative evaluation

Category/description	Comments
Patient demographics	
First name	
Middle name	
Last name	
DOB	
Sex	
SSN	May be helpful for integration
Med record number	
Age	
Visit	
Account number	
Barcode number	
Height	
Weight	
BMI	
Readiness	Data elements that are typically available in a patient-tracking module
Preop	
Patient	
X-ray	
Antibiotic	
Labs	
EKG	
Procedure information	
Patient location	
Primary procedure	
OR	
Date	
Time	
ASA class	
Procedure description	Typically truncated. May be unnecessary if primary procedure description is adequate
Diagnosis	
Comments	
Additional procedures	
Procedure	
Description	
Diagnosis	
Prescribed drugs	Drugs prescribed to be given preoperatively
Staff	
Surgeon	
Anesthesiologist	
CRNA	
Circulator	May be available with integration with ORMS
Scrub nurse	May be available with integration with ORMS
Location Hx	Typically associated with patient-tracking modules
Vitals	
BP	
Temp	
Temp mode	
Pulse	
Resp	
SaO_2	
Room air/% O_2	
NPO comment	
NPO since midnight	
NPO date/time	
Comments	

(continued)

Table 9.1 (continued)

Category/description	Comments
Labs	
Labs	
Value	
Unit	
Ref range	
Comments	
Date/time	
HISTORY	
Patient allergies	
Allergies	
Reaction	
Comments	
Status	
Patient home meds	Should be part of medication reconciliation process
Home medications	
Dose	
Frequency	
Last taken	
Route	
Anesthesia Hx	
None, problems, no problems, unknown	
Comments	
Surgical Hx	
Procedure	
Anesthesia type	
Perioperative complications (yes/no)	
Comments	
Date	
Conditions	
Cardiovascular	
Skin conditions	
Eyes, ears, nose, throat	
Gastrointestinal	
Hematologic/immunologic	
Hepatic	
Lab	
Metabolic	
Muscular/skeletal	
Neuromuscular	
Physical examination	
Renal/urogenital	
Respiratory	
Social	
Diagnosis codes	Not typically part of most preop modules but extremely useful if available
Anesthesia plan	
Preop ASA class	
Anesthesia plan	
Airway management	
Postop pain management	
Special monitors	
Risk/comments	
"Risks, benefits, and alternatives" statement and checkbox	Need electronic signature capabilities
Preop comments	

been involved in these installations is that the preoperative module should be implemented prior to the intraoperative module. One reason for this strategy is the obvious minimized impact on workflow involved in bringing the intraoperative module up after the preoperative module; more importantly, most describe a situation in which collected preoperative information makes utilization of the intraoperative product more facile. The lack of the preoperative module initially requires the redundant entry of patient clinical information into the AIMS after documentation on the paper preoperative chart. For example, entry of patient weight into the electronic preoperative module automatically provides these data to the intraoperative module and results in less data entry during a case.

Preoperative Evaluation Systems

Questionnaires to Efficiently Capture History and Review of Systems

Perhaps the most essential element of an effective preoperative evaluation is a comprehensive health history and current review of systems, which is often quite time consuming; consequently, much effort has gone into finding ways for the patient to enter as much information as possible. Multiple studies have described the benefits of a questionnaire as an effective means to obtain health histories, increase available information, reduce errors, and minimize the number of unnecessary laboratory tests.[7–9] As early as 1976, the *British Medical Journal* published a study regarding the benefit of using an automated questionnaire to obtain health histories from patients.[10] The EMR is of indisputable benefit as a longitudinal history record and provides a method by which to efficiently gather and make available information to all providers concerned, thus eliminating the frustrating practice of posing the same questions over and over again to the patient.

Historic Perspective of Automated Questionnaires

The concept of technology-based preoperative assessment is not new. In the early 1990s, Dr. Michael Roizen pioneered an automated health history for anesthesia with the introduction of *Health Quiz* (Fig. 9.1). However, the slower-than-anticipated adoption of the EMR markedly inhibited the success of Health Quiz. In 1993, when rights to Health Quiz were sold to a commercial company, early marketing efforts were successful; however, the sale of that company to another changed the company's business focus, and Health Quiz marketing ceased.[11]

Health Quiz did capture the attention of Dr. Sarah Spagnola, who wished to introduce the system at The Cleveland Clinic. The Chairman of Anesthesiology at Cleveland at that time, Dr. Fazzio Estaphanous, preferred to focus on an in-

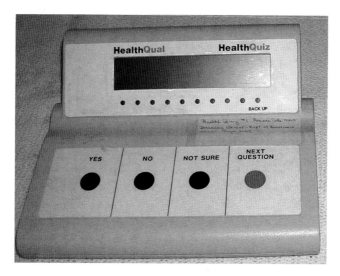

Fig. 9.1 The Health Quiz machine pioneered by Michael Roizen, MD, and used for automated collection of patient health history

house development of the Clinic's own health questionnaire, and over the course of 3 years, HealthQuest (HQ) was developed. HQ is an evidence-based, algorithmically driven tool for gathering a thorough health history, relevant family history, and complete review of systems directly from the patient via a series of yes/no questions. The questions are primarily focused on the needs of the anesthesiologist. Results are printed in an organized and standardized format (Fig. 9.2).

Additionally, HQ generates a proprietary risk score (HQ Score) similar to the ASA Physical Status. HQ uses the highest raw score for each medical condition but does not involve a physical examination; therefore, it is not completely analogous to the ASA Score. The HQ score is then "matrixed" (matched) against the surgical risk (the Pasternak or Johns Hopkins Score that stratifies surgical risk of various procedures[12]) to define the process/pathway of the patient's medical optimization (Fig. 9.3). Patients with high HQ scores who are scheduled for more complex procedures (higher risk) are directed to the hospitalists or primary care providers for additional evaluation. The importance of the scoring system is the ability to triage patients. The number of patients who need to be seen in person in the preoperative clinic (those who are healthy and/or having low-risk procedures) can be reduced by up to 40%–50%, thus improving efficiency and reducing costs in all preoperative center models.

To enhance the patient convenience of the system, HQ utilizes branch-chain logic, thereby minimizing "questionnaire fatigue." Someone who answers "no" to a question about a specific disease (e.g., diabetes) will not have to answer the same set of questions presented to someone who answers "yes." It is estimated that The Cleveland Clinic has invested more than $2 million in the development,

✚ Community Hospital   Health**Q**uestionnaire™ *Patient Report*

Name: Janice Sample	Administrator: Prompte Admin Completion Time: 00:11
Medical Record Number: 15959302	Temp MRN: Enterprise ID:
Case Id: a23222	
Home Phone: 999.555.6135	Site: Prompte Test HQS Medicine: 4
Work Phone: 999.555.5265	Physician: HQS Anesthesia: 4
Cell Phone: 999.555.1461	Surgeon: Swelle, Awls, Dr. Procedure Risk: 5
Age: 51 yrs	Evaluation Date: 05/14/2007 Procedure Cardiac Risk: High
Gender: Female	Procedure: Thoracotomy

Report reviewed and verified by Prompte Admin (8/20/2007 10:26:29 AM)

HQSm	Physical
1	Height: 168 cm / 66 in Weight: 73.03 kgs / 161 lbs BMI: 26, normal Blood pressure: 140/70 Pulse: 89 Respiration Rate: 21 Oxygen Saturation: 96% Temperature: 98.4 F / 36.89 C

HQSm	Cardiovascular System
2	METS = 4 Moderately decreased functional class
2	H/O elevated cholesterol and/or triglycerides -- treated
2	H/O hypertension, x 10 year(s) -- treated -- well controlled (<160/100mm Hg) Past cardiac studies performed: -- EKG -- -- Hospital: Community Hospital -- Echocardiogram -- Stress test -- Cardiac catheterization
3	H/O previous MI, x 1 -- Dr. Diagnosed MI -- hospitalized
3	H/O angioplasty, x 1 -- Hospital/Doctor: Community Hospital -- Cardiac Stent has been placed -- -- Cardiac Stent placed greater than 6 months ago -- -- Bare Metal Stent
3	H/O coronary revascularization, x 3
3	H/O arrhythmia -- symptomatic -- treated -- controlled

HQSa	HQSm	Pulmonary System
	3	H/O tobacco use -- cigarettes -- ex-smoker -- quit <1 year ago -- 50 pack year history
		H/O asthma
	3	H/O chronic bronchitis H/O emphysema/COPD -- untreated
	2	H/O TB or TB exposure -- +PPD or Tine test -- treated
4	4	H/O sleep apnea

HQSm	Endocrine System
	HQS has no output to report

HQSm	Neurological System
3	H/O chronic muscle weakness/wasting

HQSm	Urinary & Reproduction System
	HQS has no output to report

HQSm	Gastrointestinal System
2	H/O GERD
2	Current EtOH excess

HQSm	Blood & Coagulation System
3	Patient takes Coumadin, Lovenox, Plavix, Pletal, or Ticlid Daily ASA/NSAID use

HQSa	Anesthetic Issues
	H/O previous anesthesia
4	H/O previous difficult intubation - Requires Anesthesia Consult -- Comments: Dr. Jones told patient that he needed to use a bronchoscope.

Other Conditions
Multiple Sclerosis

------ End of Report ------

Audit History: ✚

Signature: _____   Date: _____

Printed By: Prompte Admin

Fig. 9.2 Example of HealthQuest Patient Report output

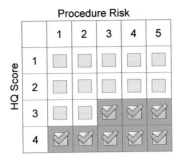

Fig. 9.3 HQ matrix used to review medical optimization

implementation, and refinement of this tool. Quality improvement and refinement are ongoing. As new evidence appears regarding certain conditions (such as obstructive sleep apnea), HQ adds or modifies questions to obtain more detailed information.

More than 350,000 patients have taken HQ since its introduction.[13] In its current form, HQ is deployed throughout the main campus of The Cleveland Clinic, with patient access to the questionnaire in every surgical office, in the preoperative assessment clinic, and via the Clinic's Web site. Physicians at the Clinic have published several studies on the benefits of utilizing a formal evaluation process that includes HQ. One such study estimated a $1.55 million reduction in laboratory costs over a 3-year period using the triage capability of HQ, equating to a per-patient savings of $30.41.[14]

Because of increased interest from other institutions, in 2005, The Cleveland Clinic licensed HQ to a Chicago-based perioperative consulting firm (Prompte, Inc.), which subsequently established a separate company to focus specifically on preoperative services. At the present time, Prompte is the only company of which we are aware that provides a commercially available, multilingual, decision-support, preoperative assessment tool.

Validity and Acceptance of Patient-entered Health History

Many authors have validated the use of automated means to gather health histories. Roizen's 1992 study compared the accuracy of an automated questionnaire with person-to-person interviews and reported a low 3% discrepancy.[7] A January 2002 study published by the American Dental Association compared a paper-and-pencil questionnaire to a handheld computer-based tool. The authors found a reliability of 93%, with an average of 5.4 inconsistent answers between paper and computer methods. Additionally, patient acceptance of the computer tool was 73%. Legibility of results and ability to import directly to clinical data systems—thus eliminating the need for tedious, costly, and error-prone provider data entry—justified the increased cost of the technology.[15]

A 2003 study cites the benefits of utilizing the automated questionnaire, including the gathering of more information, the ability to uncover more protected information, and the ability to provide more structured information for research.[16] In 1999, investigators reported a 4%–8% greater incidence of disclosure by patients of sensitive health risk behaviors (e.g., alcohol and drug use, domestic violence, tobacco use) when utilizing an automated method of gathering health information.[17]

Usability Considerations

Consideration must be given to patients who complete the HQ questionnaire, surgical office staff, presurgical testing personnel, and anesthesiologists, as well as the other caregivers involved in the optimization process (Fig. 9.4).

The system should be configured to be flexible enough for ease of use by wide patient and caregiver populations in a variety of settings. For example, in the surgeon's office or preoperative center, a touchscreen application eases patient acceptance. The phone-bank model may use either a touchscreen or a mouse system. The system output must be seamless to the end user (anesthesiologist or other caregiver), regardless of where the information was captured. A well-designed system will accomplish seamlessness in part by storing all information as discrete data elements, which also enables the development of internal decision-support tools.

Language issues must be considered. The number of patients who do not speak, read, or write English is increasing. In the US today, it is essential that a questionnaire tool have multilingual capabilities and that it be accessible to those with visual and/or other disabilities.[18] This feature is important both on the questionnaire and

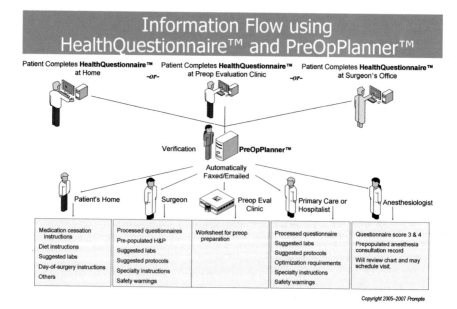

Fig. 9.4 Users and uses of the results of the HealthQuestionnaire

in all output or printed instructions given to the patient. Information technology is the most efficient way to comply with US government requirements to meet the needs of multilingual and disabled populations.

Professional Verification

Verification of the patient-entered information is often critical to system acceptance. Lacking the professional frame of reference to evaluate different symptoms and events, patients may simply err in their estimation of their own illnesses. A well-structured system requires a clinical caregiver (nurse, physician, or practitioner) to verify the information with the patient, either in person or via telephone. The system must have the flexibility to allow for the addition or deletion of information and provide an audit trail of changes.

Free Text versus Structured Data Entry

Entry of the history, present illness, and review of systems is the most difficult portion of most computerized H&P systems. Branched-chain questionnaire systems have a significant advantage in being able to deal with a wide variety of medical problems. Often (in one author's experience, as much as 25%), the patient will have one or more conditions that were not considered in the original structured problem entry system. (After all, internal medicine textbooks are generally large tomes.) Questionnaire systems (patient entry) automatically structure common patient medical problems, tagging them with at least an initial ICD diagnosis code for each problem. Caregiver-entry systems should also be structured and include automatic ICD tags for as many diagnoses as possible. Nevertheless, the accurate description of an individual patient's medical facts often requires the entry of specific information that cannot be adequately planned for with pro forma text or phrases. Almost always, the ability to add minimal free text is necessary. As much as possible, the system should allow for communication of key details, such as when platelets are planned to be given to a thrombocytopenic patient, or where a missing stress test result may be located and what process is being utilized to obtain the document. This sort of precise information often requires text entry.

Physician-entry methodology should be fast, intuitive, and simple. Physicians and other anesthesia caregivers are highly skilled and productive individuals; they may dictate up to 200 words per minute and may often type 60–70 words per minute. However, they will not be satisfied with the typical spreadsheet-styled entry screen with cumbersome drop-down menus that require an inordinate amount of selection/clicking to create a note. In one author's experience, such systems typically result in a preanesthetic clinic staffed primarily with paid nursing staff and a minimum of physician or resident involvement.

Discrete and standardized data element storage can be incorporated into a data inquiry system that can be easily searched. Free-form entry systems require more finesse. For example, in a free-form system, if one caregiver uses the term "CAD" to indicate coronary artery disease and another uses the term "heart disease," a query that did not employ both terms would miss essential patient information. The use of a coding system such as the Systematized Nomenclature of Medicine (SNOMED) captures all equivalent terms and standardizes the output to enhance searching and provide complete data recovery. An alternative solution to this vexing data storage and retrieval problem was pioneered by research that involved Kaiser-Permanente, wherein individual data dictionaries were maintained for different clinical sites (individual dictionaries for individual physicians).[19,20] This system would automatically recognize the preferred terms typically used by one group to describe a medical condition and would automatically store an additional structured description based on SNOMED. Using such a system allows the retrieval advantages of SNOMED while adapting automatically to the individual physician. To date, we are not aware of any AIMS with this level of sophistication.

Decision Support

Once verified, the automated questionnaire results can be used to drive the other processes in the optimization of patient status for surgery. Verified results can also be distributed to all caregivers in a consistent format. Success in the complex choreography of preoperative patient care depends on all concerned sharing the same information about the patient.

Standardization of stored data, using a database-driven dictionary of medical terminology, medication names, and doses, allows movement of the data to an ICD- or CPT-coded record that can be used to prepopulate an anesthesia assessment record or surgeon history form, provide accurately coded information to the billing department without the need for time-consuming and error-prone re-entry of data, and aid in creating an automated anesthesia bill. Thus, human resources are less costly, workflow is more efficient, and reimbursements are improved. Planning modules allow information to be shared by all providers, including surgeons, primary care and specialty consultants, anesthesiologists, and presurgical testing personnel, as illustrated in Fig. 9.4. The system automatically faxes or electronically forwards the preoperative evaluation report to all constituents.

Note that in Fig. 9.5 the electronic communication is sent to the primary care physician. Based on each individual patient's HQ report, the planning module identifies the appropriate evidence-based management algorithms stored in the system. For example, the report of a patient with coronary artery disease, angina, and/or dysrhythmias would activate the beta-blocker algorithm (among others), which would populate both the information sent to the primary care provider and the presurgical testing center's "to do" list. By outlining everyone's roles and responsibilities in the preparation of the patient for surgery, collectively sharing health information, and standardizing the management of comorbid disease, this system ensures that the patient receives optimal care prior to surgery.

To: <u>Dr. I. M. Fine</u>

Regarding Patient: <u>Janice Tailor</u>   Tele: <u>999.555.6135</u>

From: Pre Surgical Testing
      Community Hospital
      1212 Main Street
      Springfield, WY 53101
      999.555.9999
      999.555.9998 fax

Your patient <u>Janice Sample</u> is having a <u>Thoracotomy</u> on <u>09/08/2007</u> with <u>Dr. Awls Swelle</u> at Community Hospital.

Your patient has been noted to have certain medical conditions that may increase the patient's surgical risk. Many of these items may have been addressed in prior visits. In order to optimize your patient's outcome, please provide us with any additional information that you may have (office notes, stress tests, echo results, old ECGs or laboratory studies) which will help to minimize any risk of delay or cancellation.

If you have not seen the patient recently or if you note additional medical conditions not previously addressed, please schedule the patient for a visit to assure optimization prior to surgery. Please complete the medical risk assessment (optimization) form and fax it back to (999) 555-9998.

If you wish to dictate a note, please call (999) 555-9999 and title this note: **presurgical optimization note.** (This does not need to be a complete history and physical, only a brief statement of outstanding issues or problems related to the patient's upcoming surgery). Please make PST aware that you have dictated a note by checking the box on the medical risk assessment (optimization) form and faxing it back to (999) 555-9998.

The reasons for pre-operative medical optimization included both the invasiveness of the procedure and the following conditions recorded in the HealthQuestionnaire™:

H/O previous MI	H/O chronic bronchitis
H/O Angioplasty	H/O emphysema/COPD
H/O coronary revascularization	H/O sleep apnea
H/O arrhythmia	H/O chronic muscle weakness/wasting
H/O tobacco use	Patient takes Coumadin, Lovenox, Plavix, Pletal, or Ticlid
H/O asthma	H/O previous difficult intubation – Requires Anesthesia Consult

Please note the following required labs:

☐ Chem Panel   ☐ Hemogram
☐ CXR   ☐ PT
☐ EKG   ☐ T+C 2u

The following HealthQuestionnaire™ protocols for optimization are included:

- Hypertension   - Pulmonary Algorithm
- Stepwise Approach to Preop Cardiac Assessment   - Beta-Blocker Introduction
- Cardiac III - High Risk   - Beta Blocker Management

Please note the following medication instructions given to your patient:

Introduction
The Community Hospital Pharmacy has provided a general set of recommendations regarding the cessation of medications prior to surgery. Please review the following and discuss with your patient.

Aspirin.
Patient is taking Low-Dose Aspirin.
When to hold: Discontinue 7 days prior to surgery.
Reason: Increased risk of bleeding complications.
Note: Particular vigilance should be exercised in patients having ophthalmologic and neurosurgical procedures.
Note: Patients with CAD should be continued on Aspirin whenever possible. Patients undergoing Peripheral Vascular Surgery or Cardiac Surgery may be asked by the surgeon to continue taking Aspirin until the time of surgery.

Warfarin (Coumadin).
Patient is taking Coumadin.
When to hold: Discontinue 5-7 days prior to surgery.
Reason: Increased risk of bleeding complications.
Note: A normalized PT (INR) should be available prior to surgery.
Note: Artificial heart valve patients will need specific pre-operative managment for Coumadin.

ACE Inhibitors.
Patient is taking Lisinopril.
When to hold: Do not take on the day of surgery.
Reason: Adverse hemodynamic changes during induction and maintenance of anesthesia (i.e. hypotension).

Beta Blockers / Alpha Blockers.
Patient is taking Atenolol.
When to hold: Continue.
Reason: Reduced incidence of cardiac ischemia and death post-op
Note: Continuation of current Beta-Blocker reduces the risk of rebound hypertension and tachycardia.

Thank you,

PLEASE complete the Medical Risk Assessment review and fax to: 999.555.9999 - Pre Surgical Testing Unit (As Soon As Possible).

Fig. 9.5 Example of a primary care letter

The use of institution-approved algorithms to guide the management of comorbid conditions and to recommend diagnostic testing was validated in a 2002 report.[21] Many hospitals already use with great success such algorithms for diabetes, hypertension, coronary artery disease, aortic stenosis, asthma/chronic obstructive pulmonary disease, sleep apnea, and beta-blocker therapy. In many cases,

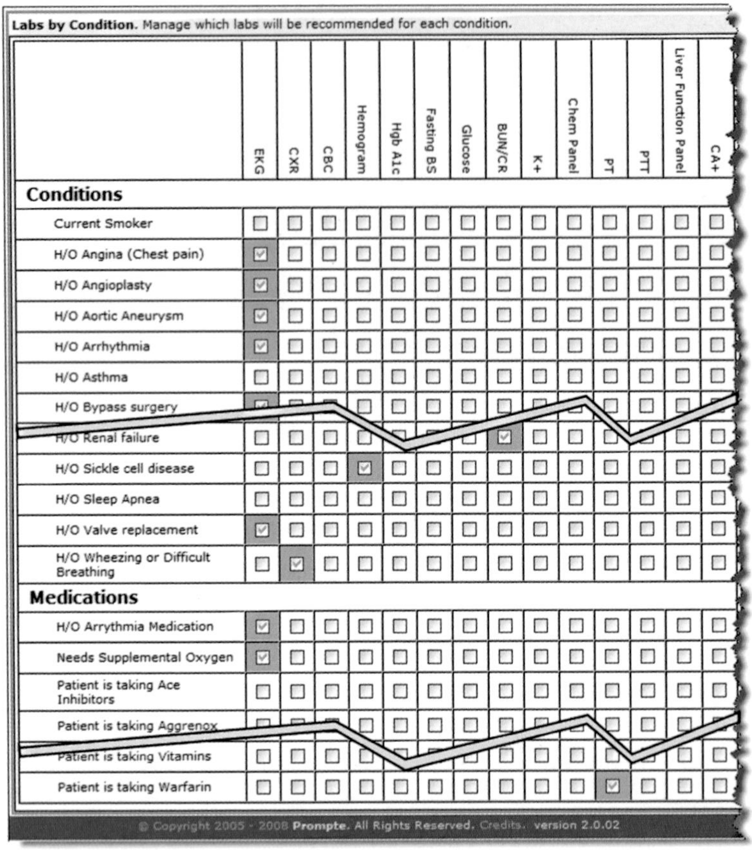

Labs by Condition. Manage which labs will be recommended for each condition.

	EKG	CXR	CBC	Hemogram	Hgb A1c	Fasting BS	Glucose	BUN/CR	K+	Chem Panel	PT	PTT	Liver Function Panel	CA+
Conditions														
Current Smoker	☐	☐	☐	☐	☐	☐	☐	☐	☐	☐	☐	☐	☐	☐
H/O Angina (Chest pain)	☑	☐	☐	☐	☐	☐	☐	☐	☐	☐	☐	☐	☐	☐
H/O Angioplasty	☑	☐	☐	☐	☐	☐	☐	☐	☐	☐	☐	☐	☐	☐
H/O Aortic Aneurysm	☑	☐	☐	☐	☐	☐	☐	☐	☐	☐	☐	☐	☐	☐
H/O Arrhythmia	☑	☐	☐	☐	☐	☐	☐	☐	☐	☐	☐	☐	☐	☐
H/O Asthma	☐	☐	☐	☐	☐	☐	☐	☐	☐	☐	☐	☐	☐	☐
H/O Bypass surgery	☑	☐		☐	☐	☐	☐	☐		☐		☐	☐	
H/O Renal failure	☐	☐	☐	☐				☑	☐	☐			☐	☐
H/O Sickle cell disease	☐	☐	☐	☑	☐	☐	☐	☐	☐	☐	☐	☐	☐	☐
H/O Sleep Apnea	☐	☐	☐	☐	☐	☐	☐	☐	☐	☐	☐	☐	☐	☐
H/O Valve replacement	☑	☐	☐	☐	☐	☐	☐	☐	☐	☐	☐	☐	☐	☐
H/O Wheezing or Difficult Breathing	☐	☑	☐	☐	☐	☐	☐	☐	☐	☐	☐	☐	☐	☐
Medications														
H/O Arrythmia Medication	☑	☐	☐	☐	☐	☐	☐	☐	☐	☐	☐	☐	☐	☐
Needs Supplemental Oxygen	☑	☐	☐	☐	☐	☐	☐	☐	☐	☐	☐	☐	☐	☐
Patient is taking Ace Inhibitors	☐	☐	☐	☐	☐	☐	☐	☐	☐	☐	☐	☐	☐	☐
Patient is taking Aggrenox	☐	☐		☐	☐	☐	☐	☐		☐		☐	☐	
Patient is taking Vitamins	☐	☐	☐	☐			☐	☐	☐	☐			☐	☐
Patient is taking Warfarin	☐	☐	☐	☐	☐	☐	☐	☐	☐	☐	☐	☑	☐	☐

Fig. 9.6 Matrix of lab tests by medical condition

primary care physicians do not fully comprehend what it means to "optimize a patient for surgery" and how this differs from their ongoing care. An effective system not only allows ease of access to the algorithms but also automatically "attaches" the appropriate algorithms to the distributed management plan for any/all captured medical conditions. When this is accomplished automatically by the system, it frees the busy preoperative staff for more clinical rather than clerical duties and promotes better patient care by providing a platform of education to the primary care providers.

Similarly, the same planning modules can "matrix" medical conditions and procedures with testing guidelines to generate the minimum laboratory and testing requirements recommended by each institution/anesthesia department (Figs. 9.6 and 9.7). This standardized approach to preoperative lab testing has demonstrated proven economic savings. Studies have shown that utilizing an algorithmic process can save up to $80,000 for every 5100 patients.[22]

Labs by Procedure Group.

Ortho	EKG	CXR	CBC	Hemogram	Hgb A1c	Fasting BS	Glucose	BUN/Cr	K+	Chem Panel
Biopsy & Mass excision (major) e.g. tumor excision	☐	☐	☐	☐	☐	☐	☐	☐	☐	☐
Biopsy & Mass excision (minor) e.g. muscle bone	☐	☐	☐	☑	☐	☐	☐	☐	☐	☐
Cast application	☐	☐	☐	☐	☐	☐	☐	☐	☐	☐
Clavicle procedure	☐	☐	☐	☐	☐	☐	☐	☐	☐	☐
Closed reduction/manipulation	☐	☐	☐	☐	☐	☐	☐	☐	☐	☐
Contracture release	☐	☐	☐	☐	☐	☐	☐	☐	☐	☐
Elbow proced...	☐	☐	☐				☐	☐	☐	
Spinal surgery (major)e.g. multi level, vertebrectomy, revision, etc	☐	☐	☐	☑	☐			☐	☐	☐
Spine surgery (minor) e.g. microdiscectomy	☐	☐	☐	☐	☐	☐	☐	☐	☐	☐
Upper arm (major) e.g. ORIF	☐	☐	☐	☐	☐	☐	☐	☐	☐	☐
Upper arm (minor) e.g. tendon repair	☐	☐	☐	☐	☐	☐	☐	☐	☐	☐
Upper extremity (major) e.g. amputation	☐	☐	☐	☑	☐	☐	☐	☐	☐	☐
Upper extremity (minor) e.g. I&D	☐	☐	☐	☐	☐	☐	☐	☐	☐	☐
Upper leg procedure (major) e.g. ORIF	☐	☐	☐	☑	☐	☐	☐	☐	☐	☐
Upper leg procedure (minor) e.g. tendon repair	☐	☐	☐	☐	☐	☐	☐	☐	☐	☐

Fig. 9.7 Matrix of lab tests by surgical procedure

Interface Capabilities in the Preoperative Process

Automated interfaces between various systems can provide tremendous benefits, including increased accuracy in data captured across systems, reduced work effort through the reduction of double data entry, and the population of coded data into multiple systems. Typical datatypes that can be exchanged include patient information, insurance information, surgical information, patient conditions, surgeries, allergies, medications, and vital signs. Information that is normally captured by hand at the beginning of the process can electronically flow through the capturing system and into downstream systems.

Successful interfacing relies on the use of discrete data elements, code-based data, and an interface broker, which acts as a traffic controller that can handle all of the steps required for exchanging data. Some of these steps include processing requests for data, processing notices that data are available, transferring the data, and error handling and processing. An interface broker brings standardization to the message or data processing and makes it easier to interface to multiple systems. The use of an HL7 integration management server with HL7 connectors further increases standardization and reduces the amount of time required to build interfaces to new systems because this server contains industry-accepted standards (Fig. 9.8). Some systems can have interfaces developed without an interface broker, but they are typically customized, one-time interfaces.

The discrete data elements and code-based data break down items to the lowest common denominator and allow for the most flexibility. Discrete data elements allow for all data to be named and ultimately referenced. The use of code-based data allows reference to other data sources, such as ICD, CPT, or medication lists. For example, information about a patient who has had hypertension for 25 years that has been treated and well controlled with lisinopril can be shared with other systems in a text string, but the other systems may only be able to treat it as text and not use the detail without parsing the detail out. The use of discrete data elements and code-based data would allow two systems to exchange the following:

- Condition: 1432—hypertension
- ICD: code if known
- Number of years: 25
- Controlled: 1 (yes)
- Drug: 6620 (lisinopril)

A receiving system that can process and store each of these discrete data elements and codes can then use these data directly within its own system for additional processing. The data can be received by an anesthesia billing system, added to other data, and used to determine candidate ICD billing codes (Fig. 9.8).

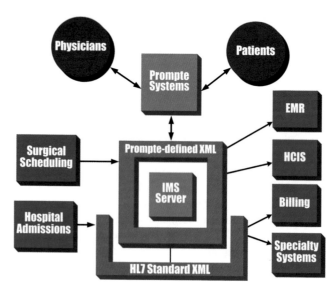

Fig. 9.8 Integration management server

The Health Information Record and Multiple Users

Discrete storage of data elements allows the system to organize each type of data into searchable components for ease of access. Multiple users who enter data can be identified by the system automatically as authors of particular components. For example:

- The technician gathers vital-sign data.
- The nurse obtains medication and allergy information.
- The nurse practitioner or physician adds review of systems and physical examination.

In addition, data from previous hospitalizations, surgeries, anesthetics, medication reactions, diagnostic tests, etc., must be incorporated from the EMR into the appropriate place in the new complete record without complicating or overwhelming the end user with information. It can be difficult to indicate the authorship/date of such information included from a previous data source. Changes in font type may assist, with provision of automated footnoting giving the details of the previous source. When data are discretely stored, all elements of one type, such as previous anesthesia records, can be accessed on demand by automated linkages.

Flexible Upkeep

All computerized EMR systems require technical upkeep of servers, security encryption, and external communication methods. A medical information system also requires ongoing clinical review and update. New drugs become available and are soon commonplace. New diseases and treatments are discovered. Risk measurements change. A records system based on Structured Query Language (SQL) usually includes methods for changing the text of questions and adding or deleting questions. A well-designed system also allows flexible changes in the management algorithms as new evidence regarding conditions and treatments becomes available. The vigilant maintenance of the system requires the close cooperation of IT and clinical personnel.

Limitations and Barriers

Billing Issues and Remuneration

Hospital administrators view preoperative evaluation as a cost-intensive operation. Historically, they have been reluctant, despite evidence of benefit, to add to these costs by investing in center improvements. For the hospital, the cost of preoperative evaluation is bundled with the surgical fee reimbursement because the third-party payers view the preoperative visit as merely part of the surgical service provided by the hospital. Although it is true that hospitals can often include in their bill a "facility fee" for the use of the preanesthetic area, because hospitals are paid one sum by third-party payers—without identification of which portions were found acceptable—it becomes difficult to prove to cost-conscious administrators that even the preanesthetic facility fee has been paid. Obtaining additional professional (physician or ARNP) reimbursement for the preanesthetic evaluation requires yet another bill and is dependent on justifying the medical necessity of the evaluation, which requires further documentation and increases the risk of billing audits.

It is easy to understand why competition among hospitals for the provision of surgical services, combined with the reimbursement issues, is driving hospital administrators to seek new opportunities to improve the financial and operational performance of perioperative services and enhance both patient and surgeon satisfaction. It is important, therefore, to continue to demonstrate that the streamlined preoperative evaluation process, driven by a well-designed information system, is actually lowering costs, justifying increased DRG reimbursements for comorbidities that would otherwise have been overlooked, reducing cancellations, and improving patient safety and satisfaction. Some hospitals do actually recognize the financial advantages of better data and actively drive the adoption of systems that are optimized from a financial perspective but may not be optimal from the viewpoint of the caregivers. In those unusual situations, the physicians must be keenly aware of their needs and continuously communicate them to hospital administration.

Moving from an Old System to a New System

Implementation of a de novo preoperative information system or changeover to an updated system poses a number of difficulties regarding already existing medical records, whether or not they are in electronic or paper form. Technologic advances are renowned for causing the obsolescence of previous systems. When faced with the complex task of trying to interface hundreds of data fields from an old system to a new one, hospital administrators may balk at the cost incurred in taking the necessary steps to ensure that all records are transferred completely and correctly. At the institution of one of the authors (GLG), the decision was made not to commit the necessary funds, and tens of thousands of electronic records simply disappeared. This kind of occurrence brings new insight to the claim that EMRs have the advantage of "instantaneous record retrieval, forever!" Designers and vendors of information systems must recognize the clinical importance of retaining and incorporating *all* health data in their products. Anesthesiology departments would be wise to obtain ironclad agreements that no data will ever be erased. Such agreements require the consideration of methods of entering old records that are not too cumbersome, the foresight to recognize the potential impact of advances in technology on current systems, and planning for all potentialities in the internal design. When transferring old records to new systems, simple text systems or scanning systems have a distinct advantage over carefully structured SQL databases—the information is far easier to migrate to a new system.

An astute hospital administration will quickly recognize that the initial purchase cost of a preoperative information system is outweighed by the advantages of far better cost accounting, the cost savings in improved staff and facility utilization, and increased reimbursements; they will sometimes even demand such systems, chosen for cost-accounting prowess. Delays and cancellations in the OR are major areas of unnecessary expense for any institution that provides surgical services. The use of an organized preoperative facility and a standardized electronic questionnaire has led to marked reductions in cancellations at The Cleveland Clinic and other hospitals. Lutheran General Hospital near Chicago, Illinois, has reduced cancellations from >5% to <1% in just 1 year following implementation of an automated questionnaire and a system that standardized the approach to preoperative preparation.[23] Preoperative nurses are able to spend more time educating patients about their surgical procedures and postoperative care than they do on gathering the health history. Even when the EMR system is not yet able to interface with the automated questionnaire, nurses report that the automated health history is useful and saves time in completing the nursing evaluation required for the intraoperative IT system.

A more difficult area is the human–computer interface. Touchscreens are becoming more familiar and are a comfortable addition to the mouse and keyboard as interface options. Preconfigured text and algorithms reduce the tediousness of data entry, but some users (especially physicians) feel a loss of individualism and professionalism. As patient demographics change, the severity of comorbid illness increases and requires more precise documentation of patient conditions. Static, formalized text has limitations in adequately conveying the situation, and the computer industry has not yet succeeded in going far beyond keyboard and mouse. In the future, handwriting and voice recognition will likely prevail. In the interim, flexible system design and collaborative staff training can help users to cope with unwieldy systems.

For some anesthesiologists, the lack of professional remuneration reduces the impetus to use and improve electronic information systems. For them, a handwritten and scanned preanesthetic evaluation is considered just as adequate and even preferable to a burdensome structured data entry system—buyers would be well advised to require the availability of this fallback method in any system considered for purchase, as user entry can prove to be much more burdensome than expected. However, anesthesiologists have historically been at the forefront of medical technology that improves patient care. Those who strive to offer the best care readily accept and investigate the use of new modalities. When faced with occasional difficulties or complications in the use of new modalities, anesthesiologists are in a unique position as clinicians and end users, to suggest possible solutions.

The Web as an Important Health-Management Tool

The Web has revolutionized many industries. However, medicine has lagged behind in its acceptance of the Web as a means for communication and, therefore, has been reluctant to enter the arena of Web-based applications. The preoperative setting, in which a variety of caregivers need the same information, demonstrates an excellent use for the Web's convenience. Although some hospitals provide management algorithms on Web sites, most continue to use a paper format due to ease of access. Use of the Web to share information with primary care physicians could help to increase adherence to institutional guidelines. In addition, anesthesiologists could review preoperative information for their patients from home and in the OR. The complex dynamics of OR management necessitate the frequent reassignment of patient rooms and personnel throughout the day. The ability to access patient information from any computer with Web access ensures better patient care and helps to prevent delays.

Web-based information is beneficial to patients as well as staff. A preoperative Web site can provide general instructions such as parking and visiting hours as well as information such as NPO guidelines. Some institutions have expanded and personalized the tool. The Geisinger Medical Center includes a link (MyGeisinger.org), where the patient can access specific health-related information.[24] The system can allow the patient to access specific personal preoperative instructions via a password-protected area within the Web site. This feature is beneficial for patients who complete the entire preoperative evaluation via the Web, for those who may lose their instructions, or for family members who need clarification.

Document-Management Systems

Even in our increasingly electronic world, we swim in reams of paper reports. Nowhere is this a reality more than during the preoperative evaluation process. Each patient typically has sheets of lab data, electrocardiographic tracings, x-ray reports, and consultant reports faxed to various offices in an attempt to collate all of the necessary documentation preoperatively. Institutions that have adopted some method of document management are attempting to provide an electronic repository for these documents. Although they are not discrete data elements that allow queries or integration with other clinical systems, these systems do provide rapid, universal access to health records. Unfortunately, even the most sophisticated of these document-management systems require a fair amount of human interaction in an effort to "index" patients' records to the appropriate patient file. Consequently, human error leads to a loss of effectiveness of these solutions. An interesting approach to this concern has been developed by My Medical File (http://www.MMF.com). This commercial vendor provides a document-management solution similar to software products that hospitals can purchase. They also employ trained personnel in India who conduct round-the-clock indexing of documents and can provide this indexing within minutes of receiving a faxed document. None of the data ever actually travel to India; rather, the operators in India have read-only access to documents and provide the indexing function within their developed system. All patient records remain in secure Web servers in the US. Additionally, My Medical File has a staff of phone operators based in Panama (all of whom speak fluent English) who remain in phone contact with surgeons' offices to help to track and manage the collation of necessary documents prior to surgery, illustrating a new era of technology profiled in the best-seller *The World Is Flat* by Thomas Freidman. Interestingly, one of the most intriguing aspects of this solution is the capability of creating the foundation of a personal health record that most recognize is a necessary component of our migration to EMRs.

Conclusion

While streamlining and standardizing the preoperative process has been shown to be of enormous benefit to hospitals and patients in terms of efficiency, safety, and cost, other areas of use for the preoperative setting may exist. Dr. Roizen has become a major proponent of the presurgical evaluation center as a center for wellness. Patients who undergo surgical procedures are vulnerable and more willing to listen to messages that relate to better health and wellness. By utilizing a modality such as HealthQuestionnaire, it is possible to add additional questions relating to colonoscopy evaluation, mammography, Pap smear screening, Zoster vaccination, and other diagnostics. Information output distributed to patients (and primary caregivers) can include helpful information about smoking cessation, as well as preventive diagnostics. The 21st century health institution must accept a proactive role in patient care in addition to its historic therapeutic role.

Key Points

- Current preoperative preparation processes vary significantly between various healthcare institutions and most are completely paper based.
- Comprehensive preoperative evaluation requires an extensive review of previous hospitalizations, medical conditions, and review of patient examination and diagnostic tests.
- Computerized patient evaluations are capable of providing a comprehensive review and correlation to rules-based algorithms for preoperative testing and preparation.
- Interfacing preoperative systems to other clinical systems provides real value and will be essential for successful adoption of these systems.

- Preoperative modules are unique components of an AIMS that frequently have multiple users with access and responsibility for data entry on each patient—a scenario that introduces new challenges and considerations.
- Improvements in hospital reimbursement remain an important driving force for the implementation of these systems.
- Incorporation of the Internet has great applicability in these systems and represents an opportunity to acquire data from patients and other healthcare providers in a timely fashion.

References

1. Parker B, Tetzlaff J, Litaker D, et al. Redefining the preoperative evaluation process and the role of the anesthesiologist. J Clin Anesth 2000; 12(5):350–6
2. Fischer SP. Development and effectiveness of an anesthesia preoperative evaluation clinic in a teaching hospital. Anesthesiology 1996; 85:196–206
3. Correll D, Bader A, Hull M, et al. Value of preoperative clinic visits in identifying issues with potential impact on operating room efficiency. Anesthesiology 2006; 105(6):1254–9
4. Gibby G. How preoperative assessment programs can be justified financially to hospital administrators. Int Anesthesiol Clin 2002; 40(2):17–29
5. Gibby GL, Paulus DA, Sirota DJ, et al. Computerized pre-anesthetic evaluation results in additional abstracted comorbidity diagnoses. J Clin Monit 1997; 13:35–41
6. Stonemetz J, Johns Hopkins Medical Institutions, Baltimore, MD. Personal Communication
7. Roizen M, Coalson D, Hayward RS, et al. Can patients use an automated questionnaire to define their current health status? Med Care 1992; 30(5 Suppl):MS74–84
8. Lutner RE. The automated interview versus the personal interview: Do patient responses to perioperative questions differ? Anesthesiology 1991; 75(3):394–400
9. Michota F, Frost S. The preoperative evaluation: Use the history and physical rather than routine testing. Cleve Clin J Med 2004; 71(1):63–70
10. Lucas RW, Card WI, Knill-Jones RP. Computer interrogation of patients. Br Med J 1976; 2(6036):623–5
11. Roizen M. Personal Communication
12. Pasternak R. *Preanesthesia Evaluation of the Surgical Patient*, Vol. 24. Philadelphia: The American Society of Anesthesiologists, 1996
13. Cleveland Clinic Foundation's PACE Clinic. Personal Communication
14. Maurer W, Borkowski R, Parker B. Quality and resource utilization in managing preoperative evaluation. Anesthesiol Clin North Am 2004; 24(1):155–75
15. Berthelsen C, Stilley KR. Automated personal health inventory or dentistry: Pilot study. J Am Dent Assoc 2000; 131(1):59–66
16. Bachman JW. The patient–computer interview: A neglected tool that can aid the clinician. Mayo Clin Proc 2003; 78(1):67–78
17. Gerbert B, Bronstone A, Pantilat S. When asked, patients tell: Disclosure of sensitive health-risk behaviors. Med Care 1999; 37(1):104–11
18. US Government. The Americans with Disabilities Act of 1990 (ADA). United States Public Law 101-336, 104 Stat. 327 (July 26, 1990)
19. Campbell KE. Distributed development of a logic-based controlled medical terminology. PhD Thesis, Stanford University, June 1997. http://www.informatics.com/Campbell-Dissertation.pdf. Accessed January 30, 2008
20. Rose JS, Kirkley D. Healthcare computer applications and the problem of language: A brief review. http://www.informatics-review.com/thoughts/cmt.html. Accessed January 30, 2008

21. Tsen LC, Segal S, Pothier M. The effect of alterations in a preoperative assessment clinic on reducing the number and improving the yield of cardiology consultations. Anesth Analg 2002; 95:1563–8
22. Vogt A, Henson L. Unindicated preoperative testing: ASA physical status and financial implications. J Clin Anesth 1997; 9:437–41
23. Weides S, Lutheran General Hospital, Park Ridge, IL. Personal Communication
24. MyGeisinger.org. Accessed January 30, 2008

Chapter 10
Intraoperative Charting Requirements

Nirav Shah and Michael O'Reilly

The first description of an automated intraoperative anesthesia recording machine was noted as early as 1934.[1] The device recorded tidal volume, FiO_2, and blood pressure. Since then, many attempts have been made to replace the paper record. One group even used video recording machines to record all of the information presented visually to an anesthesiologist from the monitor screens.[2] Despite the advances in computer and information technology, the paper record has endured as the medium of choice to document the intraoperative experience. The first modern anesthesia information systems were essentially intraoperative record keepers—with the ability to automatically capture physiologic data from monitors and other devices such as ventilators. From those humble beginnings, intraoperative record keepers have evolved into perioperative information systems that allow clinicians to manage the patient throughout the entire surgical experience.

Several drivers have contributed to this evolution in function. First, as data interfacing has become increasingly secure and prevalent, more physiologic monitoring is being automatically captured into the anesthesia record instead of being transcribed. Second, an enhanced understanding of anesthesia workflow by the AIMS vendors, in partnership with anesthesiology departments, has prompted these systems to become comprehensive anesthesia workflow tools rather than merely intraoperative record keepers. Finally, hospital leadership is looking to the ORs for revenue generation. The OR is well recognized as a financial engine that helps to drive the healthcare enterprise, and anesthesia is a key lubricant of this engine. As such, anesthesia information systems are incorporating more financially savvy functionality, and AIMS content is becoming more billing friendly.

Intraoperative charting represents an important piece of anesthesia workflow. However, without working in harmony with other pieces such as preoperative and postoperative charting, nursing documentation, billing, quality assurance, and patient tracking, AIMS do not provide a significant functional advance from their earliest systems. Fortunately, these workflow pieces are becoming increasingly integrated. The following will be discussed in this chapter: the information systems necessary to manage anesthesia workflow in the intraoperative space; the requirements for intraoperative charting to construct a comprehensive anesthesia record; modules that go beyond the charting requirements for the intraoperative record, as they are critical for intraoperative workflow; and the utility of these modules in creating an intraoperative record in a clinical scenario. Other chapters of this book will discuss charge capture, medication management, legal concerns, and decision support in more detail.

Information Systems and Anesthesia Workflow

Anesthesia workflow is designed to meet two parallel end points. Operationally, patients need to be moved efficiently throughout the perioperative system, beginning with the preoperative anesthesia consultation and continuing through the preoperative holding area, ORs, and postoperative care areas. Clinically, patients need to be adequately evaluated and managed throughout their experience. To do this, the right information must be available to the right person at the right time. Furthermore, the behaviors to meet these end points are now being reinforced at the federal level, with the inauguration of pay-for-performance metrics. Liability concerns are forcing healthcare providers to rethink how they document what they have done to protect themselves from malpractice claims. Information systems are considered valuable as risk-management tools.[3] As a result, AIMS implementations are being used to spur workflow re-engineering processes.

Several tools must work together for the re-engineering process to be successful. OR scheduling and resource utilization systems must interface or be integrated with intraoperative anesthesia systems to allow users to know when and where cases are scheduled and who is assigned to each case. Anesthesia H&P evaluations should be fully integrated with intraoperative record keepers. Ideally, surgical H&P evaluations should also be part of an integrated perioperative information system that includes anesthesia and surgical modules, as well as nursing assessments. As these evaluations contain significant overlap, common information should be shared across all of them. To optimize patient throughput and decentralize the availability of information, patient-tracking systems that display a patient's location and status are important tools that should be part of an AIMS. Interfacing with financial systems to easily generate a bill is important to make billing efficient. A reduction in charge lag and days in accounts receivable was demonstrated by the use of a system that automatically extracted billing elements from the EMR.[4] Finally, integrated quality assurance modules are necessary for quality improvement efforts. Only then will the completeness of quality assurance documentation increase. All of these systems must be integrated with the intraoperative record keeper, and they must work together to provide a common user experience. Because hospitals and other healthcare institutions will have existing systems and relationships with multiple vendors, the exact mechanisms by which these systems come together will vary, but a seamless user experience must be a common goal for all institutions that implement a system.

Intraoperative Charting: Basic Requirements

Usability

First and foremost, the electronic intraoperative charting software must be quick to learn and easy to use. The software should be touchscreen enabled. Screen design should be thoughtful—buttons must be large enough to accommodate fingers of all sizes, and layout should be designed to document with as few clicks as possible. Voice recognition has been used in the past in only limited situations but could be used more in the future as technology improves.[5] A viable standard is that a user should require approximately 1 hour of training to become familiar enough with the system to use it in a case, and 1 week to become proficient with its use and to teach someone else. Mass resistance to adoption of the system will be encountered if it is not well designed. Conversely, a well-designed and well-implemented system will be well accepted by users and can even be a recruiting and retention tool for prospective employees.

Human Factors Engineering

Although the latest generation of anesthesia machines is designed to hold monitors and keyboards in locations that facilitate charting, most anesthesia machines in use today were not built with intraoperative charting ergonomics as a top priority. However, clever use of swivel arms and keyboard trays can ensure that a keyboard and a monitor are in a comfortable location to both chart and administer anesthesia.

Anesthesia machines can accommodate hardware so that computer screens can be mounted on the left or right side of the machine, or even on top. The main advantage of mounting computer screens on the left side (nearest to the patient) of the anesthesia machine is the ability to simultaneously keep an eye on the patient (and surgeon) and document notations on the intraoperative record (Fig. 10.1). However, in many institutions, the physiologic monitors are installed on the right side of the machine because the patient is actively managed from the data on the physiologic monitor, and it is difficult to accommodate both monitors on one side. Mounting on the right side (away from the patient) allows the physiologic monitor to be on the left but makes it more difficult to actively manage the patient (i.e., mask ventilate) and document simultaneously. More important than choosing a mounting side is choosing the mounting device. Mounting arms should have enough range of motion so that users of all heights can comfortably access the screens. Arms should allow users flexibility in the lateral placement of the monitor. A mounting device with multiple joints that moves along multiple axes can make nearly any mounting location work. Ultimately, each institution will need to choose the most appropriate solution for its users.

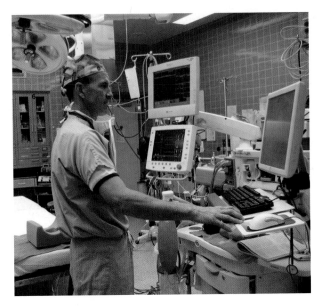

Fig. 10.1 An example of the AIMS monitor setup on the right side of the anesthesia machine, with the physiologic monitor on the left side of the anesthesia machine

Data Integration

An AIMS must be able to collect data output from the physiologic monitor. Handwritten records transcribed from the physiologic monitors have been shown to be less accurate than those generated by an AIMS and therefore less useful for research, quality assurance, and medicolegal purposes.[6,7] In addition, intraoperative paper records require more time to complete than electronic records.[8,9] At a bare minimum, basic hemodynamic and physiologic variables such as heart rate, blood pressure (both noninvasive and arterial), and pulse oximetry must be collected. In addition, gas analyzer data such as inspired and expired inhalational anesthetic concentrations, FiO_2, and end-tidal CO_2 should be interfaced. Ventilator data such as respiratory rate and tidal volume should also be interfaced. A host of other clinical variables such as laboratory results are used in anesthetic practice and would reduce transcription time if interfaced to the AIMS. A more complete list is presented in Table 10.1

Data Granularity

Data that are recorded in physiologic monitors can be either intermittent (e.g., noninvasive blood pressure taken at preset intervals) or continuous (e.g., arterial line blood pressure readings). For intermittent data, all data recorded by the monitor

Table 10.1 Interfaced physiologic variables

Heart rate (electrocardiographic monitoring and SpO_2)
Noninvasive blood pressure (systolic, diastolic, mean)
Arterial blood pressure (systolic, diastolic, mean)
$ETCO_2$
Bispectral index
Temperature
FiO_2 (ventilator)
Peak inspiratory pressure
Tidal volume
Minute volume
Respiratory rate (ventilator and $ETCO_2$)
Positive end-expiratory pressure
Pulmonary artery pressures (systolic, diastolic, mean)
Central venous pressure
Cardiac output
Cardiac index
SvO_2
Systemic vascular resistance
Nitrous oxide (inspired and expired concentrations)
Oxygen (inspired and expired concentrations)
Inhalational agents measured (inspired and expired concentrations)
Intracranial pressure
Flows—oxygen, air, nitrous oxide

should be captured by the intraoperative record keeper. If noninvasive blood pressure readings are taken every 3 minutes by the physiologic monitor, then they should be captured every 3 minutes by the AIMS. It is important that the AIMS does not collect data more frequently than does the physiologic monitor. This type of erroneous oversampling can lead to mistaken assumptions of how frequently data are captured. For continuous data, a balance must exist between the memory requirements of capturing all of the data in the AIMS and the clinical requirements of capturing enough information to present an accurate clinical picture. Arterial blood pressure readings may be sampled every second by the physiologic monitor, but the AIMS will capture arterial blood pressure readings at longer intervals. Storing every reading sampled by the physiologic monitor would consume an enormous amount of memory and provide little clinical utility. Currently, no standards have been defined, and AIMS capture data in a variety of intervals, from seconds to minutes. An institution should be aware of the interval of capture for data and satisfied that it meets clinical and/or research requirements.

Loss of Data

When data are automatically imported from the physiologic monitors to the AIMS, the expectation is that they will be imported 100% of the time. In reality, data occasionally fail to transfer from the physiologic monitor to the AIMS, either due to network or software issue. AIMS should have the ability to notify users if data are not being captured by the physiologic monitors. An icon or a message on the intraoperative screen is the clearest and most visible method by which to alert users. Automatic paging alerts are an effective alternate or supplemental technique. The user must be vigilant and aware of missing data. Failure to recognize loss of incoming data may increase medical liability.[10] In these cases, manual entry can be tedious but necessary.

Data Input

While the holy grail of interfacing every physiologic parameter is an ongoing pursuit, the necessity to manually input data continues to exist. In addition, some information that does not come from the monitors must be entered into the AIMS. Some of this information adds to the quality of the documentation; other items are mandated by regulatory or billing guidelines and must be part of the anesthetic record. A provision must be included in the AIMS to make a data item mandatory. For these items, the system should either (a) not allow the document to be completed (hard alert) or (b) allow the document to be completed but warn the user that the document is incomplete until the required item is entered (soft alert). Both types of alerts are necessary, but hard alerts should be used rarely and with extreme caution. Nothing is more frustrating for the user than encountering a hard alert when he is busy trying to manage the patient and document at the same time. On the other hand, the use of passive soft alerts, such as bolding or highlighting mandatory items, attracts the user's attention and facilitates consistent completion.

Data input falls into several categories:

1. Required documentation for billing or to meet regulatory guidelines

   (a)   Anesthesia and surgical times
   (b)   Machine check
   (c)   Confirmation of case, H&P review, and NPO status
   (d)   "Time-out" confirming patient, case, and side of surgical location with surgical and nursing colleagues
   (e)   Antibiotic dosing
   (f)   Patient disposition, such as transport to PACU or SICU

2. Routine and nonroutine clinical events that occur during the surgical case

   (a)   Induction events, such as laryngoscopic view or endotracheal tube placed
   (b)   Patient positioning
   (c)   IV lines placed
   (d)   Adverse events, such as bronchospasm and laryngospasm

3. Notes completed by the anesthetist during the case

   (a) Documentation for procedures, such as arterial lines or central venous lines

   (b) Specific documentation of difficult airway to be used for form letter to the patient

   (c) Notification of consults needed from the acute pain service for management of patient-controlled analgesia or for a patient with chronic pain

4. Clinical or physiologic data not captured by the physiologic monitors

   (a) Train-of-four counts

   (b) Fresh gas flows

   (c) Eye protection documented

   (d) Systolic pressure variation—the fluctuation of systemic arterial pressure induced by changes in intrathoracic pressure due to mechanical ventilation. Currently, physiologic monitors allow users to calculate systolic pressure variation from blood pressure waveform tracings, but typically, the number calculated must be manually entered into the intraoperative record keeper

5. Medications/fluids/infusions/blood products

   (a) Bolus medications, including antibiotics

   (b) Fluids, with amounts given and rates

   (c) Drug infusions, such as vasopressors or narcotics

   (d) Blood products, including cell-saver blood

6. Case times and modifiers

When the case is complete and all of the data have been entered into the system, the record should be closed, which can be triggered automatically by linking the closing of the record to the last item documented, such as the anesthesia end time. Alternatively, the system should have a button to close the record. After the record is closed, any additional items documented on the record should be highlighted as addendum information.

Data Display

The data that have been captured in the system, either automatically or by manual input, must be displayed clearly (Fig. 10.2). Most anesthesiologists prefer graphical views; however, tabular views must be available as well so that individual data points can be viewed.

Data Artifacts

The handling of data artifacts with intraoperative charting has been a controversial topic. An artifact can be the result of mechanical manipulation of the monitor, such as movement of the pulse oximeter, or it can be due to electrical interference (e.g., electrocautery) or equipment failure (Fig. 10.3). Certainly, if reviewers of the intra-operative chart are unaware that particular data in the AIMS are artifactual, they may have a completely different understanding of the case. Therefore, a method by which to mark an artifact and/or delete it from the record is absolutely necessary. Programs with algorithms designed to recognize artifacts and annotate clinical records have been described in the literature but are not in widespread use.[11,12] Nevertheless, an artifact must be recognized and either removed from the chart or annotated so that anyone reviewing the chart will clearly recognize it.

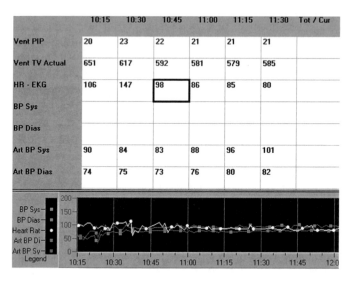

Fig. 10.2 Graphic and tabular view of data. Centricity Perioperative Anesthesia machine (General Electric Healthcare Information Technologies) (photo courtesy of GE Healthcare Information Technologies, Barrington, IL)

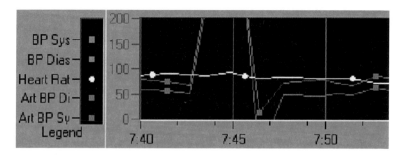

Fig. 10.3 Artifact in the blood pressure trend due to blood pressure sampling. Centricity Perioperative Anesthesia machine (General Electric Healthcare Information Technologies) (photo courtesy of GE Healthcare Information Technologies, Barrington, IL)

Audit Trails

All data entered into the intraoperative record should be time and user stamped. All commercially available systems include this capability. In addition, the user should be able to change the time of an event documented retrospectively without affecting the audit time stamp. Generally, users should not document prospectively because upcoming events cannot be documented with 100% certainty, and prospective charting is associated with medicolegal concerns.[13]

Terminology

Ideally, clinical data entered into the anesthetic record should be mapped to SNOMED CT (Systematized Nomenclature of Medicine–Clinical Terms), which is a controlled healthcare lexicon with comprehensive coverage of diseases, clinical findings, etiologies, therapies, procedures, and outcomes. Its benefits include facilitating system interoperability and allowing greater shared access to patient health information.[14] The use of standard terminology in intraoperative records allows the information (such as adverse events) to be transmitted more easily to other systems and facilitates retrospective review of data.

Intraoperative Charting: Advanced Features

Advanced features include templates, scripts, defaults, and other features that facilitate execution of practice guidelines to reduce variability and improve quality. For a system to alter behavior and truly improve clinical outcomes and prevent errors both in practice and documentation, decision-support features must be built into the software. *Decision support* refers to any information that a system provides to enable a user to better complete a task. When referring to AIMS, decision support can be as simple as a pop-up dialog box reminding users of the definition of the Malampatti classifications or as complex as dynamic protocols that change based on a patient's clinical condition.

Workflow engines are tools that allow a user to complete a task more efficiently. They can create pending work lists that tell anesthesiologists, among other things, notes that they must sign or patients whom they need to see. Workflow engines can send automatic pages to users, informing them of abnormal labs or test results for patients. They can also inform users of the status of upcoming patients (ready in preoperative holding, OR ready for patient, postoperative care area slot assigned for patient, etc.). Decision-support and workflow engines work together to analyze the data entered or interfaced and present them to the user in ways that improve clinical care or increase operational efficiency.

Decision-Support Systems

Current systems have relatively primitive decision-support systems (DSS)—usually in the scripts or templates, based on the type of case (Fig. 10.4). Cardiac anesthesia cases are managed differently from routine hysterectomies. Intraoperative templates take the various types of cases into account and enable best practices to be followed. Templates can significantly help institutions to follow practice guidelines.

Placing antibiotic dosing on case templates (in addition to physician-specific reminders) increased compliance with antibiotic administration from 69% to 92%.[15] Perhaps the most important use of decision support in the intraoperative setting is in medication delivery. Important features include:

- Dose-range checking
- Default drug doses based on patient weight
- Drug/allergy checking
- Drug/drug reaction checking

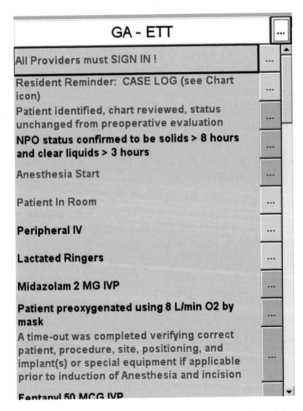

Fig. 10.4 Intraoperative case script. Centricity Perioperative Anesthesia machine (General Electric Healthcare Information Technologies) (photo courtesy of GE Healthcare Information Technologies, Barrington, IL)

AIMS should incorporate rules-based logic that actively monitors clinical variables and guides clinicians to provide standard of care. This decision support should include reminders and timers for important events such as antibiotic scheduled dosing, glucose measurement, normothermia, β-blocker therapy, and prophylaxis for deep venous thrombosis. One group demonstrated that antibiotic dosing reminders based on the specific antibiotic given increased appropriate dosing from 20% to 58%.[16] Critical conditions during procedures (e.g., light anesthesia or unstable blood pressure) can be detected using algorithms that convey messages to the user.[17] DSSs have also been used to help to predict postoperative nausea and vomiting based on clinical variables available in the electronic intraoperative record.[18] Clearly, these systems can make an enormous difference in the quality of care provided.

Workflow Engine

A workflow engine is a tool that sends notifications (based on system-created rules) to users that enable them to efficiently manage their patient. Typically, system administrators or vendors create the rules under clinical guidance. Rules are usually events that occur throughout the perioperative period, related to a patient, a provider, or both. Rules are then linked to notifications, which consist of two parts: what and who. The "what" is the type of notification—email, page, pop-up alert on screen, etc. The "who" is who is receiving it. Examples of rules with notifications include:

- If a patient's H&P is unsigned by an attending, send an email to the attending assigned to the case.
- If a postoperative note has not been documented, send a note to the pending work inbox of the resident or CRNA assigned to the case.
- If a patient's INR is >1.4 and the case is scheduled for the next day, send a page to the resident assigned to the case for the next day.
- If a user documented the need for an acute pain service consult for a patient, add the patient to the acute pain service census.

Although the output of workflow engines is not included in the intraoperative record, these tools are indispensable to the anesthetist in the intraoperative period when used judiciously. Numerous examples demonstrate that electronic reminders improve documentation compliance and professional fee reimbursement. One group demonstrated that pager reminders to document arterial line notes alone increased compliance from 80% to 98%, with an annualized incremental revenue of ~$40,000.[19] Another group showed similar success, reducing their percentage of unbillable records from 1.31% to 0.04% and increasing annual revenue by $400,000.[20] However, one must be extremely cautious when implementing alerts. When too many alerts are activated in a system, "alert fatigue" sets in, and users tend to blindly delete messages without reading them.

Patient Tracking

Perioperative environments are becoming increasingly complex, driven by an increase in the number of ORs and in level of surgical intricacy. As OR time becomes scarce, hospitals continue to add ORs as fast as they are allowed, with additional pressure to reduce turnaround times and increase patient throughput. Many times, blocks and lines are placed in the preoperative holding area to optimize OR time. In many hospitals, cases can run from complex thoracic or vascular cases on patients who are ASA 4 to straightforward urology cases on patients who are ASA 1. Thrown into this mix are practices that allow CRNAs and, sometimes, residents of varying skill levels to provide care for the patients. Added to this environment is a usually complicated system of breaks and relief.

In a facility with a relatively large numbers of ORs, managing this system can be an enormously complex task. The ability to see the real-time status of each OR and each patient within the system allows the person "running the floor" to manage cases and staffing in an efficient manner. Patient-tracking systems have developed from both OR scheduling and AIMS. At this writing, the trend is for anesthesia and scheduling systems to converge, which can allow patient-tracking software to use information from both systems.

Effective perioperative tracking systems allow the user (a) to view the location of the patient within the perioperative environment at any time during her stay and (b) to display information about the patient that allows the user to make efficient patient throughput and staffing decisions. Tracking systems can be either patient centric or location centric. Key features of an effective tracking system are listed in Table 10.2,

Table 10.2 Key features of an effective patient-tracking system

Preoperative
  View that graphically displays the preoperative holding area
  Ability to see patient's location within the preoperative holding area
  Ability to see if patient is ready for the OR
  Ability to see pending items if patient is not ready for the OR
  Automatic page to staff with patient's readiness status for the OR

Intraoperative
  View that graphically displays the operative rooms
  Ability to see in which room a patient is located
  Ability to see which anesthesia providers are assigned to the room
  Ability to see which surgeons are assigned to the room
  Ability to see the procedure that is being performed
  Ability to see stage of case (induction, incision, closing, complete but still in room, etc.)
  Ability to see if a room is open, closed, dirty, or in use
  Automatic page to staff with patient's readiness status for the PACU

Postoperative
  View that graphically displays the postoperative care area
  Ability to see patient's location within the postoperative care area
  Ability to see if a slot is open, closed, dirty, or in use
  Automatic page to staff with patient's readiness status for PACU discharge

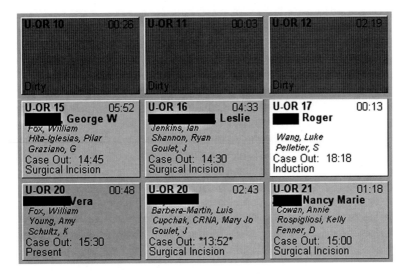

Fig. 10.5 Intraoperative tracking system. Centricity Perioperative Anesthesia machine (General Electric Healthcare Information Technologies) (photo courtesy of GE Healthcare Information Technologies, Barrington, IL)

an example of an intraoperative tracking system is provided in Fig. 10.5, and following are two examples of how tracking systems can improve efficiency.

Example 1. As experienced at most facilities, cases can substantially deviate from their predicted times. A case that is cut short or finished quickly can lead to substantial lag time in bringing the next patient into the OR area. When it is known that a case is ending early, a tracking system that allows intraoperative users to see whether the next patient is in the preoperative holding area and ready to go or still involved with pending items (arterial line, block, H&P, etc.) enables them to communicate more efficiently with the preoperative staff about what is needed to ensure that the next patient is ready on time.

Example 2. As cases start to wind down at the end of the day, many practices have developed a system of relief to send people home. A tracking system that displays each room in the operative area, with the procedure and status listed, enables the "floor runner" to begin assigning relief and determining an efficient method of closing rooms. What was previously accomplished by calling into or walking through each room is now accomplished by looking at the patient-tracking screen.

A caveat exists for these systems. The data displayed are only as good as the data entered. If providers are not diligent about entering the data, up-to-date data will not be available for viewing. Newer technology that uses radio-frequency identification is starting to be introduced in inpatient-tracking systems.[21] It is critically important that the intraoperative record keepers are integrated or interfaced to patient tracking to eliminate duplicate charting and to ensure that users are viewing accurate tracking information. When tracking systems are working well, they have been shown to increase efficiency, especially with PACU lengths of stay.[22]

Quality Assurance

Intraoperative charting can allow a user to easily describe adverse events that occur perioperatively. An integrated quality assurance (QA) module can give users a protected area to describe the exact circumstances of the event. Events documented in the intraoperative record should be listed in the QA module. The anesthesia provider can then provide exact details on the event to help the QA team in its analysis. Categories of QA occurrences should include adverse events that involve the following major categories: airway, cardiovascular, respiratory, neurologic, equipment failure, medication problems, integument problems, regional anesthesia issues.

Studies have shown that manual documentation tends to under-report the true number of adverse events that actually occur.[23] Using data that exist in the AIMS, advanced QA systems can automatically detect adverse events and enable institutions to accurately understand their complication rates. Private-practice anesthesiologists (and many academic physicians) tend to be skeptical about quality assurance programs because of the difficulty in documenting and maintaining data, the need for duplicate documentation to report adverse events (requirement to document the event in both the intraoperative record keeper and QA system), and the tendency for adverse events to be presented with no denominators. An integrated QA module can automatically gather and store data without duplicate documentation and can be an efficient source for performing outcomes research and providing feedback to individuals.[24]

Case Report: An Example of How an Automated Quality Assurance System Could Work

The patient is a 67-year-old male with history of coronary artery disease, diabetes mellitus, hypertension, chronic renal insufficiency, and peripheral vascular occlusive disease. He is scheduled for an aortobifemoral bypass. Dr. Smith enters the preoperative holding area at 6:30 a.m. and looks at the tracking screen at the nursing station. He sees that the patient is in slot 5, and the tracker indicates that the nursing assessment is complete but that the patient consent and the arterial line are still pending. He asks the clerk to page the surgeon to complete the consent form and then goes to see the patient.

Dr. Smith greets the patient and starts discussing his history. In the meantime, the nurses have already placed an IV and drawn blood. They send it to the lab to check the potassium level, which Dr. Smith ordered yesterday because of an automatic page that alerted him that the patient's potassium was 5.4. From the nursing assessment, the patient's allergies, home medications, and vital signs automatically fill in his assessment. Online, Dr. Smith can see the patient's previous H&P from his cystoscopy 2 months prior next to the current H&P, and he automatically copies the information that has not changed into the new H&P. He adds the new information to the H&P and prepares to place the arterial line. In the meantime, the surgeon completes the consent form, and the status on the patient tracker reflects this. Dr. Smith inserts the arterial line. Meanwhile, the potassium level comes back as 4.6. The patient is now ready to go. The nurse changes the status on the patient tracker to "ready."

The patient is transported to the OR. As soon as Dr. Smith walks to the anesthesia machine, he clicks "patient in room" in the intraoperative record. The status of the tracker automatically changes. Monitors are applied to the patient, and anesthesia is induced. Cefazolin is given as antibiotic prophylaxis. As it is being documented in the system, the dose checker suggests giving 2 g instead of 1 g because of the patient's weight. An extra gram of cefazolin is given per the antibiotic dosing guidelines. The anesthesia team then places a pulmonary arterial catheter in the right internal jugular vein. Surgery commences. As events occur, they are documented on the intraoperative record, usually by the user tapping on the screen or using a mouse. Physiologic variables, including heart rate, blood pressures, SaO_2, ventilator settings, and inhalational agent concentrations, are automatically captured by the system. Train-of-four counts and fluids administered must be entered manually in the record keeper.

During the case, Dr. Smith receives an automatic page stating that he did not complete the arterial line note. He completes it in the AIMS, and the department can now bill for the procedure. Later, he realizes that the patient's blood pressure and heart rate are rising. He notices that the vaporizer is empty even though he just filled it in the morning, and no warning was given by the anesthesia machine. Moreover, he can smell agent. He deduces that the vaporizer is defective. He quickly switches it with another and documents the equipment failure in the intraoperative record. It flows automatically to the QA module, where Dr. Smith can explain in detail the circumstances surrounding the failure for review by the QA committee.

A little while later, the patient begins bleeding profusely and becomes hypotensive. Dr. Smith starts the rapid infuser to deliver blood and starts vasopressors. For 20–30 min, he is busy taking care of the patient. However, all of the physiologic data are being automatically captured by the system. When the patient is stabilized, all Dr. Smith retrospectively charts is the medications that he has given to the patient. Toward the end of the case, Dr. Smith looks at the patient tracker and sees that the next patient is in the preoperative holding area but still needs an epidural placed. Dr. Smith knows that if the epidural is not placed soon, the next case may be delayed. He pages the preoperative team and apprises them of the situation. They move Dr. Smith's next patient to the top of their list and place the epidural.

As the surgeons are closing the incision, a page is automatically sent to the recovery room, stating the status of the OR. However, the nurses already know the status because the tracker indicates that the surgeons are closing. The recovery room is full, but they make an extra effort to move a patient to phase 2 and prepare a slot. After the patient is extubated without difficulty and transported to the recovery room, Dr. Smith completes the handoff to the nurses. He looks at the tracker and sees that his next patient is in slot 7. The process begins again.

Conclusion

An intraoperative charting system can be a powerful tool when it is well designed and well implemented—a tool that anesthetists realize truly transforms the way perioperative care is provided. Unfortunately, the converse is also true: these systems can be sources of constant aggravation and contribute to poor patient care when they are poorly designed and implemented. The best systems work in close conjunction with other perioperative and hospital-wide information systems, and they allow extraction of data so that institutions can use the data stored within to continually improve care. Although these types of systems have been around for several decades, only now are they beginning to achieve a critical mass of offered features, reliability, integration, and usability that allow widespread usage in both academic and community settings. Over time, electronic intraoperative charting will be as ubiquitous as propofol; however, that day is still years away. In the meantime, institutions and vendors must work closely together to continually improve these systems.

Key Points

- The prevalence of AIMS implementations is increasing because the benefits are now more widely described and ORs are seen as financial engines within the healthcare enterprise. However, paper continues to be the most popular medium of choice for the intraoperative record.
- Intraoperative record keepers are most effective in improving anesthesia workflow when they are used with preoperative and postoperative charting, nursing documentation, billing, QA, and patient tracking.
- The intraoperative record module must be easy to use. A viable standard is that a user should require 1 hour of training to become familiar enough with the system to use it in a case.
- Touchscreen monitors for documenting the intraoperative record can be mounted in any of several ways. Ultimately, it is an institutional decision.
- Data input must be possible for all types of categories (whether required documentation for billing or to meet regulatory guidelines): interfaced physiologic variables, clinical or physiologic data not captured by the physiologic monitors, confirmation of case coordination with surgical documentation, routine and nonroutine clinical events that occur during the surgical case, notes completed by the anesthesiologist during the case, medications/fluids/infusions, blood products, case times, and modifiers.
- Data must be able to be viewed in both graphic and tabular format—graphic format for trends and tabular format for individual data points.
- The system must allow artifacts to be recognized and either removed from the chart or annotated so that anyone reviewing the chart will clearly recognize them.

- Use of standard terminology in intraoperative records allows the information (such as adverse events) to be transmitted more easily to other systems and facilitates retrospective review of data.
- For a system to alter behavior, truly improve clinical outcomes, and prevent errors both in practice and documentation, decision-support features must be built into the software and work as part of the AIMS.
- Effective perioperative tracking systems allow the user to view the location of the patient within the perioperative environment at any time during her stay, and they display information about the patient that allows the user to make decisions regarding patient throughput and staffing efficiency.

References

1. McKesson EI. The technique of recording the effects of gas-oxygen mixtures, pressures, rebreathing and carbon-dioxide, with a summary of the effects. Curr Res Anesth Anal 1934; 13(1):1–14
2. Piepenbrink JC, Cullen JI, Jr, Stafford TJ. A real-time anesthesia record keeping system using video. J Clin Eng 1990; 15(5):391–3
3. Feldman JM. Do anesthesia information systems increase malpractice exposure? Results of a survey. Anesth Analg 2004; 99(3):840–3
4. Reich DL, Kahn RA, Wax D, et al. Development of a module for point-of-care charge capture and submission using an anesthesia information management system. Anesthesiology 2006; 105(1):179–86
5. Sanjo Y, Yokoyama T, Sato S, et al. Ergonomic automated anesthesia recordkeeper using a mobile touch screen with voice navigation. J Clin Monit Comput 1999; 15(6):347–56
6. Reich DL, Wood RK, Jr, Mattar R, et al. Arterial blood pressure and heart rate discrepancies between handwritten and computerized anesthesia records. Anesth Analg 2000; 91(3):612–6
7. Thrush DN. Are automated anesthesia records better? J Clin Anesth 1992; 4(5):386–9
8. Wang X, Gardner RM, Seager PR. Integrating computerized anesthesia charting into a hospital information system. Int J Clin Monit Comput 1995; 12(2):61–70
9. Edsall DW, Deshane P, Giles C, et al. Computerized patient anesthesia records: Less time and better quality than manually produced anesthesia records. J Clin Anesth 1993; 5(4):275–83
10. Vigoda MM, Lubarsky DA. Failure to recognize loss of incoming data in an anesthesia record-keeping system may have increased medical liability. Anesth Analg 2006; 102(6):1798–802
11. Gostt RK, Rathbone GD, Tucker AP. Real-time pulse oximetry artifact annotation on computerized anaesthetic records. J Clin Monit Comput 2002; 17(3–4):249–57
12. Hoare SW, Beatty PC. Automatic artifact identification in anaesthesia patient record keeping: A comparison of techniques. Med Eng Phys 2000; 22(8):547–53
13. Vigoda MM, Lubarsky DA. The medicolegal importance of enhancing timeliness of documentation when using an anesthesia information system and the response to automated feedback in an academic practice. Anesth Analg 2006; 103(1):131–6
14. Elevitch FR. SNOMED CT: Electronic health record enhances anesthesia patient safety. AANA J 2005; 73(5):361–6
15. O'Reilly M, Talsma A, VanRiper S, et al. An anesthesia information system designed to provide physician-specific feedback improves timely administration of prophylactic antibiotics. Anesth Analg 2006; 103(4):908–12
16. St Jacques P, Sanders N, Patel N, et al. Improving timely surgical antibiotic prophylaxis redosing administration using computerized record prompts. Surg Infect (Larchmt) 2005; 6(2):215–21
17. Krol M, Reich DL. Development of a decision support system to assist anesthesiologists in operating room. J Med Syst 2000; 24(3):141–6

18. Junger A, Hartmann B, Benson M, et al. The use of an anesthesia information management system for prediction of antiemetic rescue treatment at the postanesthesia care unit. Anesth Analg 2001; 92(5):1203–9
19. Kheterpal S, Gupta R, Blum JM, et al. Electronic reminders improve procedure documentation compliance and professional fee reimbursement. Anesth Analg 2007; 104(3):592–7
20. Spring SF, Sandberg WS, Anupama S, et al. Automated documentation error detection and notification improves anesthesia billing performance. Anesthesiology 2007; 106(1):157–63
21. Marjamaa RA, Torkki PM, Torkki MI, et al. Time accuracy of a radio-frequency identification patient tracking system for recording operating room timestamps. Anesth Analg 2006; 102(4):1183–6
22. Meyer MA, Sokal SM, Sandberg W, et al. INCOMING!—A web tracking application for PACU and post-surgical patients. J Surg Res 2006; 132(2):153–8
23. Benson M, Junger A, Fuchs C, et al. Using an anesthesia information management system to prove a deficit in voluntary reporting of adverse events in a quality assurance program. J Clin Monit Comput 2000; 16(3):211–7
24. Edsall DW. Quality assessment with a computerized anesthesia information management system (AIMS). Qual Rev Bull 1991; 17(6):182–93

Chapter 11
Medication Management

R. Lebron Cooper and Alan Merry

Management of medications in the OR is a topic of special interest that has surfaced in recent years. Historically, pharmacists seldom had much interaction with anesthesiologists and frequently "relinquished" control of most medications used by anesthesiologists. Controlled substances, defined as Schedule II–V by the US Drug Enforcement Agency (DEA), have been controlled in different ways at different institutions, with no standardized system established across the country. Other medications used in the OR were typically stored as "floor stock," a method of maintaining a stock of medication vials that was replenished when the stock ran low. Pharmacy (and occasionally anesthesia) technicians simply filled a bin of medications when it needed replenishing. These systems had limited inventory control, frequently inaccurate methods of billing and tracking, no automatic reordering, and few internal safeguards. Anesthesiologists retrieved the medications that they intended to administer, recorded what they gave on handwritten anesthesia records, and wasted excess drug, with no pharmacist review of the order, dispensing, or administration of the medication.

Recent advances in medication management have allowed anesthesiologists and pharmacists to work together as a team. Current systems allow pharmacists to control certain medications, track medications given, reorder stock more accurately to reduce overall inventory costs, bill accurately for medications used, and build safeguards into the system to prevent or reduce medication error and adverse drug events.

One by one, hospitals are abandoning nonstandardized, manual, medication-management systems and are looking to automation to help with the challenges faced in managing medications in the OR. Anesthesiologists are the only physicians who prescribe/order a medication, dispense the medication, and administer the medication without pharmacist review of orders before dispensing. Even a final "check" in the medication process is eliminated in anesthesia, as the prescriber (rather than a nurse, as in most other specialties) actually administers the medication. This lack of pharmacist review and nurse check results in the loss of an inherent safety feature built into most medication-administration systems, and may make medication errors and adverse drug events more likely in anesthesia. Because of the nature and potency of the medications frequently used by anesthesiologists, these errors can result in significant harm or even death.

J. Stonemetz, K. Ruskin (eds.) *Anesthesia Informatics,*
© Springer Science+Business Media, LLC 2008

The "Five Rights" of Medication Administration

The Joint Commission has defined "five rights" of medication administration, as listed below.[1] The expected outcome of following the five rights would be that the correct results are achieved. It is the responsibility of each individual involved in patient care to adhere to the "five rights" to reduce the risk of medication error:

1. Right patient
2. Right dose
3. Right medication
4. Right time
5. Right administration route

This chapter will include a discussion of the goals of medication management and solutions to the problems encountered. The goals include:

- Management of controlled substances that meets DEA requirements and reduces diversion
- Control of high-cost medications
- Reduction of medication error and avoidance of inadvertent administration of incorrect drugs or doses
- Automated alerts to notify the practitioner of an error about to be made
- "Hard stops" that prevent an incorrect medication, if selected inadvertently, from reaching a patient
- Accurate billing, inventory control, and cost reduction
- Automated reordering of medications from wholesalers

Solutions to the problems in medication management use various components of automated products, including the automated anesthesia electronic record, automated anesthesia medication-dispensing carts, barcoding technology, automated recording of medications administered, and AIMS. We will first consider the Joint Commission standards on medication management and the extent and nature of the problem of medication error and adverse drug events.

Joint Commission Standards

In 2004, The Joint Commission issued new standards for medication management in the healthcare setting that place a greater emphasis on medication safety than did the previous standards.[2] Since 2004, Joint Commission surveys have included a 1-hour review of medication-management practices with key members of the medication-management team, which typically includes pharmacists, hospital administrators, a representative from the pharmacy and therapeutics committee, a representative from the medication safety committee (if one exists), the medication safety officer (if one exists), and nursing representatives. Anesthesiologists are frequently asked to participate, as medication management in the OR belongs under their purview. Recent Joint Commission surveys have specifically targeted anesthesia medication management in the OR,[3] and if no system is in place to achieve safe medication practices at a given facility, it is at risk of losing accreditation. Twenty-five key elements of The Joint Commission standards apply to hospitals. Of these, 14 specifically relate to the responsibilities of anesthesiologists and OR medication management. They are as follows:

Patient-specific information
MM.1.10: patient-specific information is readily accessible to those involved in the medication-management system.

Selection and procurement
MM.2.20: medications are properly and safely stored.
MM.2.30: emergency medications and/or supplies, if any, are consistently available, controlled, and secured.

Ordering and transcribing
MM.3.10: only medications that are necessary to treat the patient's condition are ordered, provided, or administered.

Preparing and dispensing
MM.4.10: all prescriptions or medication orders are reviewed for appropriateness.
MM.4.20: medications are prepared safely.
MM.4.30: medications are labeled.
MM.4.40: medications are dispensed safely.

Administration
MM.5.10: medications are safely and accurately administered.
MM.5.20: self-administered medications are safely and accurately administered (IV, PCA, or PCEA).

Monitoring
MM.6.10: the effects of medication(s) on patients are monitored.
MM.6.20: the hospital responds to actual or potential adverse drug events and medication errors.
MM.7.10: the hospital develops processes for managing high-risk or high-alert medications.

Two other standards address hospital responsibilities in (a) procurement of medications based on particular criteria (MM.2.10), which is usually done by formulary committees, many of which have anesthesiologists as members and (b) the requirement that hospitals evaluate their medication-management system (MM.8.10), a task frequently completed in the OR by anesthesiologists rather than pharmacists.

In that most of the requirements of Joint Commission accreditation relative to the management of medications specifically relate to anesthesia practice, all anesthesiologists who are assigned to the OR should have a good working knowledge of these requirements to ensure that a facility retains its accreditation.[4]

Medication Error and Adverse Drug Events

A number of best practice guidelines for medication use have been published by medical societies and regulatory agencies.[5-7] Adverse drug events can result in severe morbidity and mortality, and this issue has received a considerable amount of attention in the general media, as well as in the legal arena.[8,9] In the ASA Closed Claims Project, a review of legal claims made and closed/settled cases against anesthesiologists in the US, reviewers judged the care to be "less than appropriate" in 84% of drug-error claims, a substantially higher percentage than the 35% for nondrug-error claims.[10] Payments were made to plaintiffs in 72% of the drug-error claims compared to 52% of the nondrug-error claims. Drug administration errors frequently resulted in serious problems, including death in 24% and major morbidity in 34% of cases reviewed by the ASA Closed Claims Project. It is estimated that the annual cost of drug-related errors for a 700-bed teaching hospital approaches $2.8 million.

Sources Medication Error

Bowdle reported on the different types of drugs involved in medication error, the largest category of which (22%) included insulin, heparin, protamine, and others (Fig. 11.1).[10] Succinylcholine and inhalational agents followed closely behind, with 17.1 and 13.2% of errors, respectively. Opioids were involved in nearly 12% of

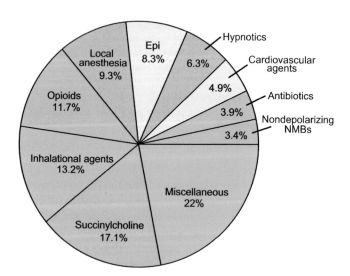

Fig. 11.1 Types of drugs involved in medication errors. The miscellaneous category includes insulin, potassium chloride, heparin, protamine, and others. *Epi* epinephrine, *NMB* neuromuscular blocker (from Bowdle TA. Drug administration errors from the ASA Closed Claims Project, *ASA Newsletter* 2003, with permission)

errors, with local anesthetics involved in 9.3%. Of note, epinephrine and other cardiovascular agents combined for a total of 13.2%. The fact that all of the drugs reported in these groups can be associated with either major morbidity or death suggests that 86.5% of all errors in these cases could have resulted in significant harm to patients. Methods to prevent these errors from reaching patients are desperately needed.

Research has shown that anesthetic records are often unreliable, contributing to anesthetic incidents.[11] A systematic review of the error-prevention literature in anesthesia regarding medication management identified the following strategies as "strongly recommended":

1. Carefully check vial/ampule before drawing up or administering drug.
2. Optimize syringe label legibility and apply standards, e.g., class color.
3. Properly label syringes.
4. Formally and orderly organize drug drawers and workspace. Manage proximity of similar and dangerous drugs.
5. Second person or device should validate drug before drawing up or administering.[12]

How Big Is the Problem?

Drug-related errors have been estimated to occur in one out of five doses given to patients in hospitals. It was estimated that one drug error was reported per 133 anesthetics when facilitated voluntary reporting was used in two academic hospital environments.[13] The most frequent errors were dose errors (20%) and drug substitutions (20%). Most errors (63%) involved IV boluses, 20% involved infusions, and 15% involved inhalational agents.

A recent MEDMARX Data Report (generated with an anonymous, Internet-accessible program used by hospitals and related institutions nationwide to report, track, and analyze medication errors) states that perioperative patients face an increased risk of harmful medication errors throughout the surgery process due to a lack of comprehensive oversight of medications.[14] The largest known national analysis of perioperative medication errors, the MEDMARX report examined more than 11,000 medication errors in the perioperative setting and revealed that 5% of the errors resulted in harm, including four deaths. This percentage of harm is more than three times higher than the percentage of harm among all MEDMARX records. Children are at higher risk than are adults for harm in the perioperative setting, with nearly 12% of pediatric medication errors resulting in harm.

Several studies have addressed the contributing factors of medication error.[13,15,16] Failure to check has been reported as the most common cause of medication error in anesthesia (17% of errors). Other causes include distraction (multitasking), inattention, haste or pressure to prepare, communication problems, incorrect labels, fatigue, unfamiliar work place or equipment, staff change/relief, similarity of vials, inexperience, and inadequate knowledge.[15]

Drug infusions may cause another host of errors. Incorrect calculations in concentration, mixing, and infusion rate, and incompatible drugs given in the same IV cannula are the most common errors.[15] It was estimated that ~50% of incidents may be caused by equipment errors (including inaccurate programming of the infusion pump), malfunctions in equipment, and poor equipment design (including lack of limits in some infusion devices).[15] Consequences of infusion errors may be grave: fatal errors with opioid infusions have been reported.[16]

Medication Errors, Adverse Drug Events, and Near Misses

An *error* is defined as the unintentional use of a wrong plan to achieve an aim, or failure to carry out a planned action as intended.[16,17] A *medication error* is defined as an error in prescribing, dispensing, or administering a medication. An *adverse drug event* is defined as any injury related to the use of a drug. A *near miss* (or "pre-error") is defined as any error that was intercepted prior to affecting the patient; an example would be attaching the wrong syringe to the IV port but realizing immediately prior to injection that it does not contain the intended drug. Pre-errors are under-reported, perhaps because of some confusion between errors and pre-errors. Picking up the wrong syringe may be considered so commonplace as not to warrant reporting.

Classification of Medication Error

A universal classification system for medication errors does not exist, and some errors may fit into more than one category. In anesthesia practice, giving a wrong drug may be a prescribing error (wrong drug was selected) or an administration error (wrong syringe was selected). Most anesthesia medication errors fit into the following few categories[16]:

- Omission (drug not given)
- Repetition (extra dose of intended drug given)
- Substitution (wrong drug)
- Insertion (wrong time – either too early or too late)
- Incorrect dose (wrong dose or infusion rate)
- Incorrect route (e.g., IV medications given in an epidural catheter)
- Incorrect patient

Reporting of Medication Errors

Voluntary reporting systems underestimate the actual incidence of medication error.[18] Participants may fail to report because of fear of malpractice litigation and punitive repercussions, or simply because they do not know that they have erred. Observational studies in critical care settings have consistently shown a higher incidence of medication error than that revealed in studies based on voluntary reporting.[19] To date, no reliable system of mandatory reporting has been found. Some AIMS have incorporated a function that requires a mandatory response in relation to medication error prior to exiting the system; however, the reporting of specific errors is still at the discretion of the provider. Educating providers may afford an outstanding opportunity to improve patient safety through reducing adverse drug events.

The Pharmacist–Anesthesiologist Liaison

Pharmacists are charged with the responsibility of all medication-management oversight and control by regulatory agencies and state licensing boards. They typically are active members of hospital pharmacy and therapeutics committees, formulary committees, and medication safety committees, and an organization's medication safety officer is frequently a pharmacist. Pharmacists order, check, acquire, track, and account for all medications administered in a hospital setting and are usually charged with the oversight of automated dispensing machines throughout the facility, which includes inventory control, managing stock, reordering drugs, and verifying reports. The facility's license to dispense controlled substances is usually issued in the name of the director of the pharmacy, who is responsible for ensuring that all controlled substances (DEA Schedules II–V) are accounted for, to the milliliter, during the entire flow throughout the medication-administration process, thus correcting discrepancies and accounting for and addressing diversions.

In addition to dispensing medications as ordered by physicians, pharmacists are important players in the verification process to ensure that a medication order is without error. However, this natural "safety net" is lost when it comes to the practice of anesthesiology. Pharmacists are seldom trained in the pharmacology of anesthesia medications, and anesthesiologists are seldom trained in pharmacy processes and regulations. However, the process of medication management can only be achieved accurately in all medication classes in all areas of the facility through collaboration between the pharmacist and anesthesiologist. Several hospitals in the US have addressed this need of collaboration by designating pharmacy–anesthesiology liaisons.[20] These individuals meet frequently to discuss situational issues and medication process flow and planning, and they work closely together to ensure any automated product, whether an AIMS or automated medication-dispensing system, is adequately designed and implemented. They focus primarily on strategies to control medications, monitor look-alike vial locations to prevent them from being located in close proximity, readjust par levels to meet clinical need without experiencing waste due to expiration of drugs, and actively manage users of the systems, supporting them with education, training, monitoring, compliance issues, and password assignments for protection and security. Pharmacists and anesthesiologists must work together to ensure maximum medication-management benefit, and the knowledge and experience of both specialists working in collaboration may result in a substantial reduction of medication errors in the anesthesia setting.

How Can Automation Solve the Medication-Management Challenge?

Computerized physician order entry is often cited as substantially improving patient safety.[19] Two inpatient studies have found that approximately half of medication errors occur at the stage of drug ordering,[21,22] although direct observation studies have indicated that many errors also occur at the administration stage.[23] The Leapfrog Group, a consortium of companies from the Business Roundtable, has endorsed computerized physician order entry in hospitals as one of the three changes that would most improve patient safety in America.[24] However, in anesthesia practice, the provider typically "prescribes" the drug by a "decision," then "dispenses" the medication by selecting it from a tray, syringe, or automated dispensing system. Because anesthesia is the only field of medicine that has neither pharmacist review of orders prior to dispensing drugs nor nursing verification prior to administering them, other ways to prevent prescribing and dispensing errors are being sought in the form of automation products.

Anesthesia Information Management Systems

The advantages of an AIMS have been described in previous chapters. One important advantage is how the AIMS can assist in medication management and the reduction of medication error in the OR. Each AIMS has its own advantages and disadvantages; however, most have not optimized their potential for medication management in the anesthesia environment. Most AIMS have been designed for automated record keeping of vital signs, documentation of medications administered, events, and provider notes with times, where relevant. Few have specifically addressed the need for facilitating medication management or the reduction of medication error, even though many have features that actually do just that.

For instance, most AIMS can generate an automated alert to the provider that a prophylactic antibiotic has not been administered within 1 hour prior to surgical incision (some systems require the user to record the surgical incision time for this purpose, but others operate on automated algorithms, such as prompting the provider if the antibiotic has not been given within 5 minutes of the beginning of anesthesia induction). Failure to administer the antibiotic during the specified window is a medication error of omission. Various automated alerts of this type can be customized to trigger action by the anesthesia provider that will reduce certain types of errors that are due to the provider simply forgetting, perhaps because of multitasking or losing concentration.

Most AIMS can provide electronic preoperative assessment tools that include patient home medications and allergies. Simple interfaces within the system allow prepopulation of these data to the intraoperative anesthesia record, reducing "transcription" error. Alerts can be customized to warn the anesthesia provider that a medication about to be administered is contraindicated due to allergy or drug–drug interactions. An EMR that can be accessed in real time or retrospectively helps to meet regulatory standards that require medication reconciliation between different areas or providers of a facility. It also allows for a consistent method of providing patients with a current medication list that also meets regulatory requirements.

Even with these advantages enabled by an AIMS, all AIMS are fraught with challenges. Only in a very few situations does full interfacing with a hospital's patient information system exist. Laboratory and radiographic data entry is still largely a manual process, and transcription errors may result. Most AIMS, although capable of providing files in such formats as PDF (portable document format) to the hospital's information system, do not interface directly with the patient's EMR. Simple interfaces, such as ADT interfaces (which provide admission, discharge, transfer data), do exist and offer the advantage of prepopulating the AIMS with vital patient data. However, these interfaces do not typically include patient clinical data, medications, or allergies. No one system yet offers all of the necessary interfacing capability to capture a complete patient experience and medication trail. Manual systems are still relied upon to complete this process.

Automated alerts can be customized to notify the anesthesia provider of drug–drug interactions, the need for perioperative or intraoperative beta blockade, or patient allergy to medications administered. One problem associated with this alert mechanism is that most AIMS require manual entry of the medication administered, which relies on the correct timing and documentation by the provider. By the time the information is manually entered into the AIMS (predominately a retrospective charting function), the administration of the medication has already occurred. Alerts designed to warn providers concerning drug–drug interactions or patient allergies to a medication may not be effective in this scenario.

Which AIMS?

Despite all of the published literature on medication error in anesthesia, only two AIMS, both of which are commercially available, have been designed specifically with medication management and reduction of medication error in mind.[25,26] The SaferSleep System (Safer Sleep, LLC, Nashville, TN) and the DocuSys System (DocuSys, Inc., Mobile, AL) offer the advantage of tracking administered medications with the use of barcode scanning devices. (Other AIMS do not currently offer a verification solution, and none has an integrated barcode scanner.) While the two systems differ somewhat in design, each involves scanning a syringe with a previously attached barcode label. The AIMS can then identify the drug administered, automatically document the drug name, amount, time of administration, and (in the case of DocuSys) dose given, and provide user prompts to assist with checking the details of the administered drug. The barcodes typically include information such as drug name and concentration, thereby reducing administration errors at the point of patient contact prior to administration and offering the possibility of computerized announcement of drug names, customized alerts of high-risk medications, and/or preprogrammed dose-range limits to prevent inadvertent overdose of a medication. To a greater or lesser degree, each system is multifaceted and includes other features designed to reduce drug administration error or to promote the safety of anesthesia in various other ways. Also, by identifying the drug administered, a patient-specific pharmacy charge can be sent to the hospital information system for accurate billing and charge capture.

Both systems rely on user compliance with the system—notably, a "manual" scan of the barcoded syringe prior to drug administration (SaferSleep) or the manual use of an additional cartridge device that holds the syringe, which allows the barcode scanner to automatically detect the amount (in milliliters) of drug administered by relative distance of syringe plunger movement (DocuSys). Although manual workarounds are still possible with either system, they both meet the goal of final verification of the medication prior to administration. Both systems also have advantages and disadvantages in relation to how the syringes are initially barcoded. The SaferSleep System uses barcoded labels, much like the current medication labels used in anesthesia practice (Fig. 11.2). These are ideally applied by the pharmacy or a registered pharmaceutical manufacturer so that drugs are provided in prefilled, prelabeled syringes; however, for flexibility and economy, an alternative is that the anesthesia provider affixes the labels to the syringes once they are filled. Obviously, user error can still occur at this stage if the medication vial or the barcoded label is misread. If a barcoded label is affixed to the wrong medication, final verification is inaccurate. Procedural practice rules can minimize this problem and must be followed.

The DocuSys System comes with a prebarcoded, syringe-loaded cartridge (SLC) that is dispensed with the vial of drug (Fig. 11.3). Although this strategy may reduce errors in reading labels, it will only do so if the SLC and the vial of drug are packaged together correctly by the pharmacy. A disadvantage is the size of the SLC. Although smaller in length than a 10-mL syringe, it is bulky, presenting storage space challenges in dispensing these syringes along with the medication vial. In addition, pharmacies are required to package the SLC and vial together prior to placing them in a dispensing location for the anesthesia provider, resulting in an increase in pharmacy labor costs. An option for off-site preparation and storage of the kits does exist. A reduction in medication error with this type of "verification" prior to drug administration has not been shown in a prospective, randomized, controlled study, but early reports based on facilitated incident reporting appear promising.[27]

Reliably prepared and labeled prefilled syringes clearly remove a significant opportunity for error. A variety of vendors offer prefilled syringes, such as the IntelliFill system (ForHealth Technologies, Inc., Daytona Beach, FL) that is used in many hospital pharmacies.[28] However, this solution may pose more problems

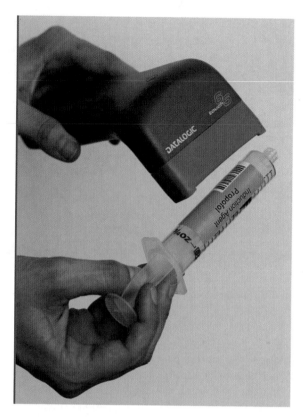

Fig. 11.2 Barcoded labels of the SaferSleep System (photo courtesy of SaferSleep LLC, Nashville, TN)

than it solves. In some cases, prefilled syringes are usually held for only 24 hours prior to their expiration, and costs will escalate with significant drug waste. In other cases (SaferSleep), stability data are available that allow a shelf-life of up to 6 months for many drugs. The dispensing system used must accommodate the filled syringe (consider the plunger length when fully extended), and it must be completely replenished and stocked by the pharmacy every day, resulting in increased pharmacy labor costs. Most centers have abandoned this approach as simply undesirable, which is unfortunate. Prefilled syringes offer a true example of engineering at least some error out of the system for drug administration in anesthesia, and the problems can all be solved to a greater or lesser degree. Currently, four premixed infusion drugs are commercially available in the US; they eliminate the possibility of a concentration "mixing" error and resultant administration (incorrect dose) error. The ideal solution is probably to provide a selection of drugs in prefilled syringes, choosing these on the basis of frequency of use, shelf-life data, and potential for harm, and incorporating the use of commercially available "premixed" infusion drugs to eliminate the possibility of a dosing error due to incorrectly

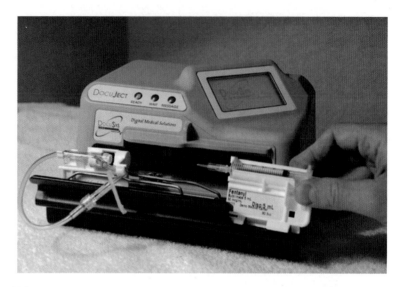

Fig. 11.3 The DocuSys System prebarcoded, syringe-loaded cartridge that is dispensed with the vial of drug (photo courtesy of DocuSys, Inc., Mobile, AL)

diluted concentrations. Certain drugs (such as concentrated potassium chloride) should probably not be provided in this format and, indeed, should be kept in a remote location from the other drugs commonly used in anesthesia. Some infusions (such as insulin) may be only provided from pharmacy-prepared stock, further reducing mixing errors.

Thus, AIMS, in general, have capabilities that help to decrease the incidence of some prescription errors (alerts or computerized announcements), some administration errors (verification of drug given, preprogrammed dose limits, etc.), and some dispensing errors (through the provision of prefilled syringes). However, none of the AIMS currently on the market completely addresses dispensing errors. The following section introduces automated products that have been designed to address this area of medication management.

Automated Medication-Dispensing Systems

Automated medication-dispensing systems were introduced into the US healthcare market in 1990, specifically designed as "dispensing cabinets" for nursing units. In 1999, after much success in this setting, these systems were introduced into the anesthesia market.[29] As more emphasis is being placed on medication management in the ORs and tighter control is being sought for unattended medications, these automated anesthesia medication-dispensing systems have made their way into many ORs across the country. Over 500 facilities now have one of the two most

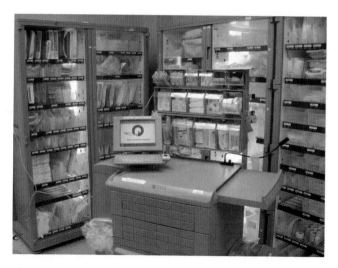

Fig. 11.4 A Pyxis anesthesia system

popular (best-selling) dispensing units in each OR,[30] and it is likely that more institutions will add them in the future.

Although initially adapted from the nursing unit design, the anesthesia medication-dispensing systems have matured to address common situations faced by anesthesiologists in the OR. The original design was marketed to pharmacists and hospital administrators as a system to lock controlled medications, control high-cost items, automate inventory and restocking, automate reordering, and facilitate capture of billing of medications used in surgery. A significant "push back" has been exhibited by many anesthesiologist users for reasons such as fear of equipment failure during emergencies. However, a small survey of trauma, cardiothoracic, and liver transplant anesthesiologists was reported in 2006 that showed that over a 12-month period of using automated dispensing systems, no delay in access to medications in emergency situations was encountered, and in the event of equipment failure, a backup system was in place so that medications were readily available.[31] Only recently have anesthesiologists begun to take interest in the dispensing systems as a method by which to not only control scheduled medications, increase billing capture, improve inventory reduction and automated reordering, but also to reduce medication errors and improve patient safety. By automating dispensing, it is theoretically possible to reduce dispensing errors.

Automated medication-dispensing cabinets are marketed by several manufacturers and have different but similar features. The Pyxis Anesthesia System (Cardinal Health, La Jolla, CA) (Fig. 11.4) and the Omnicell Anesthesia Workstation (Omnicell Corporation, Mountain View, CA) were designed to dispense medications directly to an anesthesia provider in every OR.[30,32] Both of these systems have many features in common, including user tracking by password-protected security measures, patient identification via ADT interfaces with the hospital information

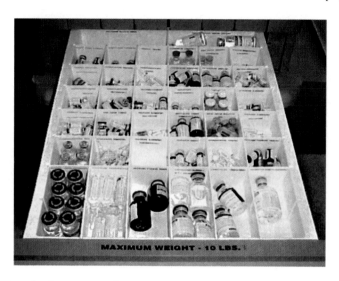

MAXIMUM WEIGHT - 10 LBS.

Fig. 11.5 Example of an open-matrix tray

system, automated charge capture and billing, accurate inventory control and automated reordering of medications, and barcode scanners for the verification and identification of medications removed/dispensed from the system. Both have single-issue drawers, which allow the removal of only one vial of a particular medication at any one time and only after specifically requested by the provider. This feature adds extra security for high-risk medications and extra control for narcotics and other controlled substances because each vial of medication removed/dispensed can be tracked to an individual provider at all times. It also allows for accurate accounting of narcotic removal, waste, and returns and can run reports for narcotic reconciliation. A recent report suggested that dispensing and administration errors *may* be reduced by the use of single-issue, minimatrix drawers, as the possibility of inadvertent removal of the unintended medication (as may occur from a free-access matrix drawer) is nearly eliminated.[33]

Both the Pyxis and the Omnicell systems have free-access matrix drawers, which are drawers that contain multiple medications stored in different "pockets" or slots that open when any one of the medications within is requested (Fig. 11.5). It is then up to the provider to remove the correct vial from the correct pocket or slot. However, this design leaves a large margin for human error. As previously noted, 17% of all medication errors in the ASA Closed Claims Project were the result of "failure to check," meaning the vial or label was misread or misinterpreted by the provider. The matrix-drawer design does not prevent the anesthesia provider from making this simple human error, which could result in a significant and possibly harmful or fatal adverse medication event. These drawers have been shown *not* to eliminate errors, and incorrect stocking (vials in the wrong place), misread labels on look-alike vials, or unnoticed manufacturer substitution of vial size or shape can still occur.[34] Some states in the US are considering eliminating their use.[35]

Error reduction may occur if medications are secured and dispensed only after specific selection of the appropriate or intended medication from a formulary list. Computer technology can intervene to confirm the medication removed or restrict the removal of certain medications to certain levels of providers.[30,32] Although none of the currently installed automated anesthesia medication-dispensing systems is marketed for the reduction of dispensing errors, it is clear that many potentially have that capability. Each of the systems has the ability to interface with hospital information systems, and some can retrieve patient data, such as medication allergies, current medications, and body weight. Automated alerts could theoretically be customized and added to the systems, thus notifying anesthesia providers that a contraindicated drug (due to allergy or drug–drug interaction), a high-risk drug (such as highly potent, undiluted vasoactive medication), or a potential overdose based on body weight, has been dispensed from the system.

The barcode scanner that is incorporated into the systems is intended to allow the anesthesia provider a quick-scan method of verification and documentation of vial removal from a free-access matrix drawer because the system itself cannot automatically identify which drug was actually removed. It also allows the pharmacy technician to ensure that the systems are restocked with the correct medication vials in their correct locations. Neither manufacturer has marketed the possibility of using this barcode scanner at the final stage immediately prior to drug administration. This feature would allow a "reverification" of the drug to ensure that it is the intended drug and is akin to the barcode features of the SaferSleep and DocuSys systems described above, thus ideally helping to reduce or eliminate administration errors and to prevent dispensing errors from reaching the patient.

Future Technologic Advances

As technology advances with automated anesthesia medication-dispensing systems, dispensing errors may be reduced further or eliminated altogether. Although these systems could soon have the ability to reduce administration errors to some extent, the likelihood is small that they will help to reduce prescribing errors. As mentioned previously, some AIMS address prescribing and administration errors but do little to address dispensing errors. The combined use of both types of automated systems may be exactly what is needed to reduce or eliminate nearly all medication errors in anesthesia. Narcotic reconciliation remains a manual process in most situations, as the two types of systems do not interface. The AIMS record may not match the total amount of controlled substance removed from the automated anesthesia medication-dispensing system. Future interfaces will solve this problem, as the AIMS will be able to (a) tell that a controlled substance has been removed from the dispensing system and (b) provide a discrepancy alert if an equal amount is not recorded by the anesthesia provider as administered or wasted. The pharmacy could be automatically notified that the discrepancy must be resolved. These interfaces may also serve as a deterrent to diversions by providing evident, closer, and tighter monitoring of all controlled substances.

At the time of this writing, two AIMS manufacturers are in contract negotiations to develop interfaces with one of the manufacturers of automated anesthesia medication-dispensing systems; successful partnerships would offer the "total solution" for reduction or elimination of error in anesthesia. Although no interface is currently complete between the various systems or manufacturers, it is exciting that the future of medication management and reduction/elimination of medication errors appears promising.

Future technologic advances may allow an AIMS to calculate drug concentration for infusion-bag mixing, calculate infusion rates based on body weight, and even program and control infusion pumps to the rate calculated. When automated anesthesia medication-dispensing systems eventually interface with AIMS, the ability to ensure that the drug administered is actually the drug removed will be realized, thereby offering a mechanism with which to track errors of omission or substitution and automating the process of tracking controlled substance discrepancies and diversions. Advances in technology (e.g., radio-frequency identification devices) and in system interfaces may be the missing elements necessary to accurately manage medications, improve patient safety, and reduce medication error in anesthesia practice.

Conclusion

Medication management represents a very real patient safety concern for anesthesiologists, as evidenced from studies that have explored this issue and the fact that anesthesia represents the only scenario in healthcare in which the five rights of medication administration are not currently implemented. Technology potentially provides some opportunities to improve this situation, possibly eliminating adverse drug events during surgery. Current technologies focus almost exclusively on barcode recognition of syringes prior to administration. Realization of tight integration with AIMS will present an opportunity to further improve the safety profile and utility of this technology.

Key Points

- Medication management represents one of the most challenging areas for anesthesia and is the only area in which the five rights of medication administration are not adhered to.
- Joint Commission standards focus significant attention on medication management, specifically in anesthesia.
- Medication errors are well recognized in anesthesia and result in significant patient harm.

- Effective medication management requires close collaboration between anesthesia and pharmacy staff.
- Automation represents an opportunity to reduce medication errors but requires change in work processes.
- AIMS may provide an improved environment to help reduce medication errors; however, they require some method of identification of medication prior to administration.
- Medication-dispensing cabinets are being utilized in an attempt to reduce medication errors; to be effective, these also require a change in practice behavior.

References

1. The Joint Commission. Accreditation essentials: Tips for addressing the "rights" of medication administration. Joint Commission Resources. http://www.jcrinc.com/6840/. Accessed February 4, 2008
2. Rich D. New JCAHO medication management standards for 2004. Am J Health Syst Pharm 2004; 61(13):1349–58
3. JCAHO Site Visit Report. Jackson Health System, Miami, FL, March 2005
4. The Joint Commission. Comprehensive Accreditation Manual for Hospitals: The Official Handbook, Section: Medication Management. Oakbrook Terrace, IL: The Joint Commission, 2007:243–7
5. Health Care Association of New Jersey—Private Nonprofit Organization. Medication Management Guideline, April 2006
6. Committee on School Health. American Academy of Pediatrics. Guidelines for the administration of medication in school. Pediatrics 2003; 112(3):697–9
7. American Society of Anesthesiologists Task Force on Acute Pain Management. Practice guidelines for acute pain management in the perioperative setting: An updated report by the American Society of Anesthesiologists Task Force on Acute Pain Management. Anesthesiology 2004; 100(6):1573–81
8. Kaufman M. Medication errors harming millions, report says: Extensive national study finds widespread, costly mistakes in giving and taking medication. *The Washington Post*, A08, July 21, 2006
9. Law offices of Kenneth N. Margolin, PC. Your legal rights as a victim of medication error. http://www.mederrorlaw.com. Accessed February 4, 2008
10. Bowdle TA. Drug administration errors from the ASA Closed Claims Project. ASA Newsletter 2003; 67(6):11–3
11. Galletly DC, Rowe WL, Henderson RS. The anaesthetic record: A confidential survey on data omission or modification. Anaesth Intens Care 1991; 19:74–8
12. Jensen LS, Merry AF, Webster CS, et al. Evidence-based strategies for preventing drug administration error during anaesthesia. Anaesthesia 2004; 59:493–504
13. Webster CS, Merry AF, Larrson L, et al. The frequency and nature of drug administration error during anaesthesia. Anaesth Intens Care 2001; 29(5):494–500
14. US Pharmacopeia. MEDMARX Data Report. A Chartbook of Medication Error Findings from Perioperative Settings From 1998–2005. http://www.usp.org/products/medmarx. Accessed February 4, 2008
15. Kahn FA, Hoda MQ. A prospective survey of intra-operative critical incidents in a teaching hospital in a developing country. Anaesthesia 2001; 56(2):177–82
16. Wheeler SJ, Wheeler DW. Medication errors in anaesthesia and critical care. Anaesthesia 2005; 60:257–73

17. Merriam–Webster's Online Dictionary. "Error." http://www.m-w.com/dictionary/error. Accessed February 4, 2008
18. Cohen M. Why error reporting systems should be voluntary. Institute of Safe Medication Practices. Br Med J 2000; 320(7237):728–9
19. Cullen D, Bates D, Leape L, and the Adverse Drug Event Prevention Group. Prevention of adverse drug events: A decade of progress in patient safety. J Clin Anesth 2000; 12:600–14
20. Heller A. Anesthesiologists and pharmacists: Trend to blend teams targets OR drug errors. Anesthesiol News 2007; 33:1
21. Hatoum HT, Catizone C, Hutchinson RA, et al. An eleven-year review of the pharmacy literature: Documentation of the value and acceptance of clinical pharmacy. Drug Intel Clin Pharm 1986; 20:33–48
22. Jenkins MH, Bond CA. The impact of clinical pharmacists on psychiatric patients. Pharmacotherapy 1996; 16(4):708–14
23. Schumock GT, Meek PD, Ploetz PA, . Economic evaluations of clinical pharmacy services— 1988–1995. The Publications Committee of the American College of Clinical Pharmacy. Pharmacotherapy 1996; 16(6):1188–208
24. Lesar TS, Briceland LL, Delcoure K, et al. Medication prescribing errors in a teaching hospital. JAMA 1990; 263:2329–34
25. DocuSys Digital Medical Solutions. DocuSys, Inc., Mobile, AL. http://www.docusys.net. Accessed February 4, 2008
26. SAFERSleep Anesthesia Safety and Record Automation. Safer Sleep, Ltd, Auckland, New Zealand. http://www.safersleep.com/index2.htm. Accessed February 4, 2008
27. Merry A, Webster CS, Larsson L, et al. Prospective assessment of a new anesthetic drug administration system designed to improve safety. Anesthesiology 2006; 105:A138
28. Intellifill IV. For Health Technologies, Inc., Daytona Beach, FL. http://www.fhtinc.com/features.html. Accessed February 4, 2008
29. Cooper L. Anaesthesia medication dispensing systems. Hospital Pharmacy Europe 2005; 19:19–21
30. Pyxis Anesthesia System. Cardinal Health, Inc., La Jolla, CA. http://www.cardinal.com/us/en/providers/products/pyxis/. Accessed February 4, 2008
31. Cooper L, Barron M, Gallagher C, et al. Patient safety in cardiac anesthesiology—Do automated anesthesia medication dispensing systems delay access to emergency medications? Abstract #SCA 97. 28th Annual Meeting of the Society of Cardiovascular Anesthesiologists, San Diego, CA, April 2006
32. Omnicell Anesthesia Workstation. Omnicell Corporation, Mountain View, CA. http://www.omnicell.com/solutions/anesthesia_providers/anesthesia_workstation.asp. Accessed February 4, 2008
33. Cooper L, Barron M, Gallagher C, et al. Automated anesthesia medication dispensing systems: Single-issue, limited-access drawers may reduce medication errors. Abstract #17AP3-7. Annual Meeting of the European Society of Anesthesia, Munich, Germany, June 2007
34. Cooper L, Barron M, Dollar B. Automated anesthesia medication dispensing systems: Current technology and design do not prevent intraoperative medication errors. Eur J Anaesthesiol 2006; 23(S37):249
35. Code of Maryland Regulations, 10.34.28.04, *Usage Requirements*, Title 10. Department of Health and Mental Hygiene, State of Maryland, September 2003

Chapter 12
Legal Aspects of AIMS

Philip Lane and Jeffrey M. Feldman

The development of AIMS and the more comprehensive EMR has focused primarily on the myriad of technologic challenges. As these challenges are met and electronic systems become the accepted method for record keeping, medicolegal proceedings will inevitably rely upon electronic data to determine liability when patient injury occurs. This chapter will address the current understanding of the legal aspects of AIMS, recognizing that in the future, the courts and legislatures will ultimately determine how these systems are used in medicolegal proceedings.

The EMR, whereby all information related to the medical care of a patient is recorded and stored, has been under development for decades, and many pioneers have implemented sophisticated systems for creating some version of an EMR.[1] Although these systems have proven themselves to be useful, few, if any, have been capable of creating a truly complete medical record that incorporates all aspects of a patient's medical care. AIMS were first introduced more than 20 years ago as computerized record-keeping systems designed to automatically record data from physiologic monitors, accept input of drug dosages and comments, and print highly legible paper records for patients' charts. Varied systems from multiple vendors have been adopted and are in use in thousands of anesthetizing locations worldwide. Although many departments have adopted AIMS, the overwhelming majority of anesthesia records are still created by hand. As a component of the EMR, the information collected by the AIMS has the potential to be a high-resolution record of the care rendered to a patient during a procedure that requires anesthesia.

Technologic limitations of computers to store and retrieve data are no longer obstacles in developing a complete EMR. However, the lack of standards for encoding and exchanging medical information between systems is an important obstacle in developing a comprehensive EMR. Although AIMS are not yet able to seamlessly share data, advanced standards for managing medical information that have the potential to facilitate information exchange between systems are now available (e.g., CPT, ICD, SNOMED, HL7). On April 27, 2004, Executive Order #13335 was created to underscore the federal government's commitment to developing and implementing a nationwide system of health information technology that would improve the quality, safety, and efficiency of healthcare.[2] The ability to deliver sophisticated, high-quality, cost-effective healthcare to a growing population may ultimately depend upon the information captured during each patient encounter that

J. Stonemetz, K. Ruskin (eds.) *Anesthesia Informatics*,

is stored and accessed using an EMR. Handwritten medical records are simply inadequate tools to meet the healthcare challenges of the future.

The development of a comprehensive EMR is inevitable. At present, every major healthcare organization is either implementing or developing a strategy to implement EMRs to capture data generated by patient encounters. Although significant progress has been made in meeting the technologic challenges to developing a complete EMR, the legal aspects of these automated systems have yet to be fully considered. The American legal system provides a fundamental foundation for society. If the EMR is to be the only legal document of a patient's care in the future, it will be routinely used by the courts. As the technology becomes more widely accepted, the legal implications will ultimately be determined by the courts and state legislative bodies.

In general, law and medicine intersect in three broad areas. *Healthcare law* is generally concerned with the business aspects of medicine, which include issues such as ownership, contracts, and billing practices. *Legal medicine* covers relationships among patients, doctors, and hospitals, as well as licensure and accreditation issues. *Medical malpractice* is the area of law that addresses conflicts involving patient injuries or adverse outcomes during medical treatment by properly accredited providers. This chapter will specifically discuss the use of an AIMS record as a legal document in a medical malpractice proceeding. The other aspects of medicine and law that relate to AIMS—healthcare law and legal medicine—are beyond the scope of this chapter. The reader is encouraged to find knowledgeable counsel if faced with making decisions regarding the legal implications of an EMR.

An understanding of the implications of AIMS vis-à-vis medical malpractice is important due to the economic, professional, and social complexities involved. Large amounts of money are spent every year in insuring, prosecuting, defending, and settling malpractice cases. Legal costs are considered to be a significant component of the financial burden of healthcare. Despite the fact that patients are older and/or sicker than ever before, juries in our society have demonstrated that a "perfect" outcome may be expected and that physicians and/or institutions will be held liable when a treatment result is less than "perfect." Therefore, legal concerns regarding AIMS are not directly related to the technology but are necessarily focused on the way that our legal system interacts with any record system that has a "public" component. A *public component* may be characterized as any situation in which a service or product is being offered to the public. Public "products and services" create duties of care, and this is particularly true in healthcare.

As long as the outcome of a surgical procedure cannot be predicted with certainty and the malpractice environment remains unpredictable and, at times, arbitrary, no record-keeping system will eliminate malpractice exposure or guarantee a successful defense. In the first part of this chapter, the evidence accumulated to date on the role of an AIMS in a medical malpractice proceeding will be reviewed. Much can be learned from anecdotal information about how to use an AIMS effectively and the limitations of the technology as a legal tool, but anecdotal experiences with the usefulness of a product or service hold little evidentiary value with the court in helping juries to determine malpractice guilt or innocence. The second part of the chapter will, therefore, examine the legal complexities that underlie establishing any records available from an AIMS as accepted legal documents. These legal complexities, and the value of an AIMS as an evidentiary tool, will become important as the AIMS evolves as the preferred method for anesthesia record keeping. We are not aware of any peer-reviewed report or study that has used commonly defined language or specifically identified parameters for development and use of an AIMS (including standardized methods for correction of errors and artifacts) that has subsequently been submitted to a legal forum for admission as evidence. Until this submission occurs, we can only speculate as to the value of the AIMS in the courtroom when prosecuting or defending a negligence claim.

What Is the Evidence that Documents the Role of an AIMS in Malpractice Proceedings?

> I remember the patient well. He was a 50-year-old owner of a successful plumbing company who suffered from severe back pain following a motor vehicle accident. I was to provide his anesthesia care for a multilevel spinal fusion. The procedure was long and surgically difficult, but the patient's anesthesia course was essentially unremarkable. I remember how I felt when the patient reported in the PACU that he was blind. How could this be? I had done everything I could think of to prevent this complication. This patient's anesthetic course was essentially indistinguishable from that of the many patients for whom I had cared during similar surgical procedures. Yet, there I stood, 5 years later, about to enter a courtroom and defend myself against allegations of negligent care that led to the permanent blindness of this patient. The monetary award for pain and suffering and loss of income was potentially enormous. More importantly, I had done absolutely nothing wrong, yet my reputation was at stake. Would the judge and jury recognize the quality medical care I had provided? Would the documentation from the case be sufficient to defend against allegations of negligence? As I took that first step into the courtroom, I knew that the ultimate outcome was not assured.

The vignette highlights the case of an essentially healthy patient who suffered a major debilitating complication during a surgical procedure. The medical professionals involved with the patient's care must convince a lay jury that this injury did not result from a failure to follow the standard of care. It is not difficult for any practicing anesthesiologist to relate to the angst of the physician entering the courtroom. Despite the quality of medical care provided, the outcome of a medicolegal suit is unpredictable. Factors that play an integral part of any malpractice trial and affect the ultimate outcome include the trial jurisdiction, the abilities of the attorneys, the composition of the jury, the expert witnesses' demeanor, the sympathy engendered by the plaintiff, the perceived credibility of the defendant, and the quality of the documentation. Risk managers and attorneys who defend physicians consistently emphasize the meticulous and accurate documentation that is essential to a successful defense. Questions may be raised by plaintiffs' attorneys about the accuracy of documentation, but no better foundation exists for a defense than a complete, legible record created at the time that care was rendered to the patient.

The handwritten anesthesia record has been the established method for documenting intraoperative anesthesia care for more than 100 years. Practitioners are taught early in their careers how to keep an anesthesia record and quickly develop a comfortable routine for documenting the process of anesthesia care by hand. The role of the handwritten anesthesia record in a malpractice proceeding is typically not appreciated until one receives a notice of intent to sue for malpractice. Unfortunately, the inadequacies of a handwritten anesthesia record become all too apparent when subjected to the scrutiny of attorneys responsible for defending the malpractice case.

Anesthesia information systems offer the ability to record data automatically during anesthesia care, to save the data electronically, and to print a complete, highly legible, paper record for the patient's medical record. Concern over the medicolegal implications of automatically recording patient data is commonly voiced by individuals who are considering the role of AIMS technology in their practice. Given the pivotal role of the anesthesia record in malpractice litigation, it is not surprising that practitioners have strong feelings about the medicolegal implications of this new form of record keeping.

How does the AIMS impact the medicolegal risk associated with giving an anesthetic when compared with the current written record? Different sources of evidence are used in an attempt to answer this question. The legal system clearly defines the criteria that must be met in a malpractice proceeding—the so-called burden of proof. The role of anesthesia information technology in meeting this burden of proof is examined with particular attention to the role of the expert witness and concerns about artifactual data. Although a small percentage of anesthesia practitioners currently utilize AIMS technology, several anesthesia departments were early adopters of this technology and have accumulated many years of collective experience. This experience is probably the best evidence to date on the medicolegal implications of these systems, and it is reviewed below. For several years, the ASA Closed-Claims Project has accumulated data on settled and closed malpractice claims in which AIMS were used, and this information is also described.

Malpractice Suits and the Burden of Proof

In a malpractice case, the main contention is that the practitioner failed to deliver medical care at the current standard of her peers. The plaintiff—typically the patient or his family—has the burden of proving that the practitioner did not meet the prevailing standard of care. If we focus on the burden of proof, it becomes easier to understand the potential of an automated anesthesia record to impact medicolegal exposure. Four elements must be satisfied to be successfully sued for negligent care. The plaintiff's attorney must show that:

- The defendant had a legal duty to care for the patient.
- The defendant breached the duty to care for the patient, i.e., did not conform to the *standard of care*.
- The breach of duty caused injury to the patient.
- The plaintiff suffered damages that are compensable.

The anesthesia record in its current handwritten form has been accepted as the documented representation of care rendered by the practitioner and is used to substantiate whether the provider did or did not meet the prevailing standard of care. The potential damages flow indirectly from this determination. If the medical standard of care has been met, there is no negligence. Without negligence, no injury or adverse outcome should result in the plaintiff receiving compensation for the problem encountered. If the standard of care has not been met, the injuries that resulted from that breach of duty, regardless of their insignificance or severity, are legally "charged" to the practitioner, and that practitioner will be at the court's mercy regarding the plaintiff's compensation for injury or outcome. The anesthesia record is absolutely critical to the determination of the standard of care given to any patient.

The primary method by which courts evaluate conformance to the standard of care is to use expert witnesses to review the medical and anesthesia records to make a determination about the care given to a patient. Expert witnesses are individuals whose credentials, training, and experience qualify them to testify about the care provided to a patient relative to an accepted community or national standard. Typically, both sides of the case will find expert witnesses so that arguments are made both for and against a breach of the standard of care and the relationship any breach has to the patient's injuries or outcome. The anesthesia record is the most objective rendition of anesthetic events that an expert witness can use to understand the care that was provided and the decisions that were made. The expert uses this record to make her case to a jury. Therefore, the most useful anesthesia record to the defense is one that (a) helps an expert witness to determine whether or not the defendant adhered to the standard of care and (b) helps to convince the jury of that fact.

In contrasting the potential of handwritten and automated anesthesia records to impact medicolegal exposure, the central issue is the role of each type of record in supporting the expert witness's case for conformance with the standard of care. From a medicolegal perspective, the ideal anesthesia record would be a contemporaneous, accurate, legible, and understandable rendition of actual events that would support an effective defense if the standard of care was met—or lead to early settlement if it was not. Records that are incomplete or difficult to decipher lead to questions about the veracity of the defendant(s). The importance of accurate and meticulous documentation is emphasized by Mr. George Gore, an experienced malpractice attorney who wrote: "…it is better to explain a problem that did occur and was properly charted than to have to defend against charges of cover-up and fraud."[3] In many ways, the AIMS record has the potential to be an ideal anesthesia record. In the best case scenario, this record should be legible, complete, contemporaneous, and readily available for evaluation. The legibility of the automated record conveys the appearance of a "credible" document when scrutinized either in the courtroom or in the process of case preparation.

Are Data Recorded by AIMS Reliable?

The legibility of the automated anesthesia record is rarely questioned, but the accuracy of the automated record has been a major concern raised by clinicians reluctant to incorporate an AIMS into their practice. One case report in the literature underscores this concern. Vigoda and Lubarsky reported a case of a patient who underwent resection of a brain tumor and was quadriplegic after the procedure.[4] In this case, a 93-minutes window of time passed during which no data were recorded from the patient monitor to the anesthesia record. The patient initiated a malpractice claim that was ultimately settled, in large measure due to the demonstration of an inordinate period of time during which the AIMS and, by extension, the anesthesiologist did not document the patient's vital signs—a period in which the patient's injury could have occurred. The plaintiff met his burden of proof by using the absent data to show that the anesthesia care team did not meet the prevailing standard of care, which currently requires documentation of vital signs at least every 5 minutes. In fact, the care providers testified that they had followed the vital signs displayed on the monitor continuously during the procedure but did not recognize the data missing from the automated record because part of the record display was obscured by a data-entry screen. However, it was the fact that no data were entered on the record that was the issue—not the fact that the AIMS had failed per se. Another important detail regarding medicolegal exposure emerged from this case. Not only had the printed copy of the record indicated missing data, but the electronic database of the case was also problematic. The plaintiff retained an expert in AIMS who reviewed the computerized data entries. Entries automatically made in an AIMS are timed, and the database reviewed in this case showed that the note indicating "presence at emergence" had been entered at the *start* of the procedure. This observation further undermined the veracity of the anesthesiologist and contributed to the decision to settle the case.

The report described here underscores not so much a fatal flaw of AIMS, but the need for careful design and protocols to ensure that an AIMS is working appropriately. In the wake of the above case, the vendor implemented an alert to the user to indicate when the recording of data from a device is interrupted. Furthermore, the authors changed the protocol for charting to eliminate prospective charting of events to the record.[5] Eliminating prospective charting represented a significant behavioral change by the physicians in a large department and required a three-step process to be successful. Educational sessions were conducted to highlight the importance of contemporaneous charting. Automated emails were generated when presence at emergence was documented more than 30 minutes before the surgery end was documented. These emails were copied to the chairman and the billing office so that personal intervention was possible with those physicians who did not comply. As a result of these interventions, correct note timing, which had been only 25% successful, exceeded 99.5%.

Gaps in recording data and timely documentation can be addressed through software design and adherence to documentation protocols. Artifactual data recorded automatically by the AIMS are another matter. Automated systems record data electronically from patient monitors and cannot reliably discriminate true from artifactual data in all cases. As a result, artifactual data from physiologic monitors will appear on the automated record and will be recorded into the electronic database. Examples of artifacts that are of concern to clinicians are the artifactually low oxyhemoglobin saturation readings from the pulse oximeter due to patient movement, or low blood pressure readings from an arterial catheter that is partially occluded by a blood clot. All automated record systems allow the clinician to edit data on the record or to enter an annotation that indicates, for example, that a period of low blood pressure was due to a clotted catheter and that readings improved after the catheter was flushed. Edited data and annotations are recorded to the database with a time stamp. What about the case in which a clinician does not recognize the artifact and does not edit or annotate the erroneous data? Does that omission increase malpractice exposure in the case of an untoward event?

Artifact is relatively easy to identify when automatically recorded data are examined. Data are printed on the anesthesia record, which appears in the patient's medical record at the 5-minute intervals typical of the handwritten record. A low oxyhemoglobin or blood pressure entry may therefore be clearly printed on the record. However, electronic data are stored by the computer at much shorter intervals—typically, every 15–30 seconds. When the electronic records are evaluated, it is often relatively easy to distinguish artifact from real data. Artifactual data typically change at a rate that is unphysiologic. Furthermore, additional electronic data can help to identify artifact. In the case of an artifactually low oxyhemoglobin saturation reading, the heart-rate measurement from the pulse oximeter will differ from the heart-rate measurement by other sources such as the electrocardiogram. In the case of low blood pressure due to a clotted arterial catheter, blood pressure changes that are recorded when the clot forms and when it is cleared are unphysiologic. Furthermore, independent measurement by an automated, noninvasive blood pressure cuff set to cycle at intervals will be recorded along with the direct arterial measurements and may help to identify the problem as artifact.

Concern that artifactual data on the automated record could lead to liability and questions about the quality of care provided is not unfounded. For artifactual data to support a case of negligence, (a) the artifactual data would have to indicate an untoward physiologic change that was misidentified as real data, (b) the plaintiff must be able to link the artifactual data or the decision(s) that resulted from using the data to an undesired outcome, and (c) an expert witness must be able to argue from the evidence that the standard of care was violated. An example would be the recording of an abnormally low blood pressure caused by a surgical team member leaning on the blood pressure cuff (or the clotted arterial line) that is interpreted as a real value and treated with a vasopressor. The subsequent hypertension (real data) that results in a stroke or myocardial infarction involves a possible breach of the standard of care. That standard might be the failure to identify and recognize artifactual data.

Although automatically recording data may not necessarily yield a completely accurate rendition of events, the handwritten record may not either. In the case of the handwritten record, the clinician has the opportunity to decide which data to include on the record. Indeed, studies that compared handwritten to automated anesthesia records documented that handwritten records do not reflect the highest and lowest blood pressures that patient's experience in the course of well-conducted anesthesia care.[6] These studies indicate that clinicians are reluctant to chart the fluctuations in blood pressure that occur during a well-conducted anesthetic. This reluctance to document variations, in itself, increases malpractice exposure, as it supports the myth that "railroad-track" vital signs are typical of all well-conducted anesthetics. Expert witnesses for the plaintiff may attempt to exploit that myth to try and link patient injury to even transient extremes of blood pressure. Conversely, "railroad-track" vital signs could be viewed as artificial documentation, and the plaintiff's attorney may argue that injury occurred due to unrecorded variations that were not recorded by the clinician. Automated systems have the potential to document in large groups of patients the blood pressure fluctuations typical of most anesthetics and erode the myth of "railroad-track" vital signs.

Real-World Experience

Departmental Experience

Speculation and individual case reports have some value in understanding the medicolegal implications of AIMS, but the proof is in the real-world experience. A number of anesthesia departments that currently use AIMS have done so for more than 5 years. Objectively, these departments would seem to be just as likely to be the subject of a malpractice suit as any other department. Their experience can be invaluable in understanding the impact of an automated anesthesia system on risk exposure. Given the fact that these systems have been in use for many years, it seems likely that data from AIMS have been used as part of malpractice proceedings. The fact that we are specifically unaware of these cases may be (a) because the legal system does not note these cases as special, (b) that these cases proceed to settlement (like the case described above) or dismissal based upon the perceived reliability of the documentation, or (c) that few if any cases have relied upon AIMS data, especially if admission of the data as evidence (see below) was hampered by the manner in which it was generated. Many of these cases may occur in state circuit courts and are not tracked by legal search engines. We simply do not know.

Although the total number of anesthesia departments using AIMS remains small, the number of cases recorded is quite extensive, as these systems tend to be installed at larger centers that perform tens of thousands of procedures annually. Therefore, it should be possible to identify cases in which automated records were used in malpractice proceedings. A survey of anesthesia departments that utilize anesthesia information systems has been completed to document the experience of these departments with these systems during malpractice proceedings.[7] Twenty-two departments out of 55 surveyed responded, and 14 of those departments had been using an AIMS for more than 5 years. Although the total number of cases recorded is not known, this survey likely represents a cumulative experience approaching one million patient encounters. The responding departments identified 41 cases since adopting an AIMS in which they had been notified of intent to sue. Of those cases, 11 actually went on to settlement or litigation. All of the respondents reported cases in which the quality of documentation supported dismissal, settlement, or defense in court. Twenty-one of the respondents felt that AIMS were either valuable or essential for risk management.

Although surveys are suspect due to the selection bias inherent in a voluntary response, the results indicate that AIMS may be beneficial in a malpractice proceeding. It is notable that all of the departments surveyed are now committed to utilizing AIMS and would not return to handwritten records. If AIMS technology had a significant potential to increase malpractice exposure, it is doubtful that these departments would remain so committed to it. Nevertheless, the results of the survey are in no way a definitive statement on the role of the AIMS in a malpractice proceeding. We simply do not have enough detail to understand the reasons why opposing counsel chose to settle a particular case, nor do we have the details of the litigation to understand how the jury viewed the information from the record.

AIMS and the Closed-Claims Database

Since 1985, the American Society of Anesthesiologists has been conducting a review of closed malpractice claims in cooperation with a number of malpractice insurance companies. This project involves standardized review of closed-claim documentation by anesthesiologists and entry of abstracted information from these cases into a searchable database (http://www.asaclosedclaims.org). In recent years, reviewers were asked to indicate if an AIMS was used and whether or not it played a role in the litigation. At this writing, the database contains 7328 claims, 38 of which have been identified as having used an AIMS record. Of those 38 claims, the AIMS was deemed by the reviewer to play a role in the litigation of four cases. The details available for these cases are as follows:

- One record indicated sustained oxyhemoglobin saturation by pulse oximetry of <60% for 1.5 hours.
- One record demonstrated no exhaled carbon dioxide for 30 minutes, consistent with an unrecognized esophageal intubation.
- One record discredited the testimony of the anesthesiologist when the record did not indicate that the patient had been preoxygenated, as claimed.
- One record indicated inadequate resuscitation of a patient with postpartum hemorrhage.

Due to the nature of the closed-claims database, it is impossible to obtain additional details about these cases. It would seem that, in these cases, the record helped to expose negligent care, but information is insufficient to be certain about the exact role of the automated record. In addition, the number of cases is insufficient to draw any conclusions about the overall impact of these systems on malpractice exposure. Also unknown is the number of cases, if any, involving an AIMS that never made it to the insurance company because they were dismissed or settled locally. The fact that the use of an AIMS is being documented in the closed-claims review should eventually help to shed more light on the role of this technology in malpractice proceedings.

When we look for real-world experience to document the role of AIMS in malpractice proceedings, the best evidence would be from actual case law precedent, which is absent. As described in the Vigoda and Lubarsky case report, problem with the AIMS was only one of the reasons that led to a decision to settle in favor of the plaintiff when no real evidence of malpractice was found.[4] However, this is no different from any other case (automated or handwritten) in which the record does not indicate any deviation from the standard of care and liability is assigned for other reasons.

AIMS technology will certainly proliferate as the efforts to establish a complete EMR gain momentum. To date, the legal experience has been accumulated by the early adopters of AIMS without a focused risk-management strategy. The survey of departments with extensive experience using AIMS indicates that automated technology may be helpful in the risk-management process. Clearly, the proper design of AIMS and discipline in record keeping, with risk management and quality control in mind, will help to make the record obtained using an AIMS to be a more accurate and complete rendition of actual events. Whether or not this quality record will serve as a better legal document remains to be seen.

How Can the AIMS Record Become a Legal Document?

An AIMS is designed to produce a highly legible printed document for the patient's chart. Our perception of that record is that it will facilitate disclosure of actual events during an anesthetic due to the increased legibility and the related aura of veracity. However, simply recreating an anesthesia record from digital data does not guarantee that the automated record is an accurate representation of actual events. These records may potentially increase liability due to the immaturity of the technology and lack of case history to recognize these records as routine business records. The requirements of admissibility and defensibility and areas of potential liability exposure involved when implementing these systems are discussed below.

Liability management is more general and encompasses a wider umbrella than the familiar term *risk management*. The purpose for enlarging the negligence/liability concept is to set some rules for understanding how the data recorded by an AIMS can ultimately be used as a legal business record. AIMS are in the infant stage of becoming universally acceptable and desirable. While many proprietary systems are available in the marketplace, fundamental standards that pertain to data collection and storage and depiction of the automated anesthesia record have yet to be established. Effective liability management using AIMS requires recognition of liability issues and the development of standards and system designs, the output of which will serve as a consistent medical record and a legal business document.

Although great advances have been made in anesthetic management, a standardized AIMS that meets the legal criteria to be considered more accurate than the handwritten record has not evolved. The printed record from an AIMS bears the same scrutiny as the handwritten record and is judged by the presence or absence of clinical data relevant to a particular case. As has been demonstrated, records from AIMS may have incomplete documentation of key clinical components, and this lack of documentation could seriously compromise the defensibility of the anesthetic record.[8]

Significant resources are required to develop and successfully deploy complex clinical automated systems. Expense and proprietary interests may be reasons why advances in system design and compatibility that would facilitate an improved defensible anesthesia record have not occurred. In addition, the industry has not made any effort to define what elements would constitute an improved defensible anesthesia record. Despite a perceived improvement in authentic data capture, we believe that significant issues with artifactual data and user error persist. Standardized form and content would greatly improve the status of the use of automated systems and of their output being used as legal business documents.

Evolution of AIMS

Stand-alone clinical systems have been used for many years. However, the ability to transmit, capture, and store real-time clinical data, and to retrieve and process this information at a reasonable cost has just recently become available. Integration now permits access to most or all of a patient's static record, which includes the gathering of data developed at the point of care—H&Ps, labs, progress notes, and records of procedures. Collection of this voluminous clinical data, integration of decision support, and the ability to provide meaningful reports are the drivers behind the anticipated value of an industry-wide migration to EMRs.

The concept of electronic anesthesia records, or AIMS, has been discussed since the advent of the personal computer in 1981. Early proprietary systems were developed within anesthesia departments and used by providers in various ways, depending on local needs. Typical use took the form of attempting to duplicate the manual anesthesia record by recording data automatically from the same monitors viewed by the anesthesia provider. These systems were basically sophisticated plotting devices. The final output was printed to a paper record, and it was up to the practitioner either to accept or physically alter the final record that was placed in the patient's chart.

Although the software "shell" for these systems has improved and the rate of transmission of data has changed, the function of the AIMS record has not fundamentally changed. However, tremendous advances have been made in the ability to store and warehouse data. The early automated systems had no requirement to "save" the data because the function of the system was to record the data from the monitors. Saving data was originally conceived as being for the purpose of printing the record and saving it for billing purposes but not necessarily for medicolegal purposes. Proprietary anesthesia record data were frequently deleted once the case was finished, depending upon the vendor's design. Recently, it has become recognized that long-term storage of these data is relevant for many reasons, as well as potentially required for medicolegal purposes. However, the storage of data and the granularity (fineness or specificity with which the data are stored) required for long-term storage and meaningful retrieval have not been standardly defined. Commercial vendors vary significantly in their storage and retrieval systems as well as their compatibility with other systems. It is incumbent upon the customer to discuss this topic with any potential vendor and to clearly understand the limitations of the long-term storage and retrievability of information. Clearly, all recorded data are now considered part of the patient's record and are therefore retrievable and potentially admissible as evidence. The academic anesthesia community became interested in actually looking at the comprehensive vital-sign data for a number of purposes, including:

- Understanding how anesthetic agents and medications used in anesthesia practice affect patients and outcomes
- Accurately documenting the conduct of anesthesia care
- Identifying the variations in practice from best-practice guidelines

To fulfill these goals, data must be stored beyond the end of the case and kept in a prescribed manner (see below) for a considerable length of time. The law is clear about this point. Data developed for any reason concerning a patient are ultimately accessible by the patient or his legal representatives and are part of the patient's medical record—and it is this accessibility to granular, comprehensive data that is deemed to be both an advantage and a vulnerability of AIMS.

Government Regulation

In anticipation of increased use and potential abuse, governmental agencies and the US Congress have mandated certain requirements for EMRs in general. In cooperation with the Department of Health and Human Services and the Institute of Medicine (IOM), it has been determined that EMR systems should have the following basic capabilities:

- Longitudinal collection of electronic health information for and about a person
- Immediate electronic access to person- and population-level information by authorized users
- Provision of information and decision support that improve patient safety and efficient patient care
- Support of efficient processes in the delivery of healthcare[9]

From these four federal mandates, the following major improvements in healthcare are anticipated:

- Improvement in patient safety
- Support of effective patient care and, where possible, movement toward an evidence-based approach
- Via accumulated information, improved identification and management of patients with chronic conditions, and identification of best practices to treat these highly morbid and expensive diseases
- Improved efficiency of care through the availability of patient information and reduced duplication of services, which will allow timely delivery of care and result in a more cost-effective healthcare system

As EMRs have proliferated, the IOM expressed an opinion that displaying the correct amount of information is important to foster both safety and efficiency.[10] Results management (presenting the results of laboratory and procedures immediately and clearly) has value. Order-entry management, decision support, and effective and accurate communication and connectivity will allow for better patient care. Patient support, administrative support, and the reporting of patient and population data will potentially improve the overall delivery of healthcare. With increased information being captured and shared, the concern over individual patient privacy rights led to the development of the government's HIPAA regulations, a full discussion of which is beyond the scope of this chapter. *In addition, the IOM was charged with calling for the development of a "functional model" with a common set of capability requirements to allow software and hardware vendors to be compared and contrasted.*[10]

Legal Proceedings, Expert Witnesses, and AIMS

Every experienced anesthesiologist is aware of continuing controversies regarding the manner of providing care to patients. An anesthetic can be successful using a variety of medications, techniques, and procedures. These differences are exploited during a legal proceeding to suggest that one approach is better than another when trying to establish liability. Certain anesthetic medications would appear to have different effects when reported by different experts. The typical malpractice case looks to find plausible experts on each side who testify to the appropriateness of the delivery and management of the anesthetic. In the final analysis, it will be the jury who decides which expert is more believable. To illustrate this point, the following two scenarios address management of the anesthetic and the anesthesia record:

1. In the first scenario, the discussion is anecdotal. The expert witness says that "in my hands" this medication works well (or does not work well) in situation X. Different experiences or disagreements that arise are most likely attributable to the fact that situations in which the drugs, patients, and conditions that are being compared are actually not the same.

2. The second scenario involves the actual veracity of the anesthetic record, which in fact, is one of the major issues of most malpractice cases. A railroad track-appearing anesthesia record, particularly in anesthetics of long duration, is a well-known phenomenon in which the patient's recorded vital signs become stable, do not vary, and look like railroad tracks on the anesthetic record. This tends to occur (a) in situations in which there is actually little change in the vital signs and (b) in relatively unstable situations in which the provider is too busy managing the patient to record contemporaneous readings every 5 minutes. Of course, during a 5-minute period, the provider may have a variety of values to record. In either event, a full and accurate automated recording of vital-sign changes could help to resolve the railroad-track issue.

In an AIMS, every vital sign, regardless of frequency, could be recorded in a database, and a 5-minute interval rendering could be made from that pool of data. The next question would be: What value should be used for the recording of vital signs? Would the recorded value come from the vital sign at the 5-minute mark or an average, a mean, or a median of the last three readings? A common event that may be problematic is the recording of noninvasive blood pressure data. Typically, monitors check blood pressure every 3–5 minutes. If the AIMS is recording a blood pressure value every few seconds, what value should be stored after the initial recording? Most AIMS will simply replicate the last value to the database every few seconds until the next reading. If the initial blood pressure measurement is erroneous, ultimately, spurious vital-sign data are recorded repeatedly to the record, which may be difficult to explain. Obviously more data do not necessarily mean a "cleaner" or a more accurate result.

Standardization of AIMS

Despite governing agencies calling for standardization of AIMS, which would allow systems to share data seamlessly and easily, the rules have yet to be established, and every system vendor has its own specifications. Standardization is necessary to allow the comparison of patient treatment and outcomes and ultimately to promote the delivery of safe and effective medical care. Furthermore, the authors are not aware of any current efforts to define precisely how data should be captured, recorded, and stored that would help to create a more defensible case in the event of a malpractice claim.[11] How can this problem be resolved? We believe a federal mandate for industry compatibility and standardization is essential to move EMRs and AIMS into the mainstream of healthcare delivery.

Medical Record, Business Record, or Legal Evidence

Many steps are required in the legal arena to make the AIMS the standard of care. First and foremost, the record must be admissible. To be admissible routinely without repeated challenges to the veracity of the record, the accepted EMR must be established as the patient medical record. Once the EMR is established as a medical record, it is, or can be considered to be, a business record. A business record (or any evidence) is not readily admitted into a court of law without adhering to legal process and rules.

How Does an AIMS Record Become Part of a Permanent Medical Record?

Regulatory bodies, including the Center for Medicare and Medicaid Services, The Joint Commission, and state and local entities, have requirements for medical records, which include (a) the information must be presented in chronologic order, (b) the information must be in a language that is customary to the intended users, (c) the information must be recorded in ink, and (d) the record must be signed and authenticated by time and date. No entry should be altered or backdated, and all additions and corrections must be specifically noted in chronologic order at the time of the corrected entry. In some cases, a small notation referring to a condition or correction can be indicated at the point of the original notation. This provision is particularly problematic for an AIMS. It is anticipated that AIMS will become accepted as the anesthesia medical record by regulatory agencies. However, establishing these records as business records is another hurdle in getting them admitted into a court of law.

Business Record

All electronic records that are under consideration for admission in court as business records (medically related or not) are subject to the same admission rules. The following characteristics are minimum legal requirements for admissibility of business documents under Federal Rules of Civil Procedure. The submitted document must be a record of acts or events made at or near the time the act or event occurred, by a person with knowledge, or from information transmitted by a person with knowledge, that is kept in the regular course of a business that has a regular practice of recording such information, and all is shown by testimony of the custodian or other qualified witness.[12] The reader should note that most states have patterned their civil procedures after the Federal Rules of Civil Procedure. Any state jurisdiction may differ significantly from the Federal Rules, and the local rules would apply unless the case is in Federal court. In general, these admissibility rules can be translated into the following common-sense criteria for any medical record:

- *Compliance*. Medical record-keeping procedures must adhere to any additional local "business-record" rules for admissibility if any of the local rules are different from the Federal Rules.
- *Responsibility*. Written policies and procedures for record storage and maintenance must be in place and must state who is responsible for the records.

- *Implementation.* All policies and procedures must be implemented and continuously followed.
- *Consistency.* Record maintenance systems must ensure that records are stored and maintained in a uniform way to assure the credibility of the records and documentation of any amendments or alterations.

All records must be:

Comprehensive. All records must be stored and maintained.

Identifiable. Specific individual records must be stored as discrete and independent transactions and must be readily identifiable and accessible.

Complete. Records under the control of the record keeper must preserve the content and structure of the entire business transaction (medical treatment) to ensure accuracy.

Authorized. Records must be developed under the auspices and control of an authorized creator (medical provider, allied professional, registered nurse, etc.) and stored with the identification of the creator readily available.

Preserved. Records must be preserved in such a way as to prevent alteration or deterioration. If a record is audited, the audit trail must be established and maintained with the record permanently.

Removable. Records can be removed only under the auspices of the authorized record keeper, and the record keeper must maintain sufficient control to ensure that the record is not altered.

Usable. The record must be something that is used in the usual course of business.[13]

If any of these elements or criteria is missing, the veracity of the records may be in question, and in fact, the record might not be admissible. These issues must be addressed at each institution where an AIMS will be installed and, in most cases, will be governed by the medical records departments as well as by any forms committees.

Admissibility

In practice, the custodian of the records, regardless of their form, would be required to provide testimony of authenticity. The custodian must be able to testify that he has personal knowledge of the hospital record storage system, that he brought the record from the repository of records, and that the record being admitted as evidence is validated, and the custodian must explain how the record was identified. The actual authentication rules are somewhat more complicated than described here, and some exceptions can be found in the Federal Rules of Evidence.

Alternate admission routes, other than the business-rule exception described earlier, would require that the actual maker of the record (in this case, the provider) certify that what was being presented was a true and accurate copy of the record. In the case of AIMS/EMR/automated anesthesia records, the maker of the record is the person(s) who electronically sign into the system and whose names appear on the record automatically. There is no characteristic to identify this maker other than an electronic "signature." There is no "handwriting" or "ink color" to assess and identify with one particular maker and link the record to that individual. All physiologic data are automatically placed on the record without effort on the maker's part. To identify a maker to attest to a true and accurate copy might be troublesome. Therefore, admission through the business-records rule is the most efficient method. The following series of questions is typical of questions that would be asked about a business medical record to determine its admissibility in a legal proceeding:

1. Was the document made as a part of the regular practice of a practitioner, hospital, clinic, office, or institution?
2. Are the records kept in the usual course of a regularly conducted business activity?
3. Were the records created at or near the time the provider cared for the patient?
4. Were the notes made by the practitioner who had personal knowledge of the patient's complaint, medical condition, diagnosis, and medical findings, or who immediately supervised those who did?
5. Are the records authentic?
6. Have the records themselves been retained according to usual applicable federal, state, and professional rules and regulations?
7. Are the records relevant to the litigation?[14]

Improvements Necessary to Enable the Use of an AIMS Record as a Legal Document

When a new technology arrives, the nature of the law requires an establishment of the new technology as reasonable and reliable a priori. In order for AIMS to become recognized as admissible from their current point in development, several things should occur. First and foremost, the AIMS must be standardized in terms of features, nomenclature, and output. AIMS should derive, process, calculate, and display numbers and graphs in a standardized way. Anesthesia governing bodies should assess these standards and approve AIMS's specific data development, reporting, and graphing functions. Unless and until these particular issues are resolved, standard admission cannot occur under the business-record exception, and as such, an AIMS record will fall short of offering any advantage over the handwritten record. Without standardization, it may be difficult for the proponent of the record to demonstrate its accuracy and veracity. Currently, no professional rules and regulations exist regarding the AIMS record—only an "acceptable" manner in which to create the paper replication.

Some individuals, including one of the authors (JF), have offered anecdotal evidence that AIMS have the potential to better document patient information than a handwritten record, but no system is perfect. The general hope in the field is that the reliance on a computer and elimination of the subjective rendering of information by hand will be sufficient to cloak the AIMS with credibility. Unfortunately, this is not sufficient in the eyes of the law. If the healthcare community wants AIMS to actually provide improved defensibility, the AIMS must be designed and utilized in a manner that adheres to the legal requirements.

Conclusion

At this writing, the use of an AIMS to document anesthetic care has not been established as the standard of care. Nevertheless, ongoing initiatives to develop a comprehensive EMR will continue, and AIMS use will continue to increase. It is likely that the record created by an AIMS will become a part of the overall EMR. Because it is likely that AIMS records will become the primary evidence in malpractice proceedings for determining whether or not the anesthesia provider(s) conformed to the standard of care regarding intraoperative anesthetic management, understanding the legal implications of a computer-generated anesthesia record is essential. Absent any standards that will ensure that the AIMS information is admissible as a business record, the utility of the information to the parties involved in a suit will remain in question. The goal in developing this technology should be to apply strict design and implementation standards to eliminate any questions about the admissibility or reliability of the information. In the meantime, when using an AIMS, as when using a handwritten record, a disciplined record-keeping practice that clearly and unambiguously documents the care that was provided should yield a complete, legible document, should help the physician's legal team to establish what the anesthesia care entailed and, at the same time, should have significant credibility in the courtroom.

Point:Counterpoint

AIMS Has the Potential to be a More Defensible Record (JF)

From a medicolegal perspective, the ideal record should be a legible, accurate, and complete rendition of the anesthetic care rendered. Creating such an ideal record depends more upon the diligence of the person keeping the record than upon the "technology" used, be it handwritten or automated. Therefore, handwritten and automated records must be compared from the perspective of how well they would serve a person who keeps a quality record. Neither approach is likely to create a defensible record if the person who is keeping the record is not diligent.

Although the documentation requirements of some procedures can be quite straightforward, the complexity of modern anesthesia care often requires that a large number of monitored variables be recorded in addition to medications, infusions, laboratory values, and annotations. It can be an almost impossible chore for the care provider to maintain a proper handwritten record when faced with the simultaneous demands of patient care. Furthermore, when a patient becomes unstable, the 5-minute resolution of the handwritten record is inadequate to capture the important physiologic changes.

The automated record inherently reduces the workload associated with record keeping by automatically recording electronic data. Further, these electronic data can be stored at a resolution that exceeds what is possible manually. Few anesthesia providers can create a handwritten record that matches the legibility of a record printed by computer. When one considers the advantages of reduced workload, increased resolution, and improved legibility, using an AIMS to create an anesthesia record is attractive. Beyond simple record keeping, the added benefits of data that can be stored and then used to support billing, practice management, quality assurance, and research activities make adoption of AIMS very compelling.

We have identified many limitations to the existing AIMS technology that reduce the effectiveness of the automated record as a documentation tool even for the most diligent of providers. Are those limitations of sufficient magnitude that handwritten records are still preferable when faced with a malpractice suit? I think not. We must recognize the limitations and use the systems appropriately. Although the AIMS technology may not be perfect, I believe it to be as good or better, even in the current iteration, than the handwritten record. By adopting the technology, we will learn lessons that will enhance the use and design of these systems so that they will ultimately serve us well from both the legal and patient-care perspectives.

AIMS Is Not a More Defensible Record (PL)

At the current level of IT sophistication, no clear-cut advantage and some very real disadvantages appear to be associated with relying on AIMS alone for anesthesia record management. The Vigoda example cited above points out a very important flaw. The purpose of manual documentation, it turns out, is not only to make a record but to ensure that the provider is actually paying attention. I think the natural human tendency is to be less attentive if the record is on "autopilot." Next, the fact that non-physiologic errors are explainable does not completely exonerate the provider in court, particularly if the plaintiff has been able to position the provider's records or actions as questionable, unreliable, or manipulative. A physician with a handwritten record that meets the standard of care, in conjunction with a professional "physician-like" demeanor of compassion and thoughtfulness, will fare much better being judged by his peers than the physician who comes in and insists that his AIMS-generated record tells all and cannot be attacked. The AIMS record does have the potential to be a more readable and more complete record if constructed properly. Alas, a warning! If the new AIMS greatly exceeds the written record in information and does become the standard, then the written record will become substandard care, and it is possible that anesthetics might be delayed or cancelled due to lack of AIMS capability. Another case of "be careful what you wish for."

Acknowledgment The authors and editors would like to thank Michael Gosney, DVM, MD, JD, MBA, Medical Director, Shoals Pain Center, Sheffield, AL, for his valuable advice regarding this chapter.

References

1. Pryor AT. Current state of computer-based patient record systems. In: Ball MJ, Collen MF, eds. *Aspects of the Computer-Based Patient Record*. New York: Springer, 1992:67–82
2. Partial testimony from the director of the office of personnel management before a House of Representatives subcommittee investigating governmental reform, July 2005
3. Gore G. Factors that influence who wins a malpractice suit. In: Gravenstein IS, Holzer IF, eds.*Cost Containment in Anesthesia*. Boston: Butterworths, 1988:135
4. Vigoda MM, Lubarsky DA. Failure to recognize loss of incoming data in an anesthesia record-keeping system may have increased medical liability. Anesth Analg 2006; 102:1798–802
5. Vigoda MM, Lubarsky DA. The medicolegal importance of enhancing timeliness of documentation when using an anesthesia information system and the response to automated feedback in an academic practice. Anesth Analg 2006; 103:131–6
6. Cook RI, McDonald JS, Nunziata E. Differences between handwritten and automatic blood pressure records. Anesthesiology 1989; 71:385–90
7. Feldman JM. Do Anesthesia information systems increase malpractice exposure? Results of a survey. Anesth Analg 2004; 99:840–3
8. Driscoll WD, Columbia MA, Peterfreund RA. An observational study of anesthesia record completeness using an anesthesia information management system. Anesth Analg 2007; 104(6):1454–61
9. Committee on Data Standards for Patient Safety. Key Capabilities of an Electronic Health Record System, Letter Report, July 200 3, p. 7
10. Committee on Data Standards for Patient Safety. Key Capabilities of an Electronic Health Record System, Letter Report, July 2003, p. 6
11. Lane P. AIS' role in anesthesiology risk management remains uncertain. Anesth Analg 2005; 100(5):1537
12. Terry v. Arkansas, 826 S.W.2d 818, citing the rules of admissibility of business records from Rule 803(6)(a) of the Federal Rules of Evidence. Records of a regularly conducted activity
13. Buckner F. Electronic records (Chap. 33). In: American College of Legal Medicine, Sanbar SS, ed. *Legal Medicine*, 6th ed. Philadelphia: Elsevier/Mosby, 2004:360
14. Oppenheim EB. *The Medical Record as Evidence*. Charlottesville, VA: Lexis Law Publishing, 1998:54

Chapter 13
Case Study: Implementation of an AIMS at an Academic Medical Center

David B. Wax and David L. Reich

The first AIMS installation at The Mount Sinai Medical Center (MSMC) occurred in January 1991 in a cardiothoracic and liver transplantation suite of six ORs. Currently, the Department of Anesthesiology at MSMC provides anesthesia care in approximately 50 ORs, 16 labor and delivery rooms, and 10 non-OR procedural areas. This growth occurred in various phases to encompass a system that uses a core AIMS vendor solution that is supplemented by various add-on applications and interfaces that were developed by departmental and institutional IT specialists. The ways in which the AIMS and the related and integrated systems have developed at MSMC are described in this chapter, including billing, physician compensation, scheduling, patient-tracking, research, and quality-improvement functions. As an academic medical center that was an early adopter of this technology and that has devoted informatics resources to enhance the core AIMS product, the successes and challenges of the department are unique, but the goal of this chapter is to illustrate principles that may be of value to others in perioperative enterprises of varying levels of complexity.

System Support and Configuration

The clinical staff of the Department of Anesthesiology consists of approximately 80 attending faculty anesthesiologists, 60 trainees (residents and fellows), and 11 CRNAs, and all are users of the AIMS. Annual turnover of clinical staff requires training of new care team members in the use of the AIMS. The AIMS vendor provides only limited training materials—a brief printed manual that is distributed to new staff and basic help built into the AIMS software. The primary training of new staff is provided through on-the-job experience that is supervised by more experienced care team members. Basic functionality is relatively easy to learn, and new staff members are always paired with more experienced AIMS users who can correct mistakes and teach more advanced functionality. Most users are comfortable with the system basics within a few days of use and master all significant aspects of the system within several weeks. "Superusers" among experienced faculty are also available for consultation, and vendor technical support is available to superusers when complex questions arise.

J. Stonemetz, K. Ruskin (eds.) *Anesthesia Informatics*,
© Springer Science+Business Media, LLC 2008

In addition to clinical staff, the department employs four full-time IT support staff members. One holds a doctoral degree in computer science and functions as the director of information systems, with systems analysis and database development roles. This individual constructs query strategies to extract pertinent information from the AIMS database for administrative, research, and quality improvement, and performs a strategic role in the development of custom applications that interface with the AIMS and other medical center systems. Another IT person is a Web developer who creates custom Web-based applications to enhance the functionality of the AIMS and the custom applications. A network engineer manages the connectivity of the hardware and software within the hospital, and a PC support technician provides day-to-day support and troubleshooting for the AIMS workstations during business hours.

Global system configuration is managed through a configuration module included in the AIMS software, access to which is limited to a group of faculty superusers and technical staff. Because changes to the configuration can produce unanticipated effects, most changes are discussed among the staff before they are implemented. Individual clinical users can also create their own set of custom configurations ("preloads") for various case types that control some aspects of the display, data entry, and printed record.

The system comprises several servers that fulfill file-storage, printing, database, and Web functions. Connectivity between the many AIMS workstations and the servers is via the hospital's Ethernet. Security is maintained with network passwords on all workstations as well as additional password protection in all AIMS applications. Antivirus and firewall software are installed, and backups of data are made regularly. Each authorized user has a unique user ID and password for the core AIMS system, and audit trails are automatically maintained to track access to and changes to protected health information.

Workstation Configuration and Ergonomics

The AIMS workstation configurations at this facility differ somewhat for each type of anesthetizing location served (Fig. 13.1). Originally, all OR workstation monitors, keyboards, and pointing devices were mounted on the anesthesia machine with articulating arms over the carbon dioxide absorber, which allowed the clinician to face the patient while entering data or reviewing trends. The CPU was positioned in a wall cabinet in the OR. The introduction of integrated monitoring and anesthesia machine equipment facilitated the placement of CPUs on the top shelf of the integrated equipment. Network cabling has always been installed in the anesthesia gas columns. A more recently introduced alternative involves freestanding computer carts positioned behind the anesthesia provider between the anesthesia machine and the drug cart. Although this configuration requires the anesthesia care team member to face partially away from the patient to enter data, it is a more practical

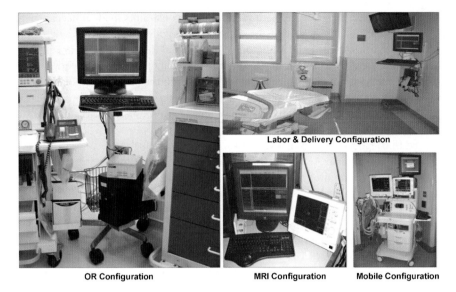

Labor & Delivery Configuration

OR Configuration   MRI Configuration   Mobile Configuration

Fig. 13.1 AIMS workstation configurations

solution in some areas, because anesthesia machines must be exchanged from time to time for maintenance or equipment replacement.

Data input to the AIMS is designed to occur via touchscreen monitors and keyboards with integrated pointing devices (trackballs or touchpads). The entry methods are designed to be redundant to facilitate entry by practitioners with different levels of keyboard proficiency and varying data entry preferences. Large virtual buttons on the touchscreen facilitate the time stamping of major events, such as anesthetic induction and tracheal intubation. The keyboard is necessary for much of the data entry, and the nearby touchpad/trackball is easier for most clinicians for navigation than is reaching for the screen. Because of the need to disinfect the keyboards for infection-control purposes, washable protective keyboard covers have been used but are troublesome to maintain. Because the trackballs cannot be covered, they accumulate debris, cannot be disinfected, and frequently malfunction. Therefore, standard keyboards are being replaced with newly available models that are hermetically sealed, have integrated touchpads, and are washable with disinfectant solutions.

A multiplexer collects physiologic and machine data from the serial outputs of the anesthesia machine and monitoring devices and feeds these into the serial input of the workstation's CPU. The data streams are decoded by vendor-specific drivers included in the AIMS software. The CPU is also connected to an Ethernet network jack to allow data exchange with the AIMS server. All connections are currently hardwired in the OR. Although wireless technology is being installed, it is unclear whether the AIMS will utilize this resource.

Some care locations require an alternate setup. Because the labor and delivery rooms at MSMC do not have anesthesia machines, the AIMS workstations are mounted to the wall on an articulating arm. Space constraints made it necessary to position the workstations so that the anesthesia provider's back would be to the patient, as in the OR. Because the current maternal–fetal monitors are incompatible with the AIMS, physiologic data must be manually recorded periodically while the anesthesia care provider is in the room with the patient. Although this is more time consuming than automated capture of vital signs, it has proven to be useful in accounting for actual face-to-face time with the patient, as required for billing for some payers. In addition, several mobile laptop-based workstations can be used in triage rooms and hallways during high-occupancy times.

In the MRI suite, an AIMS workstation is connected via a multiplexer to a wireless patient slave monitor that provides vital-sign data. Data from the anesthesia machine (e.g., tidal volumes and airway pressures) must be recorded manually. For other infrequently used radiology locations (e.g., CT, positron emission tomography), a mobile anesthesia machine with an AIMS workstation mounted on top is used. The AIMS workstation CPU can be plugged into any available network jack in the scanning rooms. If a network jack is unavailable in a remote location, the anesthesia record can be generated in an offline mode and automatically uploaded to the server once the mobile workstation is plugged into a network jack in another location. The ability to work offline (disconnect from the local area network) is also advantageous during network outages in all locations.

Perioperative Electronic Medical Record

The goal of the Department of Anesthesiology at MSMC is to integrate the AIMS into all aspects of practice to create a fully electronic perioperative medical record. While the intraoperative anesthesia record keeper is the core application of the AIMS, the preoperative and postoperative periods are also important parts of anesthesia care and ideally should be captured by an AIMS. Some of this capability is included by the AIMS vendor's suite of applications, but some are not suitable for the needs of the department. Extensive custom configuration has been made to the vendor's existing modules, and custom applications have been added to the system as needed.

The basic preoperative evaluation provides an opportunity to collect information that is needed throughout the perioperative period. It is also the basis for determining what additional evaluation is needed preoperatively and is an important component of a dataset that can be effectively mined for research purposes. Unfortunately, it also involves frequent duplication of effort, as multiple practitioners (e.g., anesthesia providers, OR nurses, and surgeons) document redundant patient information. By creating a unified preoperative evaluation instrument, the preoperative interview process may be streamlined. Some vendors offer Web-based preoperative evaluation systems. A prescreening function of the system allows patients to access the Web site to enter their own basic health information. Alternatively, a physician extender or nurse may contact the patient by telephone interview. This basic information is entered into algorithms and/or reviewed by a clinician to determine which patients require a preanesthesia clinic visit and which can bypass the preanesthesia evaluation and arrive with no further workup on the day of surgery. The system then allows various practitioners to complete their relevant sections of the full H&P exam, either during a presurgical visit or on the day of surgery. Laboratory, imaging, and consultation data can also be merged with the evaluation as they are received or reviewed. Similar systems are already used at several academic medical centers, and MSMC is in the early implementation stages of a test system.

PACU documentation capability in the AIMS is currently used only for performance improvement and administrative data. Full functionality would require an AIMS workstation or ICU EMR system, compatible patient monitors, software licenses for every location, and training of all PACU staff. At present, the PACU nurses continue to use handwritten clinical documentation. Many peer institutions have electronic critical care documentation systems that would be a functional solution for PACU EMR purposes.

The MSMC AIMS includes a generic form-management module that is flexible enough to adapt to many uses. It allows for the design of forms that can be accessed via a Web-based interface from anywhere inside the hospital firewall, from dedicated AIMS workstations, or from outside the hospital using secure connectivity solutions. Forms can also be accessed on laptop or tablet PCs, and the completed forms can be uploaded to the server in batches or via wireless connectivity. As clinicians are frequently called upon to provide services throughout the hospital in many non-OR anesthesia locations, electronic forms have been created to capture these patient encounters. Some of the forms developed include postoperative evaluation, pain management notes for both consultations and procedures, and critical care progress and procedure notes. In some cases, the electronic forms are simply administrative (i.e., electronic billing vouchers) and contain little clinical information, such as the AIMS form that is completed for urgent or emergent intubations on the hospital floors or for short cases done outside of the OR (e.g., electroconvulsive therapy) for which handwritten anesthesia records continue to be created.

Performance-Improvement Applications

Performance improvement is another area in which the MSMC AIMS has proven to be valuable. Providing safe, high-quality care is the most important goal of the anesthesia care team and is clearly mandated by various standards as well as by patients, payers, and regulators. When clear clinical guidelines are available, an AIMS can be used to promote adherence to those standards. As an example, the Surgical Care Improvement Project has been initiated and calls for administration of most prophylactic antibiotics within 1 hour before the start of the surgical procedure in a very large number of operations.[1] Compliance with this performance measure is publicly reported. In an effort to improve compliance with antibiotic guidelines, the AIMS was modified to include an antibiotic reminder icon on the AIMS

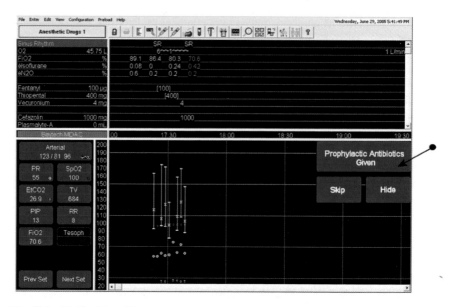

Fig. 13.2 AIMS with antibiotic performance-improvement reminder

workstation screen that appears before the icon that indicates the start of the proce-dure/surgery (Fig. 13.2). The addition of the reminder was associated with increased timely prophylactic antibiotic administration.[2] In addition to the contemporaneous reminder, data from the AIMS are extracted and analyzed to generate periodic report cards that are sent by electronic mail to all practitioners and present their personal performance related to this standard in comparison with the group as a whole, thereby encouraging the staff to improve their performance.

The aforementioned postanesthesia evaluation form allows documentation of postoperative findings and complications. Significant postoperative complications (e.g., unplanned ICU admission, neurologic injury, death) recorded in the AIMS trigger investigations by the Performance Improvement Committee to seek anesthesia-related factors that may have contributed to negative outcomes. When appropriate, this process may result in educational efforts or policy changes to prevent recurrences.

Point-of-Care Charge Capture

The healthcare industry has lagged behind other industries in its use of information systems to conduct its business. Although the health insurance industry (i.e., payers) have moved to completely electronic claims submission and back-office processing, only a minority of healthcare providers utilize electronic charge capture at the point of care or electronic submission of charges directly to payers.[3] The complexity of

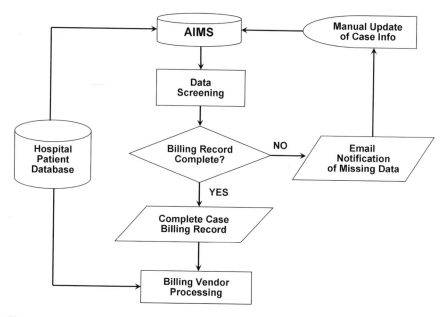

Fig. 13.3 AIMS for point-of-care charge capture

medical billing has prompted an industry of billing intermediaries that are subcontracted to optimize coding and billing and handle electronic charge submission. However, these billing vendors still receive most of the charges to be billed in the form of manual billing vouchers generated by clinicians and their office staff. These manual processes contain inherent sources of errors and omissions that may result in suboptimal reimbursement for providers or increased costs, in that reprocessing a claim incurs more in administrative expenses than one that is correctly processed the first time. Problems include illegibility, lost/missed cases, incomplete charges, inaccurate coding, discrepancies between supporting clinical documentation and billing vouchers, delays in submission, and noncompliant billing.

Because the billing module included in the AIMS was inadequate for the needs at MSMC, a custom billing application was created (Fig. 13.3). A series of automated data queries and manipulations is performed to assemble all of the data necessary for billing purposes from the existing AIMS database. An initial extraction of information from the AIMS database populates a billing worksheet for each new case. Then, each billing worksheet is processed using business rules to ensure that all necessary information for a compliant bill is present. Any deficiencies (e.g., missing electronic signature, CPT code, or teaching rule attestation) are flagged, and the responsible practitioner is alerted via electronic mail so that the problem can be remedied and the case returned to the processing queue. The data extraction and screening process is performed every business day as a batch process, and the prescreened bills are transmitted to the billing vendor for review and submission to payers. Patient demographic and financial/insurance information is transmitted to the billing vendor separately by the hospital information technology group. As a result of implementation of the point-of-care charge capture, average charge lag decreased, total days in accounts receivable decreased, and labor costs for charge entry and other billing-related duties were reduced.[3]

Additional custom features have been added to the AIMS to improve billing functions. For example, the obstetric service had a problem when laboring patients were transferred from a labor room to an OR for a cesarean section and the practitioner failed to add a cesarean-section CPT billing code in addition to the original labor and delivery code, resulting in underbilling for services. To prevent this from occurring, a real-time coding check of the AIMS data in the obstetric ORs was implemented that alerts the practitioner with a pop-up warning message on the AIMS workstation whenever a cesarean-section CPT code is missing from the record.

Compensation

Implementation of an AIMS for all clinical activities provided the necessary platform on which to add a productivity-based component to the faculty compensation system that has provided an incentive for physicians to participate fully in the point-of-care billing process. The compensation system provides financial incentives for complete base, time, and modifier unit documentation (ASA Relative Value Guide; see Chap. 14), and the subsequent increases in billing totals are most likely attributable to this process. The system accounts for participation of multiple attendings (e.g., relief by the on-call attending) and for faculty who are medically directing care in multiple locations simultaneously. This clinical productivity is then combined with other sources, including academic, research, teaching, and strategic mission-based productivity. The full compensation model is diagrammed in Fig. 13.4. To assist in monitoring personal productivity and billing compliance, a listing of all cases performed in the previous week is sent via electronic mail to each faculty member. This encourages faculty to scan for cases that may be missing or incomplete to identify and correct errors.

Operating Room Management Applications

Until recently, tracking of patient flow during the perioperative period was rudimentary at MSMC. Locating a patient scheduled for surgery was possible only by paging or telephone communication. The result was overall inefficiency and delay, and many practitioners were frustrated. To improve the situation, the team expanded upon the OR-management module built into the AIMS to create a custom, comprehensive patient-tracking system.

Currently, ambulatory and day-of-admission surgery patients are logged into the AIMS when they arrive at the hospital and register at the surgical reception area.

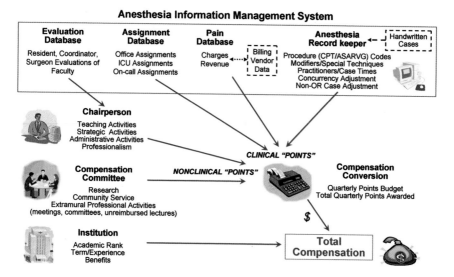

Fig. 13.4 AIMS faculty compensation system

Basic demographic data from hospital information systems and the OR scheduling system are imported into the AIMS at that time. Patient location is updated and time-stamped in the AIMS at various sites as patients move through various perioperative areas (Fig. 13.5). The AIMS module that acts as the core of the system has been modified to create administrative documentation of parameters, including assessment personnel and readiness, PACU personnel, expected recovery times, reasons for delayed discharges, and postoperative inpatient bed assignments. In all perioperative areas (except the OR itself), patients' arrival and subsequent departure are marked in AIMS records by a clerk.

For the intraoperative period, the data are more detailed. Arrival in the OR is automatically documented by the anesthesia care team when an AIMS OR record is started, as is the progress of the case based on predefined events (e.g., tracheal intubation, procedure start, extubation).

During the patient's PACU stay, nurses document progress and reasons for delay (if any) after the patient is medically ready for discharge. The hospital's bed-management staff remotely enter inpatient bed assignments and the status (e.g., awaiting cleaning) for each same-day-admission patient. All patients are logged out of the system upon transport out of the PACU. Currently, MSMC is evaluating wireless technologies (e.g., radio-frequency identification tags) to continuously track patient locations as an alternative to intermittent, manual data entry, and is considering means of integration with the wider hospital bed-board system.

Tracking data are made available to staff with real-time reporting via a variety of modalities (Fig. 13.6). Information is displayed on large-screen monitors with color-coded patient status that is suited to each display location. For example, names of patients awaiting transport to holding areas are highlighted on the screen

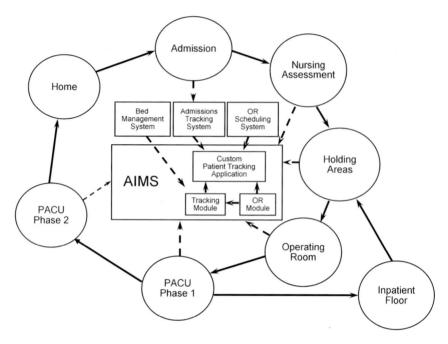

Fig. 13.5 Patient and data flow for AIMS patient tracking

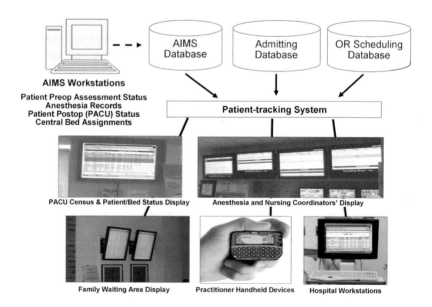

Fig. 13.6 AIMS for patient tracking

in the waiting area so that transporters can quickly be assigned to them. In the PACU, patients who are medically ready for discharge but remain in the PACU beyond that time are highlighted so that nurse managers can address the delays and minimize backups. On the OR coordinators' "big board," rooms that have been empty for excessive periods of time and "to-follow" patients who have not yet arrived are flagged, thus allowing the anesthesia and nursing coordinators to better manage the ORs by matching patients and staff with available rooms. Tracking information is also available to authorized users at all hospital workstations through a patient-tracking report that can be used to locate patients based on patient name, surgeon name, OR, procedure, scheduled time, etc. A HIPAA-compliant tracking display of limited data is also provided in the family waiting area so that relatives and friends can see when surgery begins and ends.

Tracking information can also be sent directly to clinicians (both surgeon and anesthesia care team members) via their electronic devices (i.e., text pagers, cellular telephones, and personal digital assistants). This feature provides instant notification of events that can reduce delays. For example, both the surgeon and the anesthesia care team can be notified as soon as the patient arrives in the holding area, thereby facilitating care and reducing turnover delay. Once clinicians become accustomed to receiving these notifications, even the absence of expected event messages is also helpful in alerting them that a patient has not yet arrived and may prompt efforts to mitigate inefficiencies caused by the delay.

Electronic Medical Record Integration

As in most hospitals, MSMC's information systems consist of a variety of software applications (including the AIMS) that were implemented independently over time and have limited interoperability. Recently, the importance of data integration has become a common goal, and the move toward a fully electronic medical record has received a governmental mandate.[4] Standards for structured reporting of clinical information using discrete data elements are under development for this purpose.[5] Until such a universal lexicon is established, most EMR systems allow for inclusion of mixed text and graphic documents using industry-standard image-rendering formats. Though paperless (with the inherent risks and benefits) and more easily/widely accessible to those who may need the clinical information, this alternative falls short of the ideal EMR because the data (even with optical character recognition of handwritten or typed text) are not easily categorized, extracted, or compared between patients or EMR platforms. However, in the interim, it is necessary to include the AIMS-based anesthesia records in the patient's EMR to make them readily accessible to other providers. Thus, virtual images of printed paper records are exported in tagged image file format (TIFF) to each patient's EMR data repository, which can be viewed at any hospital workstation by authorized users.

Because of the growing concern about medication-related errors in patient care, the team at MSMC felt that it was important to ensure that all drugs administered in the course of anesthesia care be visible in the EMR. As described, an image of the anesthesia record is already stored in the EMR, but most nonanesthesia practitioners seem to have difficulty understanding and locating information within an anesthesia record. Thus, it was decided that an extract of medication-administration records would be provided in discrete elements (e.g., date, time, agent, dose, route) to be exported to, and included separately in, the EMR for easy review and analysis.

Another area where discrete data are needed and may not be easily or accurately located in the anesthesia record is in quality and regulatory audits. Hospital quality benchmarking and pay-for-performance initiatives are increasingly prevalent and require accurate data to ensure maximal compliance. Hospitals must increasingly compile data from various groups to monitor and report performance. For example, the measures of the aforementioned Surgical Care Improvement Project call for antibiotic administration within 1 hour prior to the start of the procedure for most antibiotics and for a wide variety of procedures. At MSMC, rather than have auditors try to review anesthesia records, records of antibiotic agent administration and related comments taken from a controlled vocabulary (pick list) are extracted and exported directly to the hospital's quality-monitoring database.

Similarly, extensive regulatory controls have been established by various governmental agencies to prevent controlled substances from being diverted to illicit uses. Pharmacies are responsible for tracking the supply and use of controlled substances. As clinicians record all intraoperative drug administration in the AIMS, this information can be used by the in-house pharmacy to track the use of controlled substances. Using data extracted from the case records, a daily Web-based report of all controlled substances administered is created and can be accessed by authorized pharmacists to reconcile the supply and use of regulated agents.

Compliance Reporting

The training of residents and fellows in teaching hospitals is monitored by accrediting organizations such as the Accreditation Council for Graduate Medical Education (ACGME). The ACGME seeks to ensure that each trainee gains sufficient clinical experience during her training. For most programs, self-reporting by trainees with a manual "case log" is used to verify this requirement, but maintenance of case logs is burdensome to trainees and may not always be accurate or timely. As most of the information needed for such a case log is already stored in the AIMS, this reporting function has been automated. This automation provides real-time tracking, thereby allowing more frequent review by the residency program director to assess and adjust trainee scheduling toward increasing exposure in areas that may be lacking. It also ensures the availability of necessary data for ACGME audits and frees the trainees of the burden of additional documentation.

The ACGME identifies numerous categories for patient, anesthesia modality, anesthesia procedure, and surgical case type that must be tallied for each trainee.[6] Because the MSMC AIMS did not have this specific reporting feature built in, a customized query was created that extracts the necessary data from the case files for each trainee for any period of interest. Because the AIMS data structure was not specifically designed by the vendor with this in mind, the necessary data elements had to be located and assembled. For example, some information (such as patient age) is found in the basic case data but must be transformed into the ACGME-designated categories. Some experiences are identified by a record of attestation of performance of a procedure (e.g., placement of an arterial catheter) in the associated billing record. Other procedures (e.g., fiberoptic intubation) are typically documented as a comment in the narrative text of the record and must be extracted from that data structure. Tallies of surgical procedure types required the creation of a crosswalk to assign each CPT code to one of the ACGME-specified categories. Any changes to the ACGME reporting requirements, additions of new CPT codes, or changes to the AIMS data structure may require modification of the query. A system of manual adjustments to the reports is maintained, such as may be necessary to include trainee experiences in other departments or affiliate institutions that do not utilize the MSMC AIMS.

Another ACGME goal is to provide for fair and uniform evaluation of trainees to ensure competency of graduates, to provide timely feedback to trainees regarding their performance, and to help training programs improve their training methods. Similarly, trainees should have a mechanism by which to provide feedback to program directors regarding perceived strengths and weaknesses of the training program. To accomplish this, the AIMS was expanded to include a Web-based trainee evaluation report that incorporates the six ACGME-designated core competencies.[7] Faculty are encouraged to evaluate trainees based on their daily performance as well as in summary fashion at the end of each subspecialty (e.g., cardiothoracic) assignment. Because the AIMS case data contain the names of all involved practitioners, the database can be queried to determine which faculty members worked with which trainees, and this information can be matched with the evaluation data to generate reminders (via email) to those faculty to complete their required evaluations, thus improving the quantity and timeliness of feedback. A similar Web-based system was also added for the trainees to evaluate the individual faculty members, the residency program as a whole, and each subspecialty rotation.

Research and Education Applications

The vast amount of clinical and operations information stored in an AIMS provides a valuable resource for research efforts. Large amounts of data can be analyzed to answer clinical questions and to test hypotheses. Most often, this is done retrospectively, and unfortunately, the data available are limited to those that were collected at the time that care was rendered. Although including every imaginable clinical parameter at the outset of implementing an AIMS is attractive for potential future research, it is too time consuming to document a multitude of elements that may never be utilized. Of course, the AIMS data structure can be modified to include additional variables of interest, making it an excellent data-collection tool for prospective studies. Because a standard for exchange of clinical data between AIMS does not yet exist, it is not easy to combine data for multicenter studies to increase the power of retrospective analyses, though it can still be accomplished with manual mapping of variables between each system.

In the MSMC AIMS, case data are stored in flat files, and physiologic data (which are voluminous, as a multitude of measurements are recorded every 15 seconds) are compressed. For this reason, the AIMS vendor provides a research module that decompresses and extracts selected data elements from any set of existing cases and stores the results in relational database tables. Because this is a slow process and storage media have become so inexpensive, a freestanding SQL database has been created that contains all case data in an uncompressed format that is ready for extraction. Data extraction is performed by a database administrator who has been designated as an "honest broker" for the purposes of creating reports of deidentified patient information. All such reports must be related to performance-improvement projects or research projects approved by the institutional review board.

The AIMS database also provides a rich supply of cases that can be identified and used for educational purposes. Using query tools, past cases that match any search criterion of interest can be identified, whether the criterion is a procedure type, an intraoperative event, a postoperative complication, or a physiologic parameter. Cases of interest can be retrieved and used for case reports, conferences, or other educational or performance-improvement purposes. Again, a limitation is that not all such items of interest are consistently documented in the record, either because they are omitted from the clinical record or they are documented in a place or manner that is missed by the search strategy.

Conclusion

The penetration of AIMS appears to be greatest in academic institutions. The multiple applications cited earlier indicate the motivation for academic centers to become early adopters of this technology. MSMC has also created multiple linked applications that should be considered part of an AIMS but were custom add-ons that were created by the departmental programming team. Richer AIMS application packages that serve many of these needs of academic institutions and the outside pressure to adopt EMR technology will undoubtedly further increase the prevalence of AIMS in academic anesthesia departments.

Key Points

- To maximize the value of an AIMS, system functionality can be extended beyond intraoperative anesthesia record keeping to include billing, compensation, compliance, quality improvement, OR management, education, and research applications, and can encompass the entire perioperative period.
- Value-added functionality of AIMS may not be available "out of the box" with a given vendor's core AIMS software and may need to be developed in-house or obtained from third parties. Such enhancements may be made through creative use of preexisting functionality, custom development of "add-on" applications that interface with the AIMS, or development and implementation of related but independent systems.
- Realization of the full potential of an AIMS requires adequate support and training for the system and its users. User acceptance, system reliability, integration into clinical and administrative routines, integration with other hospital systems, and development and implementation of custom add-on applications require the availability of sufficient technical and/or clinician AIMS experts.

References

1. Fry DE. The surgical infection prevention project: Processes, outcomes, and future impact. Surg Infect 2006; 7:s17–26
2. Wax DB, Beilin Y, Levin M, et al. Effect of an interactive visual reminder in an anesthesia information management system on timeliness of prophylactic antibiotic administration. Anesth Analg 2007; 104(6):1462–6
3. Reich DL, Kahn RA, Wax D, et al. Development of a module for point-of-care charge capture and submission using an anesthesia information management system. Anesthesiology 2006; 105:179–86
4. Ford EW, Menachemi N, Phillips MT. Predicting the adoption of electronic health records by physicians: When will health care be paperless? J Am Med Inform Assoc 2006; 13:106–12
5. Monk T, Sanderson I. The development of an anesthesia lexicon. Semin Anesth 2004; 23:93–8
6. Accreditation Council for Graduate Medical Education. Case Entry for Anesthesiology. http://www.acgme.org/residentdatacollection/documentation/Manuals/Case_Entry_040.pdf. Accessed May 4, 2007
7. Accreditation Council for Graduate Medical Education. General Competencies. http://www.acgme.org/outcome/comp/compFull.asp. Accessed May 4, 2007

Business Case Scenario

Dr. James was the President of Northeast Anesthesia Consultants, an all-MD group of anesthesiologists practicing at a popular community not-for-profit hospital in a typical suburban environment. Dr. James was a very good anesthesiologist with an interest in the business of anesthesia and had established good business practices for his group. They had been quite successful but had seen a continual decrease in partners' income over the prior 5 years due to shrinking reimbursements and increasing clinical obligations. Dr. James was familiar with most strategies at increasing profitability; however, he had not taken any initiative to move to an electronic-record platform, primarily because he was unfamiliar with the technology and had some basic misgivings regarding the utilization and liability of these records. Regardless, the hospital had recently installed an AIMS as a module of a new Operating Room Management System (ORMS). The anesthesia module was provided for little additional charge to the hospital and was selected almost exclusively by the Chief Information Officer (CIO) and the OR Charge Nurse because of tight integration between the modules. The anesthesia department had been invited to review the product but had demonstrated little interest. Consequently, the product had been purchased, installed, and deployed with little involvement of the physicians who were primarily tasked with using the product.

Despite grumblings from almost every member of the anesthesia department, the product was, in fact, being utilized, and the CIO and CEO of the hospital mandated that this product was to be used for all anesthesia records. In an attempt to pacify the administration at their hospital, Dr. James had declared that all physicians in the group must use the record, despite his own frustration at using an electronic record that seemed much more cumbersome and difficult than the simple paper record with which he had become so comfortable over 20 years of clinical practice. That was until the day that he received a call from his business manager that would change his perception of the electronic record and result in a drastic measure that would ultimately negatively impact the tenuous relationship between Northeast Anesthesia Consultants and the hospital administration.

J. Stonemetz, K. Ruskin (eds.) *Anesthesia Informatics*,
© Springer Science+Business Media, LLC 2008

In the call, the business manager had informed Dr. James that for the first time in the history of their corporation, they would not be able to meet payroll. It seems that the receivables coming in were insufficient to cover basic expenses and employee paychecks. Consequently, the partners would have to drastically reduce their monthly draw. Investigation revealed that the reason for the shortfall was that for the prior 3 months, the billing office had been unable to process most of the anesthesia claims due to missing information. Therefore, less than one-half of the normal claims had been submitted in a timely manner. Missing from the anesthesia records were data elements such as provider names (anesthesia and/or surgeon), dates of service, start and end times (which are required to generate an anesthesia bill), and other critical clinical data that are used to generate the professional fee. Previously, this information had always been gleaned from the paper record, and the group had been very diligent about completing all of the necessary information. Every member of the group understood that this documentation was essential to their getting paid for their efforts. Unfortunately, no one from either the EMR vendor or the group had investigated the impact that going electronic would have on charge generation. Consequently, the system that had been functioning well on paper completely ceased to function when the group began generating electronic records.

Dr. James' initial response was to call an emergency meeting of the partners to discuss the ramifications of the financial crisis, and the only recommendation that resulted from this meeting was to immediately cease using the electronic record and return to paper records. This action solved the primary problem of generating claims for professional fees but created an entire cascade of acrimonious dealings with nursing and administration at the hospital. In the meantime, the group paid several employees to go through the medical records of the previous 3 months to find the missing data on the claims that had not been submitted. Ultimately, they were able to recover almost 80% of the missing data, but many of the claims were never paid because they were submitted too late to be covered by insurance. Estimates of losses were placed somewhere between $1.6 and $1.8 million dollars, and this money was never recovered. Northeast Anesthesia Consultants considered suing the vendor of the AIMS, but they were discouraged from this action by their own counsel, as the vendor had never made any type of promise or claim regarding professional fees. The financial losses were only just beginning for this corporation, however. Their refusal to use the electronic system was viewed as being uncooperative by the hospital administration, and after months of discussions, the CEO of the hospital ceased attempting to come to terms with the anesthesiologists and sent out an RFP for anesthesia services, with the intention to replace this group with one that acted with better citizenship.

Meanwhile, across town, Dr. Jones was in a similar situation as Dr. James; however, his actions yielded an entirely opposite result. Dr. Jones was President of Southwest Anesthesia Consultants, a mixed MD and CRNA group that practiced at a for-profit hospital and at a connected surgical center. Like Northeast, this corporation had also suffered lower reimbursement; however, here is where the similarity differs. Dr. Jones had always been a prolific computer user, using them primarily for email and basic applications such as spreadsheets and word processors. He had inquired into the feasibility of using an AIMS as a means of enhancing his professional-fee charge capture and had discovered that these systems could, in fact, generate more income through professional fees; however, he also learned that several issues had to be handled in advance. Because of his proactive approach, his group had been successful in convincing the hospital administration that the AIMS being offered as an add-on module from the vendor of the ORMS was not adequate for their needs. Following several months of diligent evaluations, the group settled on a particular system that demonstrated robust functionality in capturing professional-fee charges and a superior ability to interface with the ORMS. The CIO agreed to the purchase.

Dr. Jones and his group became very involved in the implementation of this system and enthusiastically supported its deployment. One of the features that the vendor agreed to at Dr. Jones' insistence was the use of "hard stops," a feature that prohibits a provider from signing out of a case and printing a record unless certain fields have been completed. This feature initially created some angst among the providers because they saw it as a disruption in their workflow. However, this initial consternation was quickly dispelled when it was illustrated how this process prevents the loss of any charges due to missing data elements. Even the loudest complainers at the beginning of the process quickly became advocates of the system when they realized that the AIMS actually decreased their workload and improved their documentation. Indeed, the most vocal advocate became the billing manager for the group. This individual was able to demonstrate, once the system became operational and the minor kinks in the processes were worked out, that the group actually realized several financial advantages almost immediately.

First, an adjudication report was generated in the manager's office that provided a daily census discrepancy report. Any cases that were recorded in the ORMS as having been done with anesthesia involvement that were not accounted for with an AIMS were highlighted in this report. Consequently, the manager would contact the anesthesia provider the next day and require her to go to Medical Records to obtain a copy of the anesthesia record for billing. One or two trips to Medical Records were usually all that was necessary to enforce completion of all future documentation. Second, the prompt collection of all billing data allowed the group to submit the professional fees in a more timely fashion. Efficiency was also enhanced by an electronic interface to the billing software system so that redundant data entry was eliminated. These improvements allowed reassignment of employees in the billing office from performing data entry for claim submission to spending more time working on outstanding claims. The end results were a faster cash turn around and higher collection percentages, which ultimately resulted in more dollars to the partners. However, the real value to the billing manager was that the AIMS provided a completely fool-proof mechanism of generating anesthesia professional fees without compliance violations. Bills could not be generated for procedures without appropriate documentation by a credentialed provider. This functionality allowed the billing manager and the partners to sleep easier at night, knowing that the group was well protected in the event of an audit by the OIG.

Improvement in professional fees and higher collections were not the only benefits of the system. Dr. Jones had effectively worked with his hospital administration at implementing a Preoperative Evaluation Clinic managed by the anesthesia group and staffed daily by nurse practitioners and one physician. The clinic was made possible by the utilization of sophisticated software that started with a Web-based health questionnaire for patients and fed directly into a rules-based engine that established a triage of patients preoperatively. The triage ranged from instructing patients to arrive at the hospital on the day of surgery, to determining which tests were needed, to informing the surgeon that specific patients would need to be seen in the clinic, either as a routine visit or an anesthesia consult. With implementation of this preoperative clinic, the hospital witnessed a significant decrease in surgical delays and cancellations on the day of surgery. More importantly, patients were effectively managed into clinical pathways preoperatively, rather than simply arriving and having surgery. For example, beta blockade was established in the at-risk population, diabetes management was started earlier, prophylaxis for deep venous thrombosis was identified preoperatively, and NPO guidelines were more effectively established. This improved patient management resulted in shorter lengths of stay, less hospitalizations for outpatients, and overall better patient care. The entire clinic's cost was covered by the hospital because Dr. Jones and his group improved their documentation of comorbid conditions to the extent that the hospital was able to improve their disease-related grouping (DRG) reimbursement, improve their health score cards, and improve their community standing.

Ironically, the group was becoming so successful that they were considering submitting a response to an RFP for anesthesia services at a hospital across town.

Chapter 14
Automated Charge Capture

Christopher Reeves and Jerry Stonemetz

Professional-Fee Charges

The primary motivation, or return on investment (ROI), for purchasing an EMR for most office-based physician practices focuses predominately on the ability to enhance and automate charge capture. In the paper world, a patient would be seen by a physician, who would create notes on paper records. The physician would then typically complete a "superbill"—a fairly standardized form that contains most of the chargeable items for that particular specialty. This superbill would be sent to the front office at checkout and form the basis for the documentation of services rendered, charges generated by the office staff, and the subsequent claim submission to the payer. Unfortunately, in this scenario, the physician filling out the superbill would frequently code or bill for a visit that was not adequately justified from the documentation in the chart. Concomitant with the passage of HIPAA, this miscoding became fraudulent billing, susceptible to fines and penalties.[1] With the advent of EMRs, the selection of charges could be generated by software algorithms based on specific rules that are incorporated into the charge functionality. These sophisticated systems could even "recommend" actions that would enhance the documentation and consequently increase the level of coding for the medical visit.[2,3] For example, an on-screen alert could indicate that if the physician would simply define the social history, the visit could qualify for an evaluation and management code that would be slightly higher than that coded without the social history. A significant proportion of the ROI cited by vendors of these systems is the ability to accurately capture all charges and potentially enhance revenue generation. Despite the obvious advantage of digitizing the clinical records and the concomitant ability to analyze these data, no business entity would decide to invest in these expensive systems unless they could generate savings, either through reduced expenses or increased revenues.

With anesthesia, the functionality of proper charge capture is even more complex. Anesthesia billing represents the single most complex billing specialty in medicine —primarily because the anesthesia charge calculation includes a time element,[4,5] which makes every single anesthetic a unique charge, and software systems that facilitate this functionality must be equally complex. However, due to this complexity,

J. Stonemetz, K. Ruskin (eds.) *Anesthesia Informatics*,
© Springer Science + Business Media, LLC 2008

anesthesia charge capture also represents an area where significant benefit can be realized through enhanced charge capture and positive financial benefits can be generated. As with all computerized systems, a system with the functionality to capture a certain data set is only a part of the solution. Other requirements—decision support, adequate usability, and appropriate system interfaces—will be expanded upon in this chapter.

We will begin with a brief description of how an anesthetic charge is generated. The primary focus of this chapter is anesthesia charges that comprise the professional fees for delivering an anesthetic for surgery in the OR, which may also include remote areas and/or office-based ORs, and the implications regarding automated charge capture within an AIMS also apply to these alternative sites, provided of course, an AIMS is available. Multiple alternative situations, such as pain management, obstetrical services, intensive-care management, and consultative services, will not be discussed here and are best handled through a professional-fee management consultant.

Calculation of the Anesthesia Professional-Fee Charge

Anesthesia professional fees are unique in that they contain a time element. Talks are underway to redesign anesthesia professional fees to more closely align with those of other medical specialists; however, it is not clear if and when these changes will be accepted by the Centers for Medicare and Medicaid Services (CMS) or the ASA. We will assume that our definitions of anesthesia charge calculation will remain germane. Essentially, the formula for calculation of professional fees is as follows:

Base Units (BU)+Time Units (TU)+Qualifying Circumstances (QCU) = Total Units,

Total Units×Conversion Factor (CF) = Anesthesia Charge (AC)

Each of the individual parameters of the equation will be explored below. However, it is sufficient to briefly describe the CF and then disregard it in the remainder of the discussion. Each business unit, whether it is an individual working in an office-based practice or a major corporation that represents hundreds of anesthesiologists, must define a CF for its local environment. An entity determines its CF based on a number of variables, including the local market and group demand, and CFs for individual business units will vary significantly. For our discussion, we will use $50 as the CF. It rarely matters in today's world in which professional-fee charges are negotiated to a much lower CF by managed-care organizations. Compounding this discount is the conspicuously low reimbursement allocated by CMS for their beneficiaries, which typically represents less than $20 per unit and frequently is in the low teens. Other issues are the extremely low reimbursement allocated to patients with Medical Assistance and the indigent population that has no insurance.

To illustrate the methodology of anesthesia professional-fee charges, the charges generated with the administration of an anesthetic for an inguinal hernia that takes exactly 1 hour of anesthesia time will be utilized as an example.

Base Unit are assigned by CMS with input from the ASA according to a rating of the complexity of the anesthetic. CMS assigns these units to individual anesthesia CPT codes (which will be described in detail below). The unit values range from the lowest of 3 units for simple cases, such as cystoscopy or carpal tunnel release, to the highest of 25 units for cardiac bypass off pump. A coronary artery bypass graft using bypass is assigned 20 units, most craniotomies are 16–18 units, major spine cases are 8–15 units, cholecystectomies are 7 units, bowel surgery cases are typically 6 units, and many orthopedic cases are 4–5 units. An inguinal hernia is assigned 4 units. The ASA publishes the Relative Value Guide, which defines the number of units for each anesthesia CPT Code. In most cases, these units are the same as those defined by CMS. Groups may choose to use the Relative Value Guide determination for charging; however, most carriers use the CMS version when differences exist in unit values for procedures.

CMS defines 1 *Time Unit* as being equal to 15 minutes. In certain states, where local insurance intermediaries have allowed an alternative system, 1 Time Unit is equivalent to 10 minutes. The tradition of "rounding" the Time Units up (16 minutes = 2 Time Units) is no longer allowed for CMS and most carriers. Consequently, most carriers now require exact minutes of anesthesia service to be reported, and the payment will represent a percentage of 1 Time Unit. In the example inguinal hernia case that lasts exactly 60 minutes, 4 Time Units would be reported. If the case were to last 65 minutes, 4.33 Time Units would be reported. A confusing but appropriate regulation by CMS has allowed the reporting of discontinuous time for the generation of anesthesia charges. In this example, if one were to begin preparing the patient for surgery and the case were delayed, the provider may add this preparation time to the total anesthesia minutes of service. However, the documentation requirements to justify this charge are so onerous that most groups simply do not bother with the attempts at capturing this additional time. With a robust AIMS, this discontinuous time should be easily captured, provided the clinical record contains sufficient documentation to indicate precisely the amount of time that was spent and what was done for the patient. In most situations in which a dispute regarding anesthesia time occurs, the presence of monitoring information is becoming an essential documentation requirement. An AIMS would potentially provide a benefit, as the vital signs would be automatically captured and recorded in the patient's record.

Qualifying Circumstance Unit alludes to special consideration for unique clinical situations, such as emergency care or the use of hypotension or hypothermia for the delivery of an anesthetic. Additionally, specific procedures that are referred to as "modifiers" are assigned specific unit values; examples are the placement of certain invasive catheters such as arterial, central venous pressure, and/or Swan-Ganz catheters; regional blocks placed in conjunction with a general anesthetic for the purpose of providing postoperative pain management; the use of fluoroscopy for placement of central lines; and possibly the use of transesophageal echocardiography during a case. As with Base Units, all of these Qualifying Circumstance Unit values are defined in the ASA Relative Value Guide. In some specific situations, the guide-book will indicate when their published values differ from CMS policies.

Returning to the inguinal hernia example, a Base-Unit value of 4 units, plus 4 units for time, with no additional units as Qualifying Circumstance Units (unless a specific block was performed in addition to general anesthesia for postoperative pain control) results in a Total Unit value of 8 units, which should be multiplied by a CF of $50 per unit to arrive at a professional-fee charge of $400. This charge would also include any time spent evaluating the patient preoperatively (completing the H&P prior to commencing anesthesia) and any care delivered postoperatively while the patient is in the PACU or hospital. This example does not include any of the possible specific situations in which routine postoperative care may not be sufficient and intensive personal management occurs, typically in the PACU or the ICU. In these situations, additional charges may apply, but the documentation requirements are substantial. As mentioned earlier, it is important to note that professional fees incur deep discounts from managed-care entities. The resultant reimbursement for the hernia example case is likely to be substantially less than the calculated $400. It is this deep discounting of professional fees that has led to a sharp reduction in total compensation to physicians and the concomitant reduction in available resources. The serious manpower shortage will continue until reimbursement is readjusted to account for the tremendous time and energy required or until a complete paradigm shift in physician reimbursement and staffing requirements occurs.

To generate professional-fee charges automatically as a byproduct of the clinical documentation, an AIMS must capture some very specific data elements.[6-8] The following section lists the minimum data elements required to generate an anesthesia charge, with the exception of the demographic data elements, as the focus here is on the discrete data elements captured as a consequence of providing an anesthetic. Some of the issues involved with the capture and integration of demographic data into a charge system are briefly discussed. These data are typically collected at the institutional level and are generally available from the hospital information system (HIS).

Data Elements Required

Patient Identifier Information

For purposes of charge capture, it is critical not only to identify the patient by name, but also to capture some discrete data elements that allow correlation of the charge data to demographic data obtained from the HIS. These data elements should be either a medical record number or a patient account number. Using the social security number is problematic, because many patients may not even have one and may be given a filler number (XXX-XX-XXXX). The relevant issue with AIMS is that typically these systems are interfaced to scheduling systems (Operating Room Management Systems, ORMS), and this may be the only interface where the medical record number or patient account number is available. Consequently, some marriage of data from the ORMS and the HIS demographic data must occur, even if the data are manually entered by the provider.

Provider Names

The anesthesia provider's name is required. Specifically, the charges must identify if CRNAs, residents, or additional physicians are involved in the anesthetic. The AIMS should supply the names of all providers present and the times that they were present, which allows the billing office to determine which name to submit as the billing physician. Typically, in supervision cases, the attending anesthesiologist who was present for most of the case will be the name used to submit a bill. Finally, the billing office needs the names of all attending surgeons for the case. Particularly important are the additional names if more than one surgical service is involved in the case.

Anesthesia Times

As defined earlier, anesthesia charges include Base Units and Time Units. It is essential that anesthesiologists have an understanding of specifically what constitutes each time stamp. The reader is encouraged to review the comprehensive listing of all essential time stamps relevant to the surgical encounter. They have been defined and described by the Anesthesia Administrators & Clinical Directors (AACD) and are available online at http://www.aacd.org. Those time stamps relevant to professional-fee charges are discussed later. Included in this discussion is the guidance outlined in the CMS Manual, where these time stamps are defined, with specific focus on what constitutes a beginning and end of each time stamp.

Anesthesia Start

Anesthesia Start corresponds to the moment the provider begins to prepare the patient for the anesthetic; it does not include the time spent performing a preoperative assessment nor the placement of lines or blocks in a preoperative area. It may include transport of the patient to the OR if it is provided personally by the anesthesia provider. As long as the provider remains in personal attendance during transport and the induction of anesthesia, this time may constitute Anesthesia Start. It has recently been recommended that any time used for billing should be accompanied with documentation of vital signs indicative of patient monitoring. If a service is provided in the preoperative area and then a hiatus occurs before the induction of the anesthetic, discontinuous time may be incorporated. Clear documentation that specifies the exact times spent with the patient preoperatively and details the services provided during this discontinued time is required.

Anesthesia End

Anesthesia End correlates to the time that the patient has been transferred to a recovery situation. Specifically, it corresponds to the time when handoff of the patient (typically, to the PACU nurse) occurs and the anesthesia provider is no longer in personal attendance. Documentation details the "sign-out" of relevant case information to the next provider (nurse or physician) and vital-sign data that indicate the stability of the patient.

The documentation of these time stamps within an AIMS should be automatically collected upon completion of specific clinical occurrences and should not require a separate action to enter time data. Some AIMS have attempted to correlate the beginning of anesthesia time and the anesthesia record with any vital-sign data that appear on a record. This functionality would be useful in trauma situations in which the provider does not have time to start a record or when the patient is not in a central scheduling system. However, the software does require significant flexibility to modify or alter this time stamp. As will be noted elsewhere, the thrust of our recommendations is that collection and determination of anesthesia-specific times for charge capture (and possibly any time that may be correlated to anesthesia efficiency) should remain the purview of the anesthesia provider, and not the circulating nurse.

Procedural Information

Procedural information comprises comprehensive descriptions of the surgical procedure, including the postoperative definition and the accompanying diagnosis. In many cases, this data element is added by selecting a prepopulated description from a drop-down box or importing the originally scheduled procedure from the ORMS interface. The problem with using either of these approaches is that frequently the preoperative procedure may change from the procedure actually performed. Additionally, prepopulated lists rarely contain all of the possible permutations of surgical procedures, and consequently, the user must edit the list, add descriptions, or simply provide inaccurate information. Using actual surgical CPT codes and their comprehensive descriptions rather than customized lists is highly recommended. The rationale for this approach will be presented below, but it is worth mentioning here that simply importing the current CPT library is not a sufficient solution, because navigation through this library is impractical. Finally, with the increased scrutiny of proper coding that resulted from the National Correct Coding Initiative, it is imperative that the postoperative diagnosis be defined in addition to the surgical procedure. Currently, providing these definitions requires the billing staff to search surgical operative notes or patient charts to capture the vital information. A more efficient alternative is for the anesthesia provider, using an AIMS that is elegant and user friendly, to provide this information.

Physician Attestations

For those groups that provide CRNA or resident supervision, it is critical to capture physician attestations or, ideally, the exact log-in of the physicians during the critical periods that require physical presence during supervision. It is not within the scope of this chapter to define the supervision requirements. Readers are urged to verify the necessary documentation with their departmental compliance officers—resources who should be involved early in the selection process of AIMS vendors to facilitate proper implementation of these systems.

Proper Procedural Coding

Current Procedural Terminology Codes

The Current Procedural Terminology codes were developed by the American Medical Association (AMA) in 1966.[5] They are copyrighted by the AMA, and this organization takes responsibility for creating and managing new codes and deleting old codes. Continual revision of these codes occurs, and new codes are released each year before the end of November. The entire CPT library comprises several sections, including evaluation and management codes, which are used for consultation and nonprocedural services; surgical CPT codes, which comprise over 5000 codes for detailed descriptions of surgical procedures; and anesthesia CPT codes, a very limited set in which one code could comprise many procedures. The surgical CPT codes constitute a more "granular" list of procedures than do the anesthesia CPT codes. For example, over 20 surgical CPT codes are offered for various types of knee arthroscopy, but only one anesthesia CPT code is available for anesthesia for all knee arthroscopies. CPT codes are used exclusively for generation of professional-fee charges for surgery and anesthesia, as well as facility fees for outpatient surgery.

A byproduct of HIPAA was the passage of the National Correct Coding Initiative, which utilizes a computerized audit function known as *NCCI Edits*.[6] On its surface, this federal bill provided legislation that enforced the requirement that surgical procedures and diagnoses between all providers (surgeon, anesthesiologist, and facility) match. The reality is that, unless all of these providers submit essentially identical procedure bills, all claims are held or rejected. These rejected claims result in delays in reimbursement at a minimum and, if observed frequently, may result in an audit under the auspices of the Office of the Inspector General (OIG), federal officers who are not known for their compassion or understanding in the disruption of a medical practice. It seems ironic, then, that the surgeon, anesthesiologist, and facility each use their own professional coders because each group feels that its needs are unique, whereas if the surgical procedure were defined at the point of care in the OR, all providers could use the same information to facilitate rapid generation of their surgical fees. One solution is to have an anesthesia provider review a comprehensive list of surgical procedures as defined by the CPT codes and obtain agreement from the surgeon of precisely what surgical procedure was performed. It is rare that a surgical procedure cannot be defined by the extensive CPT library of procedures, and even then, CPT codes exist for "unlisted procedures" in each organ system category. Although we know of no clinical group or service that practices this method of procedural agreement and billing, there is no reason why it could not be implemented. A rapid method of accessing the appropriate procedure and diagnosis codes for each procedure is necessary to make it a reality. Some AIMS exist that provide this capability (Fig. 14.1), and we feel that acceptance of procedural coding will improve as more institutions implement AIMS technology. Standardization of CPT codes rather than custom lists will augment coding efforts.

We recommend using the surgical CPT codes rather than anesthesia CPT codes to define surgical procedures. The surgical CPT code library is an extensive list of unique five-digit codes that define precise surgical procedures. As mentioned, more surgical CPT codes than anesthesia CPT codes are provided for the same procedure. Despite the requirement by some carriers to submit anesthesia CPT codes for anesthesia professional fees, the user of an AIMS should still select the surgical CPT code for each surgical procedure. Sophisticated charge-capture modules should be able to provide a crosswalk to the appropriate anesthesia CPT code. The crosswalk may require the user to make some decisions to select the exactly appropriate code, but again, the system should alert the user to this requirement and facilitate the selection of the appropriate procedure code. Another reason to use the surgical

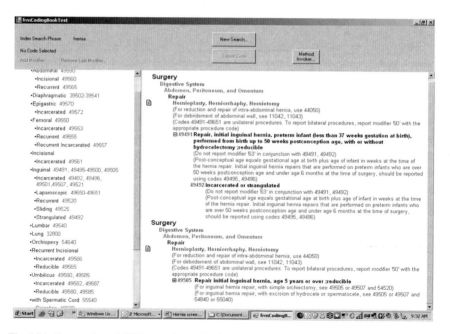

Fig. 14.1 Screen shot of CPT procedure selection screen (courtesy of DocuSys, Inc.)

CPT codes for all procedures is that using these more granular (specific) definitions enhances and facilitates outcome analysis of the data collected with an AIMS. Attempting to compare outcomes between a diagnostic knee arthroscopy and an anterior cruciate ligament reconstruction (each of which has its own surgical CPT code) would be impossible if the system only stored one anesthesia CPT code for both procedures.

For the example inguinal herniorrhaphy, the appropriate surgical CPT code may be 49505. However, this code has several derivatives, depending upon the clinical situation. The code for inguinal hernia repair on children younger than 5 years of age is 49500; for laparoscopic inguinal hernia repair, it is 49650; and for recurrent hernias, it is 49520. It is clear by this example that the possibilities are diverse, and only a system that provides rapid, easy navigation through these possibilities will facilitate an anesthesia provider defining an appropriate procedure code in the short time available during a surgical case. Ideally, the code definition should be reviewed and agreed upon by the surgeon and the anesthesia provider, who defines the code toward the end of the case, when the circulating nurse requests formal notification of the procedure and the postoperative diagnosis. Although one option may be to place coding libraries into the clinical ORMS that are used by the nurses to provide intraoperative charting, we believe that the most accurate source for anesthesia coding is the anesthesia provider. Johns Hopkins Medical Institutions is considering incorporating this function into the procedure "debriefing"—an end-of-procedure discussion that complements the time-out/briefing that occurs prior to surgical incision. This debriefing should review what happened, what went right, and what could be improved. Compliance with this debriefing has been a challenge, but initial evaluations show that incorporating the procedural and postoperative diagnoses into the debriefing seems to produce improved attention to this function.

Anesthesia Crosswalk

As alluded to above, a crosswalk conversion exists between surgical CPT codes and appropriate anesthesia CPT codes.[7] This process became formalized during the 1990s when the ASA took ownership of the creation of the crosswalk and subsequently made it available for an annual fee. The official ASA crosswalk is typically released yearly in early spring shortly after the release of new CPT codes by the AMA in January. Of particular relevance to anesthesia providers who would use a coding module within an AIMS, it is important to understand that a perfect correlation does not exist between anesthesia CPT codes and surgical CPT codes; hence, the crosswalk has notations where more than one choice of anesthesia code is available for a specific surgical CPT code. To illustrate, for an incisional hernia repair, the surgical CPT code (49560) would have a crosswalk to anesthesia CPT codes 00752 and 00832, as the first code refers to incisional hernias in the upper abdomen, while the latter refers to those in the lower abdomen. The user should be prompted to define the appropriate crosswalk code (Fig. 14.2).

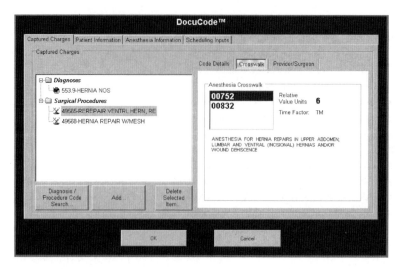

Fig. 14.2 Screen shot of anesthesia crosswalk choice (courtesy of DocuSys, Inc.)

In the scenario defined here, it would be prudent—and a recommended requirement of any compliance plan—that all procedure codes be reviewed by a professional CPT coder before submission. It would seem reasonable that review and validation of the coding selected by the anesthesia provider would be much more time efficient than a clinical coder doing the coding; in addition, one coder should be able to review most claims for an entire department. An AIMS should be capable of providing the software that facilitates the collection and identification of appropriate billing components and of handing off that information in a well-organized manner for merging with demographic data and subsequent review. It does not seem feasible that an AIMS would perform the merge and review, but it is feasible that this function would be accomplished by an office-based professional billing system. This functionality is not currently available, primarily because current billing systems are designed for manual data entry, with some limited admission/discharge/transfer (ADT) interface capabilities. We do expect that this interfacing and potential integration will develop as AIMS become more universal. The specific concerns about interfacing to these systems will be discussed in more detail below.

International Classification Diagnostic Codes

A brief discussion is warranted of the alternative set of terminology codes that are required for accurate professional-fee coding. Commonly known as *international classification diagnosis codes*, the International Classification of Diseases (ICD) codes comprise a complex set of codes that define diagnoses. The ninth revision (ICD-9) is currently being used. These codes are generally three-digit codes, with up to two additional codes after a decimal point. An example is the code that would be required for inguinal hernia, i.e., 550.9. Further definition of this diagnosis into unilateral versus bilateral, strangulation of bowel contents, and recurrence will be provided by the two additional code numbers. For example, an inguinal hernia that is unilateral, nonstrangulated, but recurrent would be coded as 550.91. Providing five-digit specificity is becoming an increasingly critical function, as the NCCI edits will reject claims when a surgical procedure does not match an appropriate surgical diagnosis. Again, defining all of these diagnosis codes is a time-consuming task for a certified coder and one that could easily be accomplished by the anesthesia provider for most cases if a system made this information available in a user-friendly manner. Obviously, cases may exist for which the diagnosis is unusual or not readily apparent, and in those cases, review of the proper documentation by a certified coder is necessary.

Besides the necessity to comply with NCCI Edits, a new requirement has also increased the urgency of correctly capturing the appropriate coding information, and that is *monitored anesthesia care* (MAC). Initially defined by CMS to assist in quantifying procedures such as cataract surgery, for which an anesthesiologist was required to provide surveillance of the patient during the procedure but not necessarily to provide anesthesia, MAC has morphed into a description of IV sedation or monitoring rather than general anesthesia. With the advent of improved pharmaceuticals that provide an enhanced plane of conscious sedation, many cases are now performed under MAC, and many carriers, including CMS, have specified that "medical necessity" be provided to justify the presence of an anesthesia provider. This medical necessity is communicated by additional diagnosis codes that are not surgical diagnosis codes; rather, they are typically comorbidity codes that define complex or unstable medical conditions that warrant the presence of the anesthesia provider. Capturing these medical-necessity diagnosis codes is a difficult process for a certified coder who may not have all of the necessary comorbid documentation. Consequently, it is imperative that the anesthesia provider have access to a user-friendly method of capturing the various and diverse ICD-9 diagnosis codes that may be encompassed by medical necessity.

Another topic of discussion worth highlighting is the use of ICD-9 procedure codes. Most physicians and office staff members are unfamiliar with this set of procedure codes. They are ubiquitously used by certified coders for inpatient hospital procedures for the hospital claim submission for all patients who require a procedure during a hospitalization. These codes are analogous to the anesthesia CPT codes in that one or two ICD-9 procedure codes are typically available to define a procedure that may have many surgical CPT codes. For example, the ICD-9 procedure code for a hernia repair would typically be 53, with up to two additional numbers after the decimal point to further define the procedure. An incisional hernia repair would be 53.51. The disparity between hospital coding requirements (ICD) and physician coding requirements (CPT) is another reason that a disconnect continues between coding efforts. However, if hospital coders were provided with an authorized listing of surgical CPT codes and diagnoses from the surgical procedure, no doubt, their tasks would be simplified.

Disease-Related Groupings

Following is a discussion of the rationale for incorporating diagnosis coding into the function of an AIMS and under the purview of the anesthesia provider. As illustrated above, hospital inpatient billing is uniquely different from professional-fee billing. Hospital bills are generated onto a "UB-92" claim form and are submitted electronically for reimbursement. These claim forms must contain information similar to the professional-fee claim form, in that surgical procedure (as an ICD-9 procedure code), date of service, and surgical diagnosis, along with provider information and other demographic data must be listed. One additional requirement, however, is the presence of secondary or "comorbid" codes. These are ICD-9 diagnosis codes that define comorbid medical conditions of patients, similar to the medical-necessity diagnosis codes defined earlier. Comorbid codes, surgical diagnosis codes, and procedural codes are entered into a software program generically referred to as a *disease-related grouping* (DRG) *grouper* to generate a DRG. Hospitals are reimbursed according to the DRG, as specified by the Inpatient Prospective Payment System (IPPS) implemented by CMS in 1984. Most states utilize a CMS DRG grouper that categorizes every surgical procedure into one of two DRG classifications—one with and one without "complications or comorbidities." Payment varies substantially between these two classifications. For example, using national average CMS reimbursement figures, a cholecystectomy that requires an overnight admission coded as a cholecystectomy without complications or comorbidities (DRG 196) results in an average reimbursement of $9115, and the same procedure coded with complications or comorbidities (DRG 195) results in a reimbursement of $17,462—almost double that of procedures without complications or comorbidities. The rationale for this increased reimbursement is the basis for the foundation of DRG, where the assumption is that patients with complications and/or complex medical comorbidities require greater resources and longer lengths of stay in the hospital. Consequently, hospital medical records departments utilize numerous certified coders to scour through charts to capture every comorbid diagnosis that may affect the DRG, and they continually plead with physicians to do a more thorough job of documenting these conditions.

One stipulation of the DRG reimbursement system is that coders may generate a comorbid diagnosis code only if a condition is documented by a provider. A perfect example of this necessity is the presence of anemia, especially hemorrhagic anemia, as may exist postoperatively. Unless a physician documents the *acute* anemia, the coders may not code this diagnosis, which could possibly alter the DRG. Additionally, the physician must specifically define the anemia as *acute* and may not simply use up or down arrows to define changes in hemoglobin. Without such comprehensive documentation of comorbid conditions, hospitals potentially lose significant revenue to which they are entitled under the current reimbursement system.

Another problem with these coding schemes is that over time, it has been determined that they are not granular enough. One DRG code to cover the diverse medical conditions is inadequate from both a reimbursement perspective and an outcomes perspective. The ubiquity of billing data has resulted in the pervasive use of administrative data as a source of outcome analysis. However, extrapolating these comorbid conditions to risk-stratify surgical patients has proven to be a poor correlation.[8] Additionally, the current DRG system provides no accounting for pediatric patients and other nontypical hospital admissions because these patients rarely have Medicare coverage. Consequently, the need to redefine the current CMS DRG system to incorporate more granular comorbid classification is incontrovertible. CMS is currently evaluating various models; one model being closely scrutinized is the all-patient refined DRG (APR-DRG) developed by 3M[9] and used extensively by all hospitals in the state of Maryland since 2005.[10] This DRG system provides two subcomponent indices known as severity of illness (SOI) and risk of mortality (ROM). Maryland hospitals are using the SOI to define granular reimbursement. For example, a hysterectomy that has four levels of SOI would be reimbursed as follows:

SOI	Reimbursement
I	$6,051
II	$7,382
III	$13,454
IV	$29,859

Understanding that CMS is budget neutral, this example clearly indicates that reimbursement will be shifted to hospitals that are able to more fully document sicker patients and that, conversely, reimbursement will decrease dramatically for hospitals that care for relatively healthy patients. Despite the purported intentions of a fairer distribution of revenue to hospitals that care for sicker patients, the true motivation behind this conversion is to reduce incentives for specialty hospitals to "cherry-pick" healthy patients and provide lucrative returns to their investors.

The CMS has notified providers that, commencing in 2008, it will adopt a newly defined DRG system known as Medicare Severity DRGs (MS-DRGs), representing one of the most comprehensive changes to the DRG reimbursement model since it was originally deployed. Modeled after, but distinct from, the APR-DRG, this new methodology will ostensibly increase the number of DRGs from 538 to 745 in an effort to recognize higher SOI between patients.[11] As described previously, this IPPS change will be budget neutral, resulting in higher payments to hospitals with sicker patients and lower payments to hospitals with lower acuity. Moreover, an additional component of these changes includes a revamping of how comorbid conditions affect DRG. Specifically, certain conditions that previously resulted in a higher DRG classification are now prevented from affecting the DRG classification. The 13 secondary conditions, or comorbid codes, that are included in this process must meet three criteria:

1. Must be high cost, high volume, or both
2. Must be assigned to a higher-paying DRG when present as a secondary condition
3. Must be reasonably preventable through application of evidence-based guidelines[12]

These secondary conditions are excluded from comorbid conditions that were "present on admission" or recognized as contributing to a patient's reason for admission. Rather, they are conditions that arise as a result of procedures or those that occur when complications arise that ostensibly should have been prevented. The adoption of a new DRG system and the focus on documentation of comorbid conditions that are present on admission represent an attempt to allow CMS to drive reimbursement toward a value-based purchasing program.

How Does This Affect Anesthesia?

The single most critical feature of the DRG code conversion will be a profound pressure on physicians to better document their patient's medical conditions. History shows that simply urging surgeons to complete a more thorough H&P is futile. Conversely, anesthesia routinely generates a comprehensive documentation of patients' medical conditions, as they have implications concerning the anesthetic chosen. Gibby et al. were the first to demonstrate that a computerized preoperative assessment could have positive benefits to DRG reimbursement.[13] The positive effects are even more dramatic in the setting of the APR-DRG, as demonstrated by Stonemetz et al.[14] The challenge, of course, is implementing a thorough documentation process into the busy workflow in the delivery of care. One possible solution is to more effectively triage complex medical patients, and in particular those scheduled for major surgery, to a preoperative assessment clinic (see Chap. 9).[15] Seeing patients in a preoperative clinic would allow for better documentation of their complex medical conditions, thereby creating a significant opportunity to improve the comorbid documentation to enhance DRG classifications. The authors propose that hospitals should subsidize the staffing of these clinics and involve anesthesia to provide better patient care and facilitate improved reimbursement through comprehensive documentation.

ICD-10 Codes

With the explosion of new technology and the need to codify diagnoses and procedures to facilitate adoption of EMRs, the current ICD-9 diagnosis and procedure system needs updating and revamping. To that end, the tenth revision of these codes (ICD-10) has been developed and is awaiting implementation. Currently in use in most countries other than the US, these codes represent an improvement over ICD-9 in that they provide for addition of information relevant to ambulatory- and managed-care encounters, expanded injury codes, creation of combination diagnosis-symptom codes to reduce the number of separate codes to describe a condition, addition of a sixth and seventh character, laterality, and enhanced specification of code assignment.[16] Not insignificantly, the ICD-10 codes provide for more than 130,000 possible codes, compared to the existing ~13,000 ICD-9 codes, which have nearly all been assigned.

It is appropriate to understand the history of the ICD system to gain a better appreciation of the function of the codes. Originally designed as a codification of causes of death, these codes had their genesis in the late 1800s as the "International Causes of Death" that were compiled and agreed upon among various countries in an attempt to better understand the causes of death and mortality. Continual revisions of these codes occurred, with the US acting as a major participant in the fifth-revision conference, which took place in Paris in 1938. Subsequent to this revision, it became apparent that in addition to causes of death, it was necessary to create a codification of causes of morbidity and other illnesses. Under the auspices of the World Health Organization (WHO), which possesses copyrighted ownership of the codes, the sixth-revision conference convened in New York City in 1946 and incorporated morbidity causes into the list to create the "International Classification of Diseases, Injuries, and Causes of Death." The seventh- and eighth-revision conferences had little effect, other than to make minor modifications to the list of codes. It was during the ninth-revision conference (convened in Geneva, Switzerland, in 1975) that the most comprehensive changes occurred. Driving most of these changes was the recognition by member countries that these codes were not only necessary for codification of diseases and statistical analysis but that they could also be used in processing healthcare information (hence, reimbursement), in particular with the advent of data processing. This increased functionality necessitated expansion of the codes; hence, the fourth- and fifth-decimal classification scheme was created. These codes have been in use by most of the international members of the WHO since that time. Shortly after the release of the ninth revision, the WHO began working with member countries to create the tenth revision, recognizing that the current structure of the ICD-9 codes is inadequate to support the expansion of medical terminology. The tenth revision has been in existence since 1989 and used primarily in Australia since 1998; Canada and most of Europe subsequently adopted this version.[17]

The US adopted the WHO classification system primarily as a tool for claim submission and reimbursement; this adoption was termed the International Classification of Diseases—Ninth-Revision Clinical Modification (ICD-9-CM) and has been in use since 1979. The diagnosis codes are contained in a two-volume set (hardbound copies), and an extensive list of procedures was added as a third volume (described above as ICD-9 procedure codes). At the request of CMS, the National Center for Health Statistics was commissioned to create the clinical modification of the ICD-10 and released a version of ICD-10-CM in 2003. Subsequent releases have been made and are available for free downloading from the Web site of the National Center for Health Statistics.[16] Additionally, CMS funded a project headed by 3M to create a revised ICD-10 procedure list, referred to as the *International Classification of Diseases-10 Procedure Coding System (ICD-10-PCS)*, which was created with four primary goals in mind:

- *Completeness.* A unique code should be available for every procedure.
- *Expandability.* New procedures should be incorporated easily into the structure.
- *Multiaxial.* Codes should consist of independent characters, with each code representing a specific function.
- *Standardized terminology.* The ICD system should not include multiple meanings for the same term.[18]

This new coding structure (procedures only) constitutes a seven-character coding structure that is alphanumeric, rather than purely numeric, and consists of 16 sections (Table 14.1). The basic structure is illustrated in Fig. 14.3. In the current configuration, the ICD-10-PCS represents over 86,000 distinct codes, a substantial increase over the number of existing procedure codes.

Even in the face of international pressure to convert to the ICD-10-CM and ICD-10-PCS systems, the US federal government has hesitated to adopt them, except to dictate that any changes will be implemented as part of the administrative simplification process of HIPAA. One major reason for the resistance is the very serious cost of these changes to existing computer systems, in both the government and the private sectors. In a report commissioned by the National Committee on Vital and Health Statistics, the RAND Corp. (Santa Monica, CA) reported that implementation could potentially cost up to $1.5 billion, with potential lost productivity of $40 million annually, although the same report also noted that eventual adoption could potentially lead to economic benefits exceeding $7.7 billion.[19] Consequently, the decision to move to ICD-10 has been a volatile political issue. Proponents of EMRs perceive migration to the tenth revision as essential to advance our ability to share standardized data, compare significant outcome data, and begin to use administrative data more effectively. Regardless of timing of the move to this new coding methodology, the potential disruption and incurred costs will be quite challenging at all levels.

Table 14.1 Sections of International Classification of Diseases-10 Procedure Coding System

0	Medical and surgical
1	Obstetrics
2	Placement
3	Administration
4	Measurement and monitoring
5	Imaging
6	Nuclear medicine
7	Radiation oncology
8	Osteopathic
9	Rehabilitation and diagnostic audiology
B	Extracorporeal assistance and performance
C	Extracorporeal therapies
D	Laboratory
F	Mental health
G	Chiropractic
H	Miscellaneous

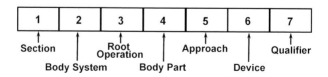

Fig. 14.3 ICD-10-PCS code structure

Professional-Fee Claim Submission

The end result of professional-fee charge capture and the beginning of the process required for reimbursement is the actual claim submission. At this writing, most healthcare charges are submitted electronically, and the tasks of most of the submission process, review process, and adjudication of charges are completed by computers. Detailed discussion of the claim submission is outside the scope of this book; however, some concerns warrant discussion for current and future prospective users of an AIMS.

We have described the primary data elements that must be retrieved from the AIMS to generate the professional fee. Additional critical data elements entail the patient's demographic data, typically reside within the HIS, and are generally made available to any authorized entity via an HL7/ADT interface. Many anesthesia billing offices or services employ an ADT interface to obtain the demographic data. Frequently, marrying the data from an ADT system with AIMS charge data is associated with data integrity and workflow issues, as discussed below. If the ADT interface is simply used to obtain a view-only copy of demographic data, the existing ADT files will suffice. If, however, one wishes to truly utilize data integration to facilitate claim submission and reduce redundant data entry, the ADT files must be closely scrutinized and the data must be cleaned; e.g., inconsistent entries must be standardized.

Before discussing consolidation of demographic and charge-capture data from the AIMS, we should review the existing workflow of an anesthesia office. Claim submission is accomplished either by an office owned by the anesthesia group or by a billing service. Both of these entities utilize sophisticated software systems that were designed to begin the claim submission process with manual entry of the patient, the procedure, and charge data. Demographic data can be entered manually or through an interface to an ADT file. Conceptually, it seems plausible and imminently feasible that these two data streams (the AIMS and the ADT file) could be integrated, removing the manual data-entry process.

We are not aware of existing billing systems that have the ability to store a consolidated batch of claims that are pending review. Additionally, editing and acceptance of the AIMS data into the claims submission process are not possible. Although most offices and billing services that utilize AIMS find their charge capture improved with enhanced readability and rapid access to previous records, we are not aware of any facilities that have proceeded to the next step of automatic integration of these two data streams, which would result in a reduction or elimination of manual data entry. This integration represents the next significant phase of improvement in the ROI of the AIMS market. The consensus of billing service vendors seems to be that the cost of billing could potentially be reduced by 25%–40% of current costs and that this savings could possibly be channeled back to groups that utilize these systems.

Manual review of all claims prior to submission is essential for two primary reasons. First, as already discussed, professional coders should review procedure codes and charges prior to claim submission. Anesthesia providers cannot be expected to remain knowledgeable on all of the subtleties of professional-fee charges;

therefore, for an effective compliance program, charges should be reviewed even if they were generated from an AIMS during the procedure. Second, experience indicates that the ADT file is frequently incomplete or erroneous. Consider the patient who arrives to the OR as an emergency case. Authentication of name, address, phone numbers, and insurance information is frequently impossible. The information for most of these cases is typically updated within 1–2 days of surgery. Consequently, in addition to the initial patient demographic information, the ADT file must provide any updates made subsequent to the surgical procedure. If no authorized entity is reviewing the updated information, then a large subset of claims will contain erroneous information, ultimately resulting in rejected or lost claims. For customers who wish to use an AIMS to augment and enhance the business end of their practices, many such issues must be reconciled.

Pay for Performance

Much of the focus of healthcare providers and administrators in recent years has been on the pay-for-performance (P4P) plans proposed by the insurance industry and in particular by CMS.[20] It is still unclear how these initiatives will actually be implemented, especially for professional-fee compensation. CMS took the lead and, based on a pilot program of voluntary reporting established in 2005, officially launched the Physician Quality Reporting Initiative (PQRI) on July 1, 2007.[21] According to CMS announcements, this initiative was undertaken in an effort to implement value-based purchasing in the Medicare program. Value-based purchasing is perceived to be a valuable tool with which to promote quality and efficiency of care, one of the cornerstones of the Value-driven Health Care initiative, which is pivotal to CMS in converting from a passive payer to an active purchaser of quality healthcare. In essence, PQRI requires physician reporting via newly enacted Category II CPT codes on the standard claim forms for specific clinical measures. In 2007, 74 measures were cited as clinical programs deemed appropriate for reimbursement. Of these, only one applies to anesthesia—*timely administration of antibiotics* (measure #30). Although controversial at this writing, a bonus may be paid for a second measure to be reported by anesthesia—*preoperative beta blockers administered prior to coronary artery surgery* (measure #44).[22] As of 2008, CMS increased the number of measures to 119 and added one more measure that is appropriate for anesthesia—*prevention of catheter-related bloodstream infections—central venous catheter insertion protocol* (measure #76). At this writing, it remains unclear if two other measures (measure #128—*measurement and documentation of body mass index* and measure #130—*verification of patients' medications*) will also be applicable. It will be important to follow the status of these measures because to qualify for the 1.5% bonus payment, a provider must report on at least three measures. Most of the surgical measures were derived from earlier efforts by the Surgical Care Improvement Project—a national partnership of private and public entities, including the ASA, whose goal was to reduce the incidence of postoperative complications.[23]

The specifics of how providers will actually submit these claims are still in discussion between the CMS and ASA leadership. As is typical with many CMS regulations, confusion exists regarding applicability. Unfortunately, the 80% reporting requirement covers the current fiscal year (2008), which is already underway without clear direction. The current plan is that on anesthesia claims submitted to CMS for surgical procedures for which a prophylactic antibiotic was administered within 60 minutes of incision, a second procedure code should be listed with a $0.00 charge. This code has been defined as 4048F—the five-digit Category II code that indicates timely administration of prophylactic antibiotics. Additionally, modifiers should be added to describe deviation from the measure. The modifier "8P" would be used when antibiotics were simply not administered. One of the major difficulties encountered when evaluating this new proposal is understanding which patients are appropriate for these measures. Clearly, not all surgical patients will require prophylactic antibiotics, and historically, the anesthesiologist primarily complies with the surgeon's request to administer these medications. CMS has proposed that specific CPT codes be used to establish the denominator for this measure and that the number of administered antibiotics (4048F) be the numerator. Providers must achieve an 80% compliance with this measure to qualify for an end-of-year bonus payment that equals 1.5% of the anesthesia fees paid for the procedures (a sum of the numerators). The proposed plan is clearly a complex formula for a very small inducement. However, as all anesthesia groups anticipate shrinking revenues, no doubt, they will carefully consider any possibilities for increased revenue.

With an AIMS, the type of reporting that will be necessary for the P4P programs will be easier and much more comprehensive. From automated reminders to administer antibiotics, to correlating the CMS list of procedures, to appropriate prophylactic patients, an AIMS has the potential to dramatically improve both compliance and reporting. Some speculate that physicians will require electronic records to participate in the PQRI program. Statements posted on the CMS knowledge page pertaining to PQRI have refuted the requirement of an electronic clinical system,[24] but clearly, physicians and administrators realize that it will be very difficult to take advantage of incentives using a paper-record system. As was alluded to at the beginning of this book, P4P, regardless of presentation, will probably require adoption of electronic records.

Professional-Fee Compliance Plans

Health Insurance Portability and Accountability Act

HIPAA became mandated as Public Law 104–191 in 1996 as a result of the broad changes espoused by the Clinton administration. Essentially a three-pronged approach, the changes attempted to improve healthcare by:

1. Ensuring that preexisting conditions were no longer a valid reason for denying health insurance to any patient. These changes also introduced medical savings accounts as a valid option for patients.
2. Simplifying administration—based on the recognition that at least 25% of the total healthcare dollar is spent in nonvalue-added administrative costs, this legislation attempted to mandate standards that would simplify claim submission. To date, the only real result of these changes has been the increased attention and focus on patient security and privacy. No significant gains have been achieved from simplification.
3. Increasing funding to combat fraud and abuse of fraudulent Medicare billings.

Recommendations for the third arm of the legislation came from the results of Operation Restore Trust (ORT), an initiative launched during the Clinton administration that examined fraudulent Medicare billings and aggressively sought, found, and prosecuted violations, resulting in heavy fines and penalties. It was determined that for every dollar spent on this initiative, $23 were recovered into the Medicare Trust, making it one of the few government projects that ever made money. Consequently, with the passage of HIPAA, over $1 million was allocated to combat Medicare fraud and abuse. The money was utilized to facilitate the OIG in investigating claims of fraudulent billing and predominately went to reward whistle blowers who reported episodes of fraud and abuse.

Anesthesia billing is typically one of the highlighted areas of the yearly OIG Workplan, a document released by the OIG that indicates the specific areas that the OIG will heavily investigate in the coming year.[25] Anesthesia is highlighted primarily because the billings are very complex, and areas that receive perennial review by the OIG involve time discrepancies and supervision lapses of the Anesthesia Care Team.[26] One particular concern is the stance of CMS that mistakes in billings constitute an attempt at fraud. If a mistake is made that results in fewer charges, no consequence or penalty is levied. However, a mistake that results in increased charges is considered to be a fraudulent claim, and the claimant may be subjected to a $10,000 fine per occurrence plus the requirement to reimburse the charges with any interest that may have accrued. Based on heavy criticism and feedback, CMS modified the approach to assigning penalties. If an entity can demonstrate that it makes a concerted effort to combat fraud and abuse, then mistakes are not penalized as heavily. Charges and interest still apply, but the onerous assignment of penalties is removed. For this reason, it is imperative that all groups generate and follow a robust compliance plan. Well-delineated and well-executed compliance plans are essential, regardless of whether a group uses an AIMS or paper records. It is essential for practices with AIMS to understand how this technology should be incorporated into the compliance plan. AIMS should augment the ability to meet documentation compliance, ideally providing real-time feedback to providers on documentation that is missing or practice patterns that should be adjusted (see illustrations below). Another advantage of an AIMS is that it facilitates a better representation of the Anesthesia Care Team model. For example, in groups where supervision concurrency is an issue, an alert that informs the provider at the start of the case that it may represent a concurrency violation would allow that provider to find another supervising physician, delay the case briefly, or decide to proceed, recognizing the implications of her decision. This method of notification is preferable to the retrospective chart review that demonstrates a concurrency violation when the primary provider was completely unaware. One specific feature of an AIMS that has relevance to a compliance plan is its ability to indicate the precise time that documentation is made.[3] For example, a provider indicating "present at emergence" at the *beginning* of the case could potentially be viewed as a compliance violation. The data in an AIMS database have great potential to substantiate compliance documentation, provided that documentation occurred at the appropriate time of the procedure. Conversely, it can also be used to substantiate compliance violations.

Examples of Improved Reimbursement Using an AIMS

The documentation necessary for billing as outlined above must be complete and clear in order for payment to be received for services. These elements include the evaluation prior to anesthesia, intraoperative management, and postanesthesia care. The AIMS provides an opportunity to capture these billing elements and potentially prompt the provider to input or complete any missing or incomplete data. Up to 10% of potential revenue may be lost by billing omissions and errors made by providers. AIMS have the potential to simplify the billing process and reduce costs. It is estimated that the cost to follow-up and correct billing errors may be up to six times more than if the data were submitted correctly the first time.[27] Many AIMS must be modified to meet the specific needs of individual institutions and practices to produce a completed bill for submission. With the development of a charge-capture module, groups would be able to recover lost revenue by decreasing documentation errors and omissions. We now describe three charge-capture modules that were developed and implemented at academic centers in the US.

Massachusetts General Hospital

In 2003, the department of anesthesiology at Massachusetts General Hospital installed an AIMS. Shortly after its implementation, the department noted that many of the records could not be submitted for billing due to documentation errors. Spring et al. developed an Anesthesia Billing Alert System (ABAS) to recognize and alert providers to missing or incomplete data in the AIMS.[28] A secondary AIMS server was populated with data from the primary AIMS server. Each of the required billing elements was assigned an alphanumeric identifier. The ABAS scanned the secondary AIMS server every 10 minutes, looking for the billing identifiers and their associated time stamps. The identifiers were coupled with 58 validation rules that checked to ensure that all clinical and documentation elements required for billing had been completed. If an error was detected, a text message was sent via the hospital paging system, alerting the provider of the documentation error. The ABAS sent a reminder page after 15 minutes and on postoperative days one and three. Email reminders were sent on postoperative days 2 and 4 for any unresolved documentation errors.

The data from the ABAS were compared to historical data for the 3 months prior to the implementation of the system, with four performance metrics used in the analysis: (a) the number of records not submitted for billing due to documentation errors, (b) the percentage of documents with errors at the end of each day, (c) the number of days it took to correct these errors, and (d) the average number of days it took to release the records for billing. In the 3 months preceding the implementation of the ABAS, 1.31% of the total records were never submitted for billing due to documentation errors. After the implementation of the ABAS, only 0.04% of records were not submitted for billing due to documentation errors. The percentage of records with documentation errors at the end of the day increased from 3.8% to 5.4%; however, this increase was not statically significant ($p = 0.0724$). The time required to correct billing errors decreased from an average of 33 days prior to the implementation of the ABAS to 3 days after implementation. The amount of time it took to release records for billing decreased from 3 to 1.1 days after the full implementation of the ABAS.

The authors concluded that the ROI for the ABAS was favorable. Based upon the case volume at their institution, the ABAS can potentially save their department $390,000 per year by recouping funds from records with uncorrected billing errors. Assuming a 2-day reduction in billing and accounts receivable and using a 4% short-term investment rate, an additional $10,000 per year could be generated. The ABAS cost $180,000 to develop and requires an ongoing cost of $37,500 for 50% of one full-time programmer/analyst for ongoing maintenance. In addition to the financial benefits of the ABAS, the authors also noted an overall improvement in documentation. Moreover, satisfaction surveys of the faculty and providers concluded that the new system was better than the previous system and relatively user friendly. Another benefit was that as the number of documentation errors decreased, quality increased and one full-time billing staff member was reassigned from data-entry tasks to recouping payment from records with missing documentation.

Mount Sinai School of Medicine

Reich et al.[29] developed a customized charge-capture module for their institution and examined days in accounts receivable and charge lag as primary outcomes. Their institution began implementing an AIMS in 1991 and completed implementation by 1998. The AIMS contained all of the data elements necessary to generate a bill. Anesthetic procedures were assigned numeric identifiers that were used in the charge-capture database, and most data required to generate a bill were made available in drop-down menus. In addition, complete listings of CPT codes were made available by a searchable database for diagnosis and procedures. These features were updated on a regular basis and could be edited by the department coders. The customized program would generate reports that included the billing worksheet, missing data worksheet, incomplete and complete billing archives, an incomplete progress report, and added cases. Several data extractions from the AIMS were performed daily to populate these reports: the first to generate the billing worksheet, the second to check for missing information, and the third for additional information that became available after the initial extraction. An email was sent to the provider for any incomplete records. Reports were sent to the billing vendor, where manual entry was made concurrent with the electronic voucher for the first 2 months of the program, after which the vendor began to accept only the electronic voucher.

As mentioned, the primary outcomes were charge lag and days in accounts receivable. *Charge lag* is the time from the date of service until the bill is submitted to payers. When the authors compared the results with the 7-month period prior to the implementation of the electronic charge voucher system, they reported a 7.3-day decrease in the charge lag. With respect to total days in accounts receivable, the authors found a 10.1-day decrease. This represented a *one-time* revenue gain of 3.0% of total annual receipts.

Similar to results with the ABAS system at MGH, the Mount Sinai authors reported a decrease in the requirement for manual entry of billing data. They reported a decrease in one full-time equivalent for billing, which resulted in a savings of $32,000 per year, along with a $10,000 savings for ancillary costs associated with manual billing entry and voucher development. Additional benefits were noted in the improved documentation and potential savings from compliance penalties.

University of Michigan

Kheterpal et al.[30] at the University of Michigan developed an automated reminder system for documenting the placement of peripheral arterial catheters. The authors randomized residents and CRNAs to experimental and control groups. Each group and the departmental administrators were blinded to the objectives of the study. It was presumed that once the study began, the awareness that certain individuals were being sent reminders for documentation would become manifest. In phase II of the study, the entire department would receive reminder pages to document the placement of arterial catheters. Only catheters that were placed in the OR were included in the study, as some catheters may have been placed by other services in the hospital. The authors found that during the 2-month trial, the experimental group that received reminders documented 88% of all lines placed, compared to 75% for the control group ($p < 0.001$). This result was compared to a baseline documenting compliance rate of 80%, as determined from a retrospective review of the AIMS for 1 year prior to the study. During phase II of the study, when all staff members were sent reminder pages, compliance increased to 99%.

According to the authors, the professional-fee charge for the placement of a peripheral arterial catheter is $310, with a reimbursement of $83. When they extrapolated the 99% compliance rate achieved after full implementation of the reminder system, they found that professional-fee charges increased by $151,000, with an associated $40,500 increase in reimbursement for previously unbilled services. Development of the system was associated with a one-time cost of $1111, yielding a positive ROI within the first year of implementation.

In conclusion, the availability of automated charge-capture modules in existing AIMS is limited. In the examples provided above, custom modules had to be developed to meet the specific needs of the respective institutions, requiring additional financial and human resources. Despite the costs associated with the development of a simple reminder program for minor procedures or a fully automated charge-capture/reminder system, the ROI is notable. AIMS manufacturers have included some charge-capture features in their systems, but with the wide range of billing regulations and unique provider settings, a "one size fits all" module may prove difficult. As more institutions implement automated charge-capture modules, critical elements necessary for calculating ROI will become available (e.g., days in accounts receivable, professional-fee charges, and reimbursement). Other chapters in this book discuss the business case for implementing an AIMS. Automated charge capture is a feature that should be a part of every AIMS to fully realize its economic potential. Additionally, the intangible benefits of improved documentation and compliance may avoid penalties and risk-management issues.

Conclusion

An AIMS has the potential to substantially impact the professional-fee charge capture and implementation of a compliance plan. It is essential that groups understand the business models of their practice and analyze integration or interface opportunities with the billing division to optimize this potential. As we move forward into an arena of payment for performance, an AIMS should far surpass the paper world in automating the capture of discrete measures and the ability to report these measures in real time.

Key Points

- Improved charge capture with an AIMS is possible, but the customer must focus on the comprehensive capture of all essential data elements.
- Proper procedural and diagnosis coding is essential to ensure effective charge capture.
- Diagnosis coding provides an opportunity to enhance revenue for hospitals and provides anesthesiologists with potential tools to align financial incentives with hospitals.

- Coding efforts will inevitably change when the US converts to ICD-10 codes.
- Professional-fee claim submission requires detailed analysis of data interfaces and interactions between the AIMS and the billing software system.
- Pay for performance is a reality in the current healthcare environment—and almost impossible without an AIMS.
- All groups need a comprehensive compliance plan, and it is especially critical with the implementation of an AIMS.
- The literature contains accounts of clearly improved charge capture and professional-fee billings secondary to implementation of an AIMS.

References

1. Shuren AW, Livsey K. Complying with the Health Insurance Portability and Accountability Act. Privacy standards. AAOHN J 2001; 49(11):501–7
2. Kawamoto K, Houlihan CA, Balas EA, et al. Improving clinical practice using clinical decision support systems: A systematic review of trials to identify features critical to success. Br Med J 2005; 330:765
3. Vigoda MM, Lubarsky DA. The medicolegal importance of enhancing timeliness of documentation when using an anesthesia information system and the response to automated feedback in an academic practice. Anesth Analg 2006; 103:131–6
4. Blue Cross & Blue Shield, Medicare Part B Reference Manual, Anesthesia Billing Guide, April 2004
5. AMA Web site for CPT codes. http://www.ama-assn.org/ama/pub/category/3113.html. Accessed December 19, 2007
6. National Correct Coding Initiative Policy Manual for Medicare Services. Chicago: American Medical Association, 2005. Chap. 2, Anesthesia Services CPT Codes 00000–09999
7. American Society of Anesthesiologists, 2007 Crosswalk. Park Ridge, IL: ASA Publications, 2007
8. Wynn BO, Beckett MK, Hillborne LH, et al. Evaluation of Severity-Adjusted DRG Systems: Interim Report. Santa Monica, CA: Rand, 2007
9. Averill R, Goldfield N, Hughes J, . What are APR-DRGs? An Introduction to Severity of Illness and Risk of Mortality Adjustment Methodology. Salt Lake City, UT: 3M Health Information Systems, 2003
10. Health services cost review commission fact sheet on transition to APR-DRG for Maryland hospitals. http://www.hscrc.state.md.us/current_policy_papers/documents/fsr_apr_drg_transition.doc. Accessed December 19, 2007
11. CMS Payment System Fact Sheet. http://www.cms.hhs.gov/MLNProducts/downloads/AcutePaymtSysfctsht.pdf. Accessed February 8, 2008
12. CMS Fact Sheet on FY2008 IPPS Proposed Rule Improving Quality of Hospital Care, released 04/13/07. http://www.cms.hhs.gov/apps/media/press/factsheet.asp?Counter=2119&intNumPerPage=10&checkDate=&checkKey=&srchType=1&numDays=3500&srchOpt=0&srchData=&keywordType=All&chkNewsType=6&intPage=&showAll=&pYear=&year=&desc=&cboOrder=date. Accessed July 2007
13. Gibby GL, Paulus DA, Sirota DJ, et al. Computerized pre-anesthetic evaluation results in additional abstracted comorbidity diagnoses. J Clin Monit 1997; 13(1):35–41
14. Stonemetz J, Pham JC, Marino RJ, et al. Effect of concurrent computerized documentation of comorbid conditions on the risk of mortality index. J Clin Outcomes Manage 2007; 14(9):499–503

15. Stonemetz J. Establishment of an anesthesia consult service. Annual Meeting of the American Society of Anesthesiologists, San Francisco, CA, October 13–17, 2007. Anesthesia 2007; 107:A1871

16. National Center for Health Statistics. http://www.cdc.gov/nchs/about/otheract/icd9/abticd10.htm. Accessed August 2007

17. World Health Organization. http://www.who.int/classifications/icd/en. Accessed January 8, 2008

18. Averill RF, Mullin RL, Steinbeck BA, et al. Development of the ICD-10 Procedure Coding System (ICD-10-PCS). http://ncvhs.hhs.gov/020409p2.pdf. Accessed January 8, 2008

19. Libicki M, Brahmakulam I. *The Costs and Benefits of Moving to the ICD-10 Code Sets.* Santa Monica, CA: Rand, 2004. http://www.rand.org/pubs/technical_reports/2004/RAND_TR132.pdf. Accessed January 8, 2008

20. Medicare "Pay For Performance (P4P)" Initiatives. http://www.cms.hhs.gov/apps/media/press/release.asp?Counter=1343. Accessed January 8, 2008

21. CMS Physician Quality Reporting Initiative (PQRI). http://www.cms.hhs.gov/pqri/. Accessed January 8, 2008

22. Bierstein K. Pay for Participation in Medicare's Physician Quality Reporting Initiative. http://www.asahq.org/Newsletters/2007/05-07/pracMgmt05_07.html. Accessed January 8, 2008

23. Bierstein K. Anesthesia is in the P4P Game. ASA Newsletter, 2006. http://www.asahq.org/Newsletters/2006/12-06/pracMgmt12_06.html. Accessed January 8, 2008

24. CMS PQRI FAQ page. http://questions.cms.hhs.gov/cgi-bin/cmshhs.cfg/php/enduser/std_adp.php?p_faqid=8451&p_created=1180632624&p_sid=JYI3jsDi&p_accessibility=0&p_lva=&p_sp=cF9zcmNoPTEmcF9zb3J0X2J5PSZwX2dyaWRzb3J0PSZwX3Jvd19jbnQ9MTkmcF9wcm9kcz04LDYxLDk0NSw5NjgmcF9jYXRzPSZwX3B2PTQuOTY4JnBfY3Y9JnBfc2VhcmNoX3R5cGU9YW5zd2Vyc2VhcmZ1bGwmcF9wYWdlPTEmcF9zZWFyY2hfdGV4dD0w/p_li=&p_topview=1. Accessed January 8, 2008

25. Office of Inspector General. Work Plan: Fiscal Year 2007. Department of Health and Human Services. http://oig.hhs.gov/publications/docs/workplan/2007/Work%20Plan%202007.pdf. Accessed January 8, 2008

26. Bourdreaux A. Committee on anesthesia care team: A committee for all. ASA Newsletter, 2005. http://www.asahq.org/Newsletters/2005/03-05/boudreaux03_05.html. Accessed January 8, 2008

27. Garrity C. Automated charge capture at the point of care increases revenue. Healthc Financ Manage 2001; 55:66–71

28. Spring SF, Sandberg WS, Anupama S, et al. Automated documentation error detection and notification improves anesthesia billing performance. Anesthesiology 2007; 106(1):157–63

29. Reich DL, Kahn RA, Wax D, . Development of a module for point-of-care charge capture and submission using an anesthesia information management system. Anesthesiology 2006; 105:179–86

30. Kheterpal S, Gupta R, Blum JM, et al. Electronic reminders improve procedure documentation compliance and professional fee reimbursement. Anesth Analg 2007; 104(3):592–7

Chapter 15
Decision Support

Michael M. Vigoda, Michael O'Reilly, Frank J. Gencorelli, and David A. Lubarsky

Work Environments: Anesthesia and Aviation

Dr. Jones, an anesthesiologist, boards a plane to visit her ailing father who is scheduled to have a colectomy after recently being diagnosed with colon cancer. She is worried about his cardiac status and long-standing history of diabetes. Having been in practice for 20 years, she is also concerned about a number of aspects of his care. Will he receive his usual dose of insulin despite the fact that he is NPO? Will he receive prophylactic antibiotics within an appropriate time frame? Will his β-blockers be continued? Will the anesthesia team monitor his glucose during his procedure? Will he become hypothermic? Will he suffer any cognitive dysfunction as a result of his anesthetic?

Glancing through the door at the cockpit as she boards the plane, Dr. Jones considers the often-cited similarity of the work environments of pilots and anesthesiologists. She imagines that the pilot would be as bewildered by the array of physiologic/ventilatory monitors as she is by the myriad of aircraft monitors. However, as she takes her seat, she realizes that a profound difference exists between their work environments. Dr. Jones is not concerned about the pilot or the air traffic controller (both of whom she has never met). She is not concerned about this particular aircraft (on which she has never flown). The length of her flight is not dependent on which particular pilot is in charge of the aircraft or which individual air traffic controller is involved in transferring the aircraft from one geographic zone to another. She does not worry about whether the plane has enough fuel to get to her destination, whether the plane will land on the runway (and not before or after), whether the plane will come too close to another plane, or whether the takeoff speed will be sufficient to get the plane airborne.

Yes, their work environments are similar but the pilot's monitors assist in standardizing task completion. They anticipate exceedences and help to detect overlooked conditions, while the anesthesiologist's monitors simply tell her when a parameter is out of range. While every aviation accident is analyzed to determine the cause, errors in healthcare frequently go undetected. Only when a catastrophic event (e.g., medication overdose resulting in death) makes the front page of major newspapers[1] do changes in healthcare delivery occur. Major changes came following both the Libby Zion[2] and

Dana-Farber[3] cases. The former ultimately resulted in a limit on residents' work hours; the latter heralded a total system redesign of a world-famous cancer center.

Decision Making in Anesthesiology

When initially designed over 100 years ago, the anesthetic record documented a patient's condition by recording only a few physiologic parameters (e.g., heart rate, blood pressure, respiratory rate). With the increase in scope of surgical procedures, patient selection, and anesthetic techniques, came a concomitant increase in the number (and sophistication) of monitors. Standard monitoring now includes temperature, O_2 saturation, and end-tidal CO_2. Processed electroencephalographic monitoring is becoming more common, and frequently, anesthesiologists use additional invasive monitors to measure blood pressure and O_2 extraction.

The safety profile of anesthetic care has improved, despite an aging population and an increase in both the number and the complexity of procedures performed each year. This increased safety is, in part, due to our ability to more fully assess a patient's condition. However, the proliferation of devices and the need to integrate multiple data streams to provide information have perhaps challenged our ability to assimilate all of these data. Are we able to gather data, interpret them, and design our therapies effectively and efficiently? In fact, we may not be.

Fallibility of Human Decision Making

More than a quarter century ago, Tversky and Kahneman[4] demonstrated (in a now-classic paper) that the presentation of information can have a large impact on how decisions are made. How a scenario is framed (e.g., 80% probability that an event will occur versus 20% chance that it will not occur) can affect which option is chosen. Kahneman's work in the area of "behavioral economics" was recognized by the mainstream academic world when he won the 2002 Nobel Prize in economics (despite his claim that he had never taken a single economics course). A key feature of behavioral economics is that a higher value is placed on avoiding a loss than on making a gain, even if both choices are of equal magnitude.

Emotion can play a role in decision making. Patients with lesions in the ventromedial sector of the prefrontal cortex have impairment in making decisions but retain cognitive functions.[5] Even those whose livelihoods depend on quantitative decision analysis (e.g., experienced financial traders) are not immune to the emotional component of decision making.[6] During periods of increased market activity relative to periods of normal volatility, traders had statistically significant differences in ectodermal responses and cardiovascular parameters. Studies in both psychology and economics have demonstrated human fallibility in everyday decision making.[7] Thirty years ago, it was shown that physicians (serving as their own controls in a crossover design study) detected and responded to events (e.g., ordering a test, prescribing a medication) twice as often when they had computerized reminders as compared to when they relied on their own memory.[8] Investigators hypothesized that errors in medical diagnosis and judgment reflect the limited abilities of humans to process information rather than a deficiency in knowledge.

The concept that people have limitations in incorporating all available information in decision-making processes is not new. Our ability to store information in short-term memory is limited to approximately seven data elements.[9] Three well-described bottlenecks that can impair our ability to recognize (i.e., attentional blink), store (i.e., visual short-term memory), and act (i.e., psychologic refractory period) upon visual information have been localized to specific regions of the brain.[10]

What are the implications of these possible causes for faulty decision making? The clinical practice of anesthesiology may benefit from experience gained in three environments (i.e., nuclear aircraft carriers, nuclear power plants, and air traffic control centers) that share several key elements[11]:

- The environments are complex, internally dynamic, and, intermittently, intensely interactive.
- Personnel perform exacting tasks under considerable time pressure.
- Demanding objectives are achieved with low incident rates and an almost complete absence of catastrophic failures over several years.

Given the pivotal role that decision-support systems (DSS) serve in these areas, their applicability to our working environment may be very relevant.

The Value of Decision-Support Systems

As a specialty, anesthesiology has come a long way in the past half century from the time when "...death from anesthesia [was] of sufficient magnitude to constitute a public health problem."[12] However, both the aviation and the nuclear power industries have far better safety records. Unlike these industries, the practice of anesthesia (and the delivery of healthcare in general) is characterized by tremendous variation in patient care. Much of this variation occurs at the level where individual physicians diagnose and/or treat a specific medical condition. From a systems perspective, this variability translates into a poor-quality product. Early efforts to address this fundamental problem can be seen in the emergence of pay-for-performance programs. These initiatives, directed at evaluating whether physicians provide specific treatments, are not meant to assist physicians at the point of care. In some ways, their design is reminiscent of the difference between alarms in aviation and anesthesiology. The programs identify when something has gone wrong; they do not warn the physician beforehand.

DSS have the potential to standardize some clinical practices, reduce errors of omission/commission, and assist anesthesiologists in their patient-care responsibilities. Their design can range from minimal (if any) control to total control so that the decision aid acts autonomously (Table 15.1).[13]

Table 15.1 Levels of automation

1. The computer offers no assistance: human must make all decision and take all actions
2. The computer offers a complete set of decision/action alternatives, OR
3. Narrows the selection down to a few, OR
4. Suggests one alternative, AND
5. Executes that suggestion if the human approves, OR
6. Allows the human a restricted time to veto before automatic execution, OR
7. Executes automatically, then necessarily informs humans, AND
8. Informs the human only if he is asked to be notified, OR
9. Informs the human only if it, the computer, decides to
10. The computer decides everything and acts autonomously, ignoring the human

From Sheridan TB, Thompson JM. People vs. computers in medicine. In: Bogner MS, ed. *Human Error* in Medicine. Hillsdale, NJ: Lawrence Erlbaum, 1994:141–59, with permission

Use of Decision Support in Other Industries

Aviation

The genesis of DSS in the airline industry came about as a result of a fortuitous meeting between the president of American Airlines and a top-level IBM salesman. American Airlines' manual reservation process was time consuming, had a limited ability to adapt to changing business models, and was not scalable. IBM saw an opportunity to use its product (computational machines) to address a business need. The collaboration between vendor and customer launched the SABER (Semi-Automatic Business Environment Research) project. Initially designed to automate the reservation process, the goal expanded to include equipment maintenance, food deliveries, and planning of new routes. Years later, the name was changed to SABRE, and American Airlines later spun it off as a separate company. Currently, 200 airlines (as well as car-rental companies, hotels, railways, and cruise lines) use the system for optimizing their operations.

DSS have other benefits—planning air routes and predicting weather hazards (while aggregating data from radar, satellite, and surface observations). After fuel costs increased, airlines developed software tools to identify less-expensive flight paths[14] and economical locations to purchase fuel. The Traffic Alert and Collision Avoidance System (TCAS), a computerized system designed to reduce the possibility of midair collisions between aircraft, is an example of level 4 automation in which the system suggests a course of action. Due to the high reliability of the system, the Federal Aviation Administration has instructed pilots to follow the directions specified in any TCAS message.

Other Industries

Decision-support tools are also used when computational speed or power is required. Computational speed is needed when decisions are made in a short period of time, as with computerized trading of stocks and futures. Computational power is required when large amounts of data must be processed. Examples include the oil and gas industry (to maximize the probability of drilling productive wells) and the pharmaceutical industry (to minimize the risk in new drug development). Industries that have a time-sensitive product (e.g., hotels and restaurants) use decision support to optimize their business processes. Their incentive to maximize the use of a consumable product (time) is similar to a clinical director's desire to maximize the utilization (or contribution margin) of OR time.

Decision Support in Healthcare

Existing healthcare DSS can be categorized as (a) software applications that control medical devices through a feedback mechanism or (b) reminders/alerts/prompts that assist the physician at the point of clinical care.

Software Protocols

Software protocols that use decision support to standardize managing and weaning ventilated patients have been used in the ICU. The proof of concept was demonstrated in patients with trauma-induced acute respiratory distress syndrome.[15] Subsequent studies established that computerized weaning resulted in fewer days of mechanical ventilation and reduced lengths of stay in the ICU.[16] In light of the national shortage of intensivists, the equivalence of protocol-based and physician-directed weaning can be viewed as one possible solution to standardizing ICU care.[17]

Reminders

Randomized trials have shown the efficacy of computerized reminders in the inpatient setting. In hospitalized patients who received nephrotoxic or renally excreted medications and had rising creatinine levels, computerized alerts prevented renal impairment and were accepted by clinicians.[18] Prompts were designed to increase ordering rates for preventive measures (pneumococcal vaccination, influenza vaccination, prophylactic heparin, and prophylactic aspirin administration at discharge) that had not been ordered by the admitting physician. With over half of the 6371 patients (total of

10,065 hospitalizations) having at least one indication, computerized reminders increased ordering rates for all four measures in a statistically significant manner.[19] Prevention of deep vein thrombosis and pulmonary embolism was achieved using computerized alerts, which increased the use of prophylaxis in high-risk hospitalized patients and markedly reduced the rates of both morbidities.[20] Although generally efficacious for hospitalized patients, the use of electronic reminders to improve out-patient care in patients with chronic conditions (e.g., diabetes and coronary artery disease) has been less positive.[21]

Computerized Physician Order Entry

Currently, the most frequent use of clinical decision support is computerized physician order entry (CPOE). CPOE holds great promise for reducing many of the medication errors that have been implicated in a large percentage of adverse drug events. Implementation has been limited to <10% of institutions, which is similar to the market penetration of AIMS. Studies with first- and second-generation CPOE systems that were based on homegrown systems have reported positive results. Medication errors that were not intercepted by nursing or pharmacy personnel were reduced by >50% when physicians used CPOE in the inpatient setting.[22] In children's hospitals, where medication errors are more common due to weight-based dosing, reductions in harmful adverse drug effects were achieved.[23,24]

At this writing, some commercial CPOE systems are available; however, they have not yet achieved the generally positive results reported by homegrown systems. A number of factors might explain these differences, including a more customized approach, a more in-depth knowledge of physician-ordering patterns, greater enthusiasm for the technology, and the nature of the hospital culture where these systems were adopted. While deployment of commercial systems is still relatively rare, reports have been published of unanticipated increases in mortality in a PICU[25] and facilitation of medication ordering errors.[26]

Lessons Learned from Decision Support in Medicine

User Participation

A meta-analysis of 100 studies found that clinical DSS (CDSS) improved practitioner performance in two-thirds of studies. Automatic prompts (as opposed to systems requiring user-initiated requests) were more successful.[27] Studies in which evaluated systems were developed by the authors (as opposed to those that were not developed by the authors) showed a significant improvement in practitioner performance (74 vs. 28%; $p = 0.001$).

Although CPOE can play a role in encouraging patient-safety efforts, successful implementation usually requires a paradigm shift in hospital policies and processes.[28] User buy-in is particularly important, and physician participation in both the planning and the rollout of the application is critical. One overlooked but significant determinant of the success of any DSS is its degree of integration into the clinician's workflow, which requires physician involvement in the customization process. However, in general, budgets for these projects do not include compensation for physician involvement. A physician who participates in these endeavors may experience a reduction in his compensation (from decreased clinical productivity). This situation potentially creates a vicious cycle, with limited physician involvement leading to lack of acceptance by physicians of the application, leading to a general lessening of physician interest.

Design Considerations

Design considerations are important to ensure smooth integration into the clinician's workflow. Barriers to using computerized reminders are lack of flexibility and poor interface usability, while features that facilitate use include (a) limiting the number of reminders, (b) strategic location of computer workstations, (c) integration of reminders into the workflow, and (d) the ability to document system problems and receive prompt administrator feedback.[29] One institution with a long-standing use of CDSS found that computerized standing orders were more effective than computerized reminders for increasing the rates of vaccine administration.[30]

In one study that lasted 3 months and reviewed almost 8000 alerts, it was found that 80% were overridden for a variety of reasons (i.e., physician was aware of alert condition but did not consider it relevant, patient did not have the allergy or tolerated the medication, patient was taking the recommended medication already).[31] While 6% of the overridden alerts were associated with an adverse drug event, it was felt that the overrides were clinically justified and thus not the cause of the adverse drug event. To aid in their implementation, some pioneering physicians have created tenets for effective decision support (Table 15.2).[32]

Unintended Consequences

Unintended consequences of using CPOE include more/new work for clinicians, unfavorable workflow issues, never-ending system demands, problems related to paper persistence, untoward changes in communication patterns and practices, negative emotions, generation of new kinds of errors, unexpected changes in the power structure, and overdependence on the technology.[33]

Table 15.2 Ten commandments for effective clinical decision support

1. Speed is everything
2. Anticipate needs and deliver in real time
3. Fit into the user's workflow
4. Little things can make a big difference
5. Recognize that physicians will strongly resist automated guidelines
6. Recognize that changing direction is easier with defaults
7. Simple interventions work best
8. Ask for additional information only when you really need it
9. Monitor impact, get feedback, and respond
10. Knowledge-based systems should be managed and maintained

Adapted from Bates DW, Kuperman GJ, Wang S, et al. Ten commandments for effective clinical decision support: Making the practice of evidence-based medicine a reality. J Am Med Inform Assoc 2003; 10(6):523–31

Implementation Considerations

The social, political, and organizational aspects of implementation cannot be ignored. In the US, objections by physicians and nurses led to the deinstallation of a $34 million computer system only 3 months after its implementation. The main criticisms were a lack of physician involvement in the planning process and the significant workflow changes associated with use of the system.[34] Sometimes, the cultural environment is the determinant in the success or failure of these systems. The same CPOE system was installed in two Dutch hospitals (one academic and the other a large, regional, nonacademic facility). Whereas implementation was halted in the academic hospital, it succeeded in the other.[35]

Unanswered Questions

As so few institutions have implemented these systems, the cumulative experience has been limited to those evangelists who are dedicated to designing the models and improving their shortcomings. A number of questions have yet to be answered. Will decision support be accepted by experienced anesthesiologists? Will a certification process be established to exempt some physicians from using it? Will use of these systems generate dependence on them (much like calculators or word-processing spell checkers appear to lessen students' capabilities)? What mechanisms could be put in place to ensure that incorrect advice is not given?

Situational Awareness

The introduction of high-fidelity aviation simulators led to a more complete understanding of how pilots make decisions and, perhaps more importantly, characterization of their decision-making errors. Endsley's model of situational awareness is the most commonly used model of aviation decision making and is applicable to the working environment of the anesthesiologist.[36] Situational awareness is the:

- Perception of the environmental elements within a volume of time and space (level 1)
- Comprehension of their meaning (level 2)
- Projection of their status in the near future (level 3)[37]

Situational awareness can be disrupted by a variety of factors, including focusing attention on a single piece of data to the exclusion of other relevant data, failing to consider other hypotheses, workload demands, anxiety, fatigue, lack of appreciation for the changing dynamics of a situation, and inaccurate mental models. The failure to process information at any level can disrupt one's situational awareness. This would include a failure to correctly perceive the information (level 1), failure to comprehend the situation (level 2), or failure to project the situation into the future (level 3). Analysis of situational awareness errors in aviation reveals that three-quarters of errors are level 1 errors.[38] Level 1 errors occur when relevant data are not available, when it is difficult to discriminate or detect data, when a failure to monitor or observe data occurs, when presented information is misperceived, or when memory loss occurs.

Decision Support in Anesthesia

Current

Broadly defined, decision support includes any aid that lessens the chance that an anesthesiologist will forget to do something that is required in providing anesthetic care; this can include both clinical and operational decision support. Using closed-loop control of propofol (with manual adjustments of remifentanil), investigators demonstrated that automated control of consciousness using the bispectral index (BIS) is clinically feasible and outperforms manual control.[39] Sufficient agreement was found between plasma and exhaled propofol concentrations to permit real-time monitoring of propofol via end-tidal mass spectrometry analysis.[40] Point-of-care systems that require the user to explicitly access information provide a passive form of decision support. In a simulated environment, these systems improve management of anesthetic crises.[41] Clinicians with experience using AIMS have augmented their systems with these features (Table 15.3).

Table 15.3 Example of available point-of-care decision support

- Advanced cardiac life-support protocols
- Malignant hyperthermia protocols and location of supplies, blood tests, and tubes required
- Current clinical protocols for kidney, liver, and heart transplants
- Guidelines and doses for subacute bacterial endocarditis prophylaxis
- Guidelines and doses for preoperative antibiotic
- Automated retrieval of prior anesthetic records to identify patients with a known difficult airway
- Drug dose calculator, with weight imported from application
- Automatic generation of form-letter templates that can be given to patients for:
  ○ Difficult airway events, how the problem was solved, and recommendation to obtain a Medic Alert bracelet
  ○ Possible drug reactions (to be communicated to an allergist)
  ○ Dental trauma (with instructions on how to contact the anesthesia business office to arrange for follow-up care)

Richard Epstein (personal communication)

Early work focused on detecting light anesthesia and lability of blood pressure.[42,43] Although not yet used in clinical practice, this long-term goal would be equivalent to position specification in the aviation industry. Timely feedback[44] and intraoperative reminders[45] have been used to increase rates of preincisional administration of prophylactic antibiotics.

Decision support can provide significant value in reminding providers about documentation omissions, which are essential for billing purposes but are often overlooked by providers. Software designed to automatically scan the anesthesia EMR to detect documentation omissions was implemented at one facility.[46] Scanning the record every 10 minutes, the application automatically notified the provider of missing entries, relieving her of the need to remember (or check) which elements had not yet been documented. The percentage of nonbillable records declined from 1.31% to 0.04%, and the median time to correct documentation errors decreased from 33 to 3 days. Based on historic data, the institution anticipates an increase in department collections of approximately $400,000 per year.

Embedding decision support in an existing AIMS has been used to automate point-of-care charge capture and submission and to increase compliance rate for documentation of invasive procedures.[47,48] Reminders have been used to audit anesthetic records for required fields (ASA status, diagnosis, procedure, and similar entries that are required by the Center for Medicaid and Medicare) and to notify providers of the anesthesia end time for a prior case to avoid a possible overlap with the start of anesthesia care for the next case (Richard Epstein, personal communication). Decision support may play an increasing role in managing patient flow. Scheduling procedures that require an anesthesiologist's participation can be automated so that patients arrive just in time for non-OR anesthesia, surgery, or regional block placement.[49]

In the future, these design features will no doubt be extended for additional functionality in the preoperative (Table 15.4), intraoperative (Table 15.5), and postoperative (Table 15.6) phases of patient care.

Table 15.4 Possibilities for future preoperative decision support

- Identification of specific herbal medications that patients are taking, as one-third of patients take them and anesthesiologists often do not ask about herbal supplements

- Identification of a patient seen at the preanesthesia clinic as a candidate for a clinical study

- Identification of patients with, or at risk for, coronary artery disease who are candidates for β-blocker therapy

- Automatic retrieval of past anesthesia records to identify significant events that occurred with past anesthetics, such as difficult mask ventilation or laryngoscopy, difficulty with line placement, sensitivity/resistance to medications

- Calculation of body mass index; estimation of ideal body weight

- Automation of the American Heart Association/American College of Cardiology algorithm for evaluation of patients with cardiac risk factors

- Identification of patients at risk for postoperative nausea and vomiting

Table 15.5 Possibilities for future intraoperative decision support

- In the case of multiple-room supervision, setting of parameter limits so that attending is automatically notified by PDA/text pager about changes in patients' conditions

- Identification of possible episodes of light anesthesia and/or awareness

- Automated calling for help (i.e., code)

- Deciding which cases to move to optimize OR efficiency on the day of surgery

- Use of automated systems to recommend the ordering of fresh frozen plasma and cryoprecipitate based on blood loss, patient's estimated blood volume, and laboratory values

- Recommendation to consider a diagnosis of malignant hyperthermia based on interpretation of heart rate, end-tidal CO_2, and minute ventilation

- Prediction of wake-up time based on pharmacokinetic analysis of propofol infusion history

Table 15.6 Possibilities for future postoperative decision support

- Standardization of postanesthesia orders:
  - For particular types of procedures
  - By accounting for body mass index and ideal body weight, as well as intraoperative medication administration
  - Based on patient's weight (especially for children) and age (especially for elderly)

Medicolegal Implications of Using Decision Support

CDSS may be used in a voluntary manner, so that a physician can access context-sensitive information, or they might be implemented in such a manner that they serve as software embodiments of "guidelines," which is the model for CPOE implementations. As CDSS become more commonplace, questions about the appropriateness of their use may become a factor in malpractice claims. Two issues arise. Should physicians use them? What are the consequences for using (or not using) a CDSS when a patient has a bad outcome?

While the role of a CDSS in the context of patient care will be an evolving issue in malpractice litigation, it is important to note that determination of negligence is typically based on community standards of care. In this context, the definition of "community" will be important. Vendors are not necessarily enthusiastic to offer CDSS enhancements to their existing systems, as the FDA would most likely consider them to be medical devices. With the current level of interest in any type of EMR, vendors will not need to add "value" to their products to encourage sales. As a result, CDSS may continue to be home grown, and the "community" standard of care may be restricted to a single institution. (The experiences of commercially available CDSS were described above.)

Very little case law exists regarding the impact of computer-assisted decision-making programs in malpractice claims, principally because they are available in only a small number of institutions. Furthermore, data are limited concerning how the public regards the role of computers in clinical practice. A recent study sheds some light on how the public might regard their use by physicians.[50] In the first experiment, undergraduates (who would have more education than the average juror) were presented a scenario in which a physician made a correct or an incorrect diagnosis with and without the use of a decision aid. If a physician made the correct diagnosis using a decision aid, she was viewed less favorably than if she had not used one. In a second experiment, undergraduates and medical students were presented a scenario in which a negative outcome occurred. The physician in the scenario (a) agreed with the decision aid, (b) did not use the aid, (c) agreed with the aid over his initial opinion, or (d) disagreed with the aid and chose his own opinion. In the context of a negative outcome, the physician who agreed with or went along with the aid was perceived as being at less fault. The physician who disagreed with the aid and went with his initial impression was perceived to be at similar fault as the one who did not use the aid.

Another dimension to the medicolegal context pertains to the so-called meta-data, or data concerning data. When using a CDSS, a physician may choose to act upon the software's alert/reminder or she may ignore it for a variety of reasons (e.g., the alert is not sufficiently specific to the patient's condition, or the patient's condition warrants a certain medication despite the risks). In either case, the software will record the physician's actions. Should this data element be considered part of the medical record? The question is further complicated, because while the federal government is strongly encouraging the use of EMRs, state law governs the composition of medical records. The determination as to whether CDSS metadata are part of the medical record may depend on the manner in which the data are stored.[51] If, as is the case these days, a CDSS is a creation of individual institutions, it may be possible to segregate and deidentify the data if they are to be used for research purposes. If the CDSS is a component of a commercially available EMR, the metadata may be considered to be part of the record.

The significance of metadata in this context is relevant because in one study, physicians overrode 80% of drug allergy alerts when using a CPOE system.[52] Currently, it is unlikely that any data that compare individuals' methods of use (similar to pay-for-performance data) would be admissible (either for the plaintiff or for the defense) in a tort claim.[53] Whether data about how a physician used (or did not use) a CDSS are admissible remains an open question.

Conclusion

DSS have been incorporated into business processes in other industries with significant improvements in safety (aviation) and operational efficiency (aviation and financial). CPOE is the most prevalent form of a CDSS in healthcare. The most advanced CPOE systems had their origins more than a decade ago and have undergone many refinements. Reports of unintended consequences from the use of CPOE call attention to the need for careful consideration as to how these tools can best aid physicians in providing clinical care.

Some existing AIMS have rudimentary tools that allow users to specify conditions that can trigger alerts or reminders. However, development of decision-support tools has been undertaken by relatively few institutions. These in-house efforts are most likely the result of reluctance on the part of vendors to add "smart" features, which might require FDA approval for medical devices. Institutional cultures and practices may also be a factor in the development of such tools. With no centralized developmental process, individual institutions are duplicating the work of others. More rapid progress (as well as standardization of decision aids) might occur if development of decision-support initiatives was commissioned by the ASA.

Key Points

- Some industries (e.g., aviation, financial) have undergone significant changes in safety and efficiency as a result of DSS.
- DSS are in their infancy, primarily because <10% of institutions have anesthesia EMRs.
- DSS are often developed by individual institutions, reflecting their own specific procedures and processes.
- Experiences with CPOE have demonstrated that user interface and speed of processing are key factors in the successful implementation of a DSS.

- The deployment of some commercially available DSS has had unintended consequences, including facilitation of order entry errors.
- The medicolegal consequences of using, ignoring, or not using CDSS are still an open question.

Acknowledgment The principal author would like to thank Lou Vigoda for enthusiastically supporting my educational endeavors and Joan and Sophie Leonard for their suggestions during the writing of this manuscript.

References

1. Dosing errors kills 2 preemies; 3rd critical: Infants accidentally given adult amount of drug, Indiana hospital says. Associated Press. http://www.msnbc.msn.com/id/14883323/. Accessed February 5, 2008
2. Doctors' accounts vary in death of Libby Zion (January 1, 1995). http://query.nytimes.com/gst/fullpage.html?sec=health&res=990CE4DC1230F932A35752C0A963958260. The New York Times. Accessed February 5, 2008
3. Organizational change in the face of highly public errors. I. The Dana-Farber Cancer Institute Experience. AHRQ, Morbidity and Mortality Rounds on the Web. http://www.webmm.ahrq.gov/perspective.aspx?perspectiveID=3. Accessed February 5, 2008
4. Tversky A, Kahneman D. The framing of decisions and the psychology of choice. Science 1981; 211:453–8
5. Bechara A. The role of emotion in decision-making: Evidence from neurological patients with orbitofrontal damage. Brain Cogn 2004; 55:30–40
6. Lo A, Repin D. Psychophysiology of real-time financial risk processing. J Cogn Neurosci 2002; 14:323–39
7. Gilovich T. *How We Know What Isn't So: The Fallibility of Human Reason in Everyday Life*. New York: The Free Press, 1991
8. McDonald CJ. Protocol-based computer reminders, the quality of care and the non-perfectability of man. N Engl J Med 1976; 295:1351–5
9. Miller GA. The magical number seven, plus or minus two: Some limits on our capacity for processing information. Psychol Rev 1956; 63:81–97
10. Marois R, Ivanoff J. Capacity limits of information processing in the brain. Trends Cogn Sci 2005; 9(6):296–305
11. Reason J. Human error—models and management. Br Med J 2000; 320:768–70
12. Beecher HK, Todd DP. A study of the deaths associated with anesthesia and surgery: Based on a study of 599,548 anesthesias in ten institutions 1948–1952, inclusive. Ann Surg 1954; 140:1–34
13. Sheridan TB, Thompson JM. People Versus Computers in Medicine. In: Bogner MS, ed. *Human Error in Medicine*. Hillsdale, NJ: Lawrence Erlbaum, 1994:141–59
14. Carey S. Calculating costs in the clouds: How flight-planning software helps airlines balance fuel, distance, wind, "overfly" fees. *The Wall Street Journal*, March 6, 2007:B1. http://online.wsj.com/article/SB117314795095227844.html
15. McKinley BA, Moore FA, Sailors RM, et al. Computerized decision support for mechanical ventilation of trauma induced ARDS: Results of a randomized clinical trial. J Trauma 2001; 50(3):415–24
16. Lellouche F, Mancebo J, Jolliet P, et al. A multicenter, randomized trial of computer-driven protocolized weaning from mechanical ventilation. Am J Respir Crit Care Med 2006; 174(8):894–900
17. Krishnan JA, Moore D, Robeson C, et al. A prospective, controlled trial of a protocol-based strategy to discontinue mechanical ventilation. Am J Respir Crit Care Med 2004; 169:673–8

18. Rind DM, Safran C, Phillips RS, et al. Effect of computer-based alerts on the treatment and outcomes of hospitalized patients. Arch Intern Med 1994; 154:1511–7

19. Dexter PR, Perkins S, Overhage JM, et al. A computerized reminder system to increase the use of preventive care for hospitalized patients. N Engl J Med 2001; 345:965–70

20. Kucher N, Koo S, Quiroz R, et al. Electronic alerts to prevent venous thromboembolism among hospitalized patients. N Engl J Med 2005; 352:969–77

21. Sequist TD, Gandhi TK, Karson AS, et al. A randomized trial of electronic clinical reminders to improve quality of care for diabetes and coronary artery disease. J Am Med Inform Assoc 2005; 12:431–7

22. Bates DW, Leape LL, Cullen DJ, et al. Effect of computerized physician order entry and a team intervention on prevention of serious medication errors. JAMA 1998; 280:1311–6

23. Upperman JS, Staley P, Friend K, et al. The impact of hospital wide computerized physician order entry on medical errors in a pediatric hospital. J Pediatr Surg 2005; 40:57–9

24. Potts AL, Barr FE, Gregory DF, et al. Computerized physician order entry and medication errors in a pediatric critical care unit. Pediatrics 2004; 113:59–63

25. Han YY, Carcillo JA, Venkataraman ST, et al. Unexpected increased mortality after implementation of a commercially sold computerized physician order entry system. Pediatrics 2005; 116;1506–12

26. Koppel R, Metlay JP, Cohen A, et al. Role of computerized physician order entry systems in facilitating medication errors. JAMA 2005; 293:1197–203

27. Garg AX, Adhikari NKJ, McDonald H, et al. Effects of computerized clinical decision support systems on practitioner performance and patient outcomes: A systematic review. JAMA 2005; 293:1223–38

28. Upperman JS, Staley P, Friend K, et al. The introduction of computerized physician order entry and change management in a tertiary pediatric hospital. Pediatrics 2005; 116:634–42

29. Saleem JJ, Patterson ES, Militello L, et al. Exploring barriers and facilitators to the use of computerized clinical reminders. J Am Med Inform Assoc 2005; 12:438–47

30. Dexter PR, Perkins SM, Maharry KS, et al. Inpatient computer-based standing orders vs. physician reminders to increase influenza and pneumococcal vaccination rates. JAMA 2004; 292:2366–71

31. Hsieh TC, Kuperman GJ, Jaggi T, et al. Characteristics and consequences of drug allergy alert overrides in a computerized physician order entry system. J Am Med Inform Assoc 2004; 11:482–91

32. Bates DW, Kuperman GJ, Wang S, et al. Ten commandments for effective clinical decision support: Making the practice of evidence-based medicine a reality. J Am Med Inform Assoc 2003; 10(6):523–31

33. Campbell EM, Sittig DF, Ash JS, et al. Types of unintended consequences related to computerized provider order entry. J Am Med Inform Assoc 2006; 13(5):547–56

34. Clancy TR, Delaney C. Complex nursing systems. J Nurs Manag 2005; 13(3):192–201

35. Aarts J, Berg M. A tale of two hospitals: A sociotechnical appraisal of the introduction of computerized physician order entry in two Dutch hospitals. Medinfo 2004; 11(Pt 2):999–1002

36. Endsley MR. Situation Awareness Global Assessment Technique (SAGAT). Proceedings of the National Aerospace and Electronics Conference (NAECON). New York: IEEE, 1988:789–95

37. Endsley MR. Design and evaluation for situation awareness enhancement. Proceedings of the Human Factors Society 32nd Annual Meeting. Santa Monica, CA: Human Factors Society, 1988:97–101

38. Jones DG, Endsley MR. Sources of situation awareness errors in aviation. Aviat Space Environ Med 1996; 67(6):507–12

39. Liu N, Chazot T, Genty A, et al. Titration of propofol for anesthetic induction and maintenance guided by the bispectral index: Closed-loop versus manual control: A prospective, randomized, multicenter study. Anesthesiology 2006; 104(4):686–95

40. Takita A, Masui K, Tomiei K. On-line monitoring of end-tidal propofol concentration in anesthetized patients. Anesthesiology 2007; 106(4):659–64

41. Berkenstadt H, Yusim Y, Ziv A, et al. An assessment of a point-of-care information system for the anesthesia provider in simulated malignant hyperthermia crisis. Anesth Analg 2006; 102:530–2

42. Reich DL, Osinski TK, Bodian C, et al. An algorithm for assessing intraoperative mean arterial pressure lability. Anesthesiology 1997; 87(1):156–61

43. Krol M, Reich DL. Development of a decision support system to assist anesthesiologists in operating room. J Med Syst 2000; 24(3):141–6

44. O'Reilly M, Talsma A, VanRiper S, et al. An anesthesia information system designed to provide physician-specific feedback improves timely administration of prophylactic antibiotics. Anesth Analg 2006; 103:908–12

45. Wax DB, Beilin Y, Levin M, et al. The effect of an interactive visual reminder in an anesthesia information management system on timeliness of prophylactic antibiotic administration. Anesth Analg 2007; 104(6):1462–6

46. Spring SF, Sandberg WS, Anupama S, et al. Automated documentation error detection and notification improves anesthesia billing performance. Anesthesiology 2007; 106(1):157–63

47. Reich DL, Kahn RA, Wax D, et al. Development of a module for point-of-care charge capture and submission using an anesthesia information management system. Anesthesiology 2006; 105(1):179–86

48. Kheterpal S, Gupta R, Blum JM, et al. Electronic reminders improve procedure documentation compliance and professional fee reimbursement. Anesth Analg 2007; 104:592–7

49. Dexter F, Xiao Y, Dow AJ, et al. Coordination of appointments for anesthesia care outside of operating rooms using an enterprise-wide scheduling system. Anesth Analg 2007; 105(6):1701–10

50. Pezzo MV, Pezzo SP. Physician evaluation after medical errors: Does having a computer decision aid help or hurt in hindsight? Med Decis Making 2006; 26(1):48–56

51. Rollins G. The prompt, the alert, and the legal record: Documenting clinical decision support systems. J AHIMA 2005; 76(2):24–8

52. Hsieh TC, Kuperman GJ, Jaggi T, et al. Characteristics and consequences of drug allergy alert overrides in a computerized order entry system. J Am Med Inform Assoc 2004; 11(6):482–91

53. Kesselheim AS, Ferris TG, Studdert DM. Will physician-level measures of clinical performance be used in medical malpractice litigation? JAMA 2006; 295(15):1831–4

Chapter 16
Perioperative Process Improvement

Paul St. Jacques and Michael Higgins

Imperative for Change: Efficiency and Safety

Data collection and analysis is the cornerstone and first step toward process improvement. Through integration of multisource data and delivery of processed data to multiple users in a real-time, near real-time, or periodic fashion, an AIMS has several distinct advantages over traditional paper-based record-keeping systems. For example, data collection can be handled in a manual process in which codification occurs by the user at the time of entry, or in an automated fashion in which data are collected and codified by the electronic system without user intervention. Improving the accuracy and completeness of data collection produces improvements in the quality and quantity of data available for subsequent analysis. Improvements have been shown in detection of adverse events, in which the rates of reporting are notoriously low when the data are self-reported.[1] Data processing can also be immediate, yielding potentially important on-the-fly decision-support information. These data can then be relayed to clinicians in the field via alphanumeric pagers, wall-mounted computer displays, or handheld computers. Alternately, data can be queued for offline multiphase review and analysis. Reports can be produced in a standardized format through monthly reports delivered to decision makers, or they can be produced via database queries or on-demand data aggregation at the level of granularity that is required.

Efficiency gains result in multiple benefits to the perioperative suite. Revenue is improved through increased charge capture, better schedule management, and more efficient patient flow. Patient satisfaction and expectations are more successfully met through decreased delays and case cancellations due to better management of patient disease-related issues, better scheduling of manpower and OR facilities, and a decreased need for the patient to endlessly repeat the same medical and demographic information to multiple staff members. These same efficiency gains can also decrease staff frustration with the inefficiencies so common to the OR, such as those related to room turnover, instrument availability, staff availability, and even patient availability.

It is important to remember that beyond efficiency and satisfaction, the paramount goal of process improvement is to achieve the highest levels of patient safety possible. Although safety has always been a goal of the medical community, the Institute of Medicine focused national attention on this issue in the year 2000 with the release of the landmark report *To Err is Human: Building a Safer Health System*, which recommends such action items as the creation of tools, protocols, and research to enhance the knowledge base of patient safety.[2] Additionally, developing both mandatory- and voluntary-reporting systems to encourage quality improvement was recommended. Later, a second Institute of Medicine report, *Crossing the Quality Chasm: A New Health System for the 21st Century*, designated six aims for an optimal healthcare system: safe, effective, patient-centered, timely, efficient, and equitable.[3] The report noted that information technology has enormous potential for transforming healthcare and presented specific suggestions (e.g., automated order-entry systems, automated reminder systems, clinical decision-support systems, and alignment of financial incentives for both patients and practitioners with quality improvement) as potential methods for using electronic information systems to provide a substantial improvement in healthcare quality.[3] Additionally, other groups such as the Leapfrog group, Institute for Safe Medication Practices, and The Joint Commission are encouraging the use of electronic systems to improve efficiency of patient care, cost effectiveness, and safety.[4]

Data Analysis

In a traditional perioperative suite that lacks an AIMS, paper-based data collection or chart abstraction presents multiple impediments to a process-improvement program. Every clinician has experience with paper-based records that are often incomplete or missing. Even when available, they frequently must be physically obtained from a distant medical records repository for analysis. While the paper records are out for analysis by one group, they are unavailable for use by anyone else for either clinical or administrative purposes, unless they are photocopied. The security and the integrity of the medical records are also at risk while they are out for analysis, as it is entirely possible for the records to be lost, stolen, inadvertently misplaced, or discovered by nonauthorized staff or visitors. Additionally, it is relatively easy for a paper-based medical record to be altered without discovery or audit capability of who made the changes and at what time.

EMRs support data discovery. Manual review or chart abstraction is a very labor-intensive process. It is not uncommon, therefore, to dedicate a large portion of a project's effort toward gleaning and coding data from paper charts. Also, due to the amount of labor involved in manual extraction, it is common to only survey a sample percentage of charts and extrapolate those data to the entire chart population or to base statistics on a much smaller sample size, with resulting decreases in statistical power. Lastly, the manual chart extraction process is quite inflexible. For example, if after the review of 100 charts, it is found that an additional data field is required to complete a study, it is necessary to re-review all of those charts to gain access to that one additional data field. In contrast, review of electronic data allows for massive numbers of charts to be reviewed, up to the limit of the number of patients or encounters in the system. Often times, an EMR-based study will present data from tens of thousands of cases. Also, any modifications to the dataset specifications are relatively straightforward to obtain by rerunning a modified data query, something that can often be accomplished in a matter of seconds to minutes.

Electronic data query is not completely without effort. It requires a support structure for both the server hardware on which the database relies for management and storage and for a team of IT professionals. The database analysts in this structure may fulfill many roles. In the building of a data warehouse, data must be secured, backed up, and cleaned of spurious entries (Fig. 16.1). Additionally, depending on who has access to the data, it may be necessary (depending on local laws or standards) to have a separate section with data that are deidentified to protect patient privacy. In a more developed system, the analysis team can structure the data [e.g., into online analytical processing (OLAP) cubes] to create a mechanism whereby the end users can access and develop queries to the data using common-sense wizards and tools. This last function greatly enhances access to and utility of the data set, as any authorized clinical or managerial user can then generate data reports on demand to their specification without the intervention of an IT professional.

Improving the Preoperative Process

An efficient surgical day results from bringing together properly prepared patient, staff, and equipment to the same place at the same time. Typically, many of these factors are arriving "just in time" for the scheduled surgery. As such, efficiency on the day of surgery can be greatly affected by processes that are in place for preoperative scheduling, patient evaluation, and equipment availability. Computerized surgical scheduling has a long history of successful implementation and is frequently the only use of information management in many operating suites Allocating surgical time based on "block time," whereby cases are assigned to an individual surgeon or surgical service, increases efficiency by grouping similar types of case and/or cases by the same surgeon into predictable time periods. For example, block-time allocation can be displayed on a computer screen at the time of scheduling, and limits can be placed so that only appropriate cases are scheduled in a given block. Block-time release can also be programmed into the scheduling paradigm so that when a surgeon does not fill an assigned block by a certain time (e.g., 24 or 48 hours prior to the day of surgery), the time can be released for other surgeons to utilize. The electronic system aids surgical schedulers by keeping an up-to-date database of all of the scheduled cases, surgical blocks, and block-time releases. Additionally, as the time to complete a surgery may vary by surgeon, surgical time estimation can be based on the historic time required to complete surgery by the same surgeon performing the same or similar procedure. This feature is greatly facilitated by an electronic system that can keep a running average, based

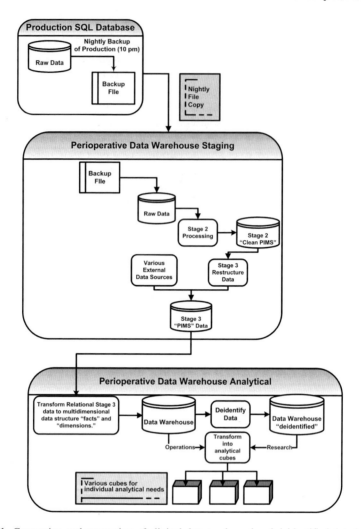

Fig. 16.1 Conversion and processing of clinical data to cleaned and deidentified data in a data warehouse. The data pass through several computerized steps. Each iteration serves to clean out-of-range data or restructure data to novel formats for analysis. Data are ultimately transformed into multidimensional data cubes for online analysis, referred to as *online analytical processing* (OLAP) cubes. To facilitate research and protect patient privacy, deidentification processes are applied to irreversibly separate the clinical data from any individually identifiable personal data such as names, social security numbers, and medical record numbers. *SQL* Structured Query Language, *PIMS* perioperative information management system

on management specifications, of the past times to complete a particular surgery. Electronic scheduling improves efficiency related to instrument availability. Scheduling systems may also enable electronic reservation of key pieces of equipment (e.g., microscopes) and tracking of individual instruments and instrument trays to ensure that two surgeries that both require a limited resource are not scheduled simultaneously. Electronic scheduling allows groups of surgical scheduling staff to easily view all known aspects of the surgical schedule for any given day so that as new cases are added to the schedule, they are placed into the appropriate OR to maximize the efficiency of the day of surgery as it relates to the surgeons, patients, OR staff, and instruments. Follow-up review by clinical management staff is also simplified as cases are moved for the purposes of gap reduction and load balancing among the ORs.

Staff assignment is also facilitated in an electronic system. Typically, due to the dynamic nature of the OR as it relates to case complexity and staff availability, schedules become obsolete almost immediately. Computerized entries of staffing information into particular work locations reduce management's need to issue multiple updated paper schedules and calendars. Additionally, the ability to access the schedules from any computer workstation allows staff members to "self-service" their assignment for a given shift, thereby reducing the load on managers.

Since they were first described in 1949, outpatient preoperative evaluation clinics (PECs) have provided significant financial and efficiency gains to the operating suite.[5,6] Benefits include a decrease in the number of cancelled surgical cases on the day of surgery due to inadequate patient preparation or previously unknown medical issues, as well as a decrease in the number of case delays due to unexpected testing or consultation on the day of surgery.[6,7] Among ASA type 3 and type 4 patients, delays caused by the need to obtain a preoperative electrocardiogram or laboratory analysis are reduced by ~50%.[6] Reducing these delays and cancellations results in significant cost savings and noticeable improvement to staff morale and patient satisfaction.

Implementation of a well-designed AIMS can streamline data acquisition in the PEC and ease access to collected data by subsequent clinicians. In the PEC, informatics solutions provide scheduling, demographic, and process-related data, such as time tracking to PEC visits. In this way, management can demonstrate utilization and efficiency of the clinic and potentially advocate for additional resources or space when necessary to best serve the surgical clinic's needs, which include seeing patients before surgery whether they are scheduled PEC visits or unscheduled walk-in visits. Additionally, an electronic PEC system can receive data in an automated fashion from the hospital patient database, which is particularly important for items such as a problem list, medications, or allergies. Also, as many patients who are seen for surgery are repeat patients, the PEC system can retrieve a detailed history from the patient's last visit to the PEC, allowing the practitioner to enter only interval change data and automatically electronically transcribe existing data into the current PEC record. The resulting PEC database may provide a rich data set by which hospitals can extract patient comorbidity data, which can be added to billing data for the purposes of justifying increasing reimbursement based on increased costs of caring for sicker patient populations.

The preoperative evaluation form prepared in accordance with standards set by an anesthesiology group is one of the most complete patient summaries in the medical record. In a paper-based system, a record is available in only one place at any given time, and clinicians must undertake a paper chase and travel from their site of work to the site of the report, typically the PEC, in order to review the form. To make matters worse, the preoperative charts may be difficult to find, as they are passed from person to person in the PEC and mixed with multiple other patient charts for multiple days of surgery. In an electronic system, this report is available through an electronic interface via Web browser or similar technology. This ability provides clinicians with an easy-to-access snapshot-type summary of the medical history. Clinicians no longer need to go to the PEC or other clinic to review these data; they come to the clinician in a concise, easily readable format. Similar to a paper report, an electronic report can have a standard clinically relevant format, either in SOAP (Subjective, Objective, Assessment, Plan) or another format. However, unlike a paper report, a computer-generated report will always be legible, reducing errors from missed or omitted information due to the inability to read the information. Even more important, it is always available and easily accessible.

Preoperative case review is facilitated by the electronic availability of preoperative reports. Because accessing reports is rapid and easy from virtually any location, clinicians are more likely to review patient data when they are presented in an electronic format. This review, coupled with investigation and possible resolution of potential causes of case cancellation or delay on the day of surgery, provides significant financial value to the hospital.[6] Additionally, as patients often have to make significant arrangements prior to surgery (time off from work, accompanying family members, travel, etc.), patient satisfaction may be improved due to the decreased number of case cancellations and delays on the day of surgery.[8–10] Time delays are a frequently cited negative comment, even among patients who are satisfied with their care. Online case review also provides a significant benefit to the resident education process. Training programs typically encourage or require a preoperative discussion between a resident (or other class of trainee) and the attending physician (or other class of teacher) of the salient features of a particular case and formulation of an anesthetic plan prior to the day of surgery. Having the patient's record available electronically for simultaneous review by both parties—even if they are at separate computer workstations—is a great improvement upon the heretofore standard scenario of two people discussing a case using a note or photocopy that frequently is in the possession of only one provider.

Improving the Day-of-Surgery Process

As we have seen with the preoperative process, electronic systems lend themselves to improving processes that occur on the day of surgery. One of the most critical aspects of efficiency on the day of surgery is ensuring "just in time" arrival of patients, staff, equipment, and OR staff. Electronic tracking of all of these elements allows management to adjust schedules and enables automatic electronic prompts and reminders that indicate patient readiness, surgical staff presence, documentation completeness, and other key elements that are necessary to proceed with surgery. Tracking of patients can begin at the front door of the hospital. Electronic systems can be in place whereby greeters have access to a current OR schedule and can direct patients to the proper admitting area or waiting area, thereby decreasing delays due to "missing" patients. Additionally, the greeter can log the patient into the system, notifying downstream staff that the patient has arrived. In this manner, patients are able to be brought to the OR suite early if necessary due to a previous case cancellation, early finish, or room change.

Patient-tracking indicators for transition between two locations such as from the admitting area to the preoperative holding or prep area can also be electronically relayed. Likewise, status changes, such as an intraoperative status change to case closing or similar state, can be electronically propagated from the OR to the OR suite charge nurse for notification that the room will soon be ready for the next patient. Depending on procedure, the charge nurse can then coordinate the correct time of transfer of the next patient to the holding area to begin preparation for surgery. In a similar fashion, the holding area itself can be notified electronically via a page, a message, or an icon placed on a tracking board that the OR will soon be ready for the next patient and that preparations should begin.

Other elements must be brought together for surgery. As in the previous example, an instrument room or equipment preparation area can be updated on the course of ongoing surgeries and soon-to-start surgeries either via electronic messages or tracking screens. On-time arrival of the necessary instruments and equipment is facilitated by this distributed knowledge of the state of the operative system. Surgeons, who are often not physically present in the OR or OR suite between cases, can also be notified of case status. Pages can be sent to surgeons through centralized integrated IT systems to notify them of the status of the patient relative to entry to the OR, the status of previous cases in the event of case over-runs, a previous case cancellation, or an early finish.

New technologies such as radio-frequency identification (RFID) are emerging, allowing for electronic tracking of patients through the hospital. These systems, which are becoming commonplace in many industries and retail locations, provide for tracking objects (equipment, staff, patients, etc.) by placing a computer chip "tag" on the item or patient. Often, this tag is embedded into a wristband, badge, or similar physical device. The chip generates a radio-frequency response when it is brought into proximity with a particular transmitter that is issuing a radio query to matching RFID chips in the area. By triangulating the response times and received signal intensity from the chips to an array of transmitters, a computer system is able to generate a three-dimensional location of that object. The location can then be relayed to a second computer with a programmed facility map, thereby identifying in which room the particular RFID tag is located and reporting that location to the host application or OR personnel.

RFID-equipped facilities track the flow of patients by relaying the patient location information from the RFID system to the patient-status indicators and graphic display components of the perioperative IT system. This design allows a nonuser interactive update of patient status based on location. Even with this type of automated tracking in place, some time-based events such as anesthesia ready time, surgical incision, and case closing must still be manually entered as the patient remains in the same physical location. RFID can also increase OR safety, for example, by ensuring that the correct patient is brought to the correct location. Sandberg et al.[11] have demonstrated this feature by using a combined RFID/infrared location system. In their study, the computerized location system compared the actual location of a test subject to the scheduled location of where the subject was supposed to be. In the event of a mismatch between subject and location, a page was sent to the operating team to notify them of the potential danger. Location and patient/item flow data can also be aggregated and presented in visual fashion for later management analysis on workflow process changes and improvement.[12]

Surgical instrumentation preparation and delivery to the OR is a continual source of frustration for many surgical teams. A large hospital may have hundreds of thousands of individual instruments. This vast number of instruments and numerous instrument types make organization and tracking of them very difficult. Additionally, the instruments must pass through several sets of hands between individual uses. A single instrument is passed from the OR team, to a decontamination team, to a set- or pan-assembly team, to teams for sterilization and storage, and finally, to the OR. Electronic-tracking systems that use barcode scanners and instruments etched with individual identification numbers can track these instruments through all phases of their use and maintenance. Implementing such tracking systems can improve the efficiency of the OR by ensuring that instrument trays are delivered there on time and in a complete form. Additionally, audit of the instrument-tracking systems can reveal each staff member who has been responsible for the instrument during its last use and identify issues related to proper handling of missing or broken instruments. This auditing can provide a basis for reporting on exceptions to standard processes and form the basis for improvement.

Even well-managed operating suites will be subject to unpredictable delays. As part of a process-improvement program, these delays should be analyzed by management teams and changes in processes should be implemented to correct or eliminate sources of delay. An electronic system greatly enhances this process. Delays can be tracked electronically by incorporating integrated delay-tracking frameworks into perioperative applications. Thus, in the course of normal documentation, delays are identified either by the users or the systems, which can track times and other data points and automatically identify to the user when a delay has occurred. The clinical user can then verify and categorize the delay without leaving the primary charting application. This maximizes efficiency for the user and enables the system to capture an increased amount of delay data. Additionally, delays can be assessed over a cross-section of OR staff. For example, the same delay event may be perceived differently by staff in two disciplines. By building the delay tracking into the software of multiple groups of clinicians, it becomes possible to improve validity of the quantity and quality of delay tracking through comparing the reporting of the different groups. Delay-reporting systems must aggregate and analyze delays on a recurrent basis. A monthly report delivered to management or reviewed at an OR committee meeting provides a powerful tool for process improvement. Delays can be sorted into type—categorical, time based, subjective or objective, location, surgical service, stage of care, and individual clinician. By reporting the delays in both aggregate and specific contexts, management is able to drill down to improve root-cause identification of delays and best effect process improvement.

Additionally, electronic delay and time tracking allows for detailed analysis of all phases of operative care. One of the most commonly analyzed perioperative time periods is the time between cases, commonly referred to as *turnover time*.[13] Although reduction of turnover time is the focus of many OR-related process-improvement projects, studies have shown that decreasing turnover time does not provide enough efficiency gain to provide time for an additional OR case to be completed.[14] However, reduction of turnover time may correlate to a decrease in over-run of the daily schedule, a persistent problem that typically results in staff overtime, poor morale, and frequent complaints voiced by surgeons and other staff members. Utilizing an electronic system for tracking key time periods through the perioperative process enables large-scale data analysis of these time periods. Electronic systems can be used to prompt users to correctly enter time fields, provide additional definition of the various time fields through the use of context-sensitive help screens, and aid in error correcting by checking for out-of-sequence time entries and incorrect date entries. Additionally, it is possible to combine and analyze any of the various components of any given procedure such as "in room" to "anesthesia ready" time, "in room" to "incision" time, or "anesthesia ready" to "incision" time. In doing so, management can examine the contribution of individuals and individual processes to the total case time. By having these different times available, it becomes possible to focus initiatives for process improvement on those items that are most likely to yield benefit.[15] Subsequently, by having the ability to track changes at regularly repeating intervals over a longer time period, it is also possible to gauge the effect of implemented process-improvement strategies so that those efforts that yield minimal results can be redesigned. Finally, the ability to generate and publish reports on efficiency possibly provides the most effective method of establishing control mechanisms to facilitate persistence of the process-improvement effort.

Electronic Quality Assurance Tracking

Quality assurance (QA) and *continuous quality improvement* (CQI) are buzzwords of modern medicine. As has been mentioned, while always a goal of the medical community, improving safety and quality of delivered care was once again brought to national attention via the Institute of Medicine's reports in 2000 and 2001. Perioperative informatics systems greatly improve the ability of clinicians and management to identify, track, and analyze issues to enable process improvement. As with manual QA processes, the cornerstones of event detection, analysis, peer review, reporting, and process change also apply to an electronic process. However, the electronic process can enhance and streamline many of these steps.

Manual, self-reporting, QA processes are notoriously poor in capturing quality-related data.[1] Quality data can be electronically identified in several ways. Computer systems can provide behind-the-scenes scans of electronic records for missing clinical data such as vital signs that fall outside of given ranges.[16] These scans can be performed on a continual, automated, nonuser-interactive basis, thus providing a rich data set for reporting and analysis. Alternately, user self-reporting of data can be used to identify critical events, "near misses," and nonsafety-related delay items.

Once captured, data can be analyzed and distributed via several methods. For example, medical- or safety-related events (reintubation, anaphylaxis, etc.) can be electronically reported to a peer-reviewed database, either in an automated fashion, as described earlier, or by a manual process via data entry to a postoperative database by clinicians on postoperative rounds, or by other staff members who call or email discharged patients. Depending on local laws and regulations, this database can be kept separate from the central patient data repository to maintain nondiscoverable protection of the peer-review process from possible subsequent litigation. Follow-up often begins with generation of a standardized electronic report of QA events to QA leaders. Events can then be reviewed in a peer-review process, with the results and recommendations codified and entered into the database for summary tabulation and reporting. In this way, data are available to provide feedback to clinicians about the group's performance on these indicators. Deviations from standards are then identified, and when necessary, changes to policy and procedures can be enacted by the clinical administration. It also becomes relatively straightforward to track the results of the corrective measures by continuing to measure the incidence of the deviations.

Secondarily, efficiency from the patient's and practitioner's perspective can be a measure of quality. Perioperative systems are complex, and what appear to be unavoidable delays may be regularly recurring and avoidable with changes to process, thereby precluding "reinventing the wheel" every time. For example, instrument-related delays are frequently cited as causes of delay either before or during a surgical procedure. By analyzing the frequency of the delays and the types of instruments or equipment involved in the delays, it may be possible to redesign the process to provide a faster turnaround of key instruments or to recommend the purchase of additional sets of instruments or certain individual instruments required to complete a set. However, as with other improvements, this one begins with careful capture and analysis of data. As seen with other systems, transforming from a paper-based delay-analysis system to a computerized delay-tracking system offers several key advantages. Compared to a computerized record, paper record-keeping systems are labor intensive on an ongoing basis. Additionally, paper QA reports are more likely to be lost and less likely to be completed by clinicians. Computerized record-keeping systems can gather data automatically or prompt users for entry of the reasons for delay when delay is noted. Additionally, the delay-related fields can be made mandatory so that users are required to enter sources of delay. Lastly, multiple system users (i.e., nursing, surgery, anesthesiology, or technical staff) can be polled for reasons for a given delay, providing management with multiple perspectives from which to analyze data and create improvement programs.

Patient satisfaction is perhaps the paramount goal of all QA processes, as a satisfied patient is likely to return for further care. Satisfied patients also serve as a source of referral for friends and family members and are less likely to seek legal action when an unanticipated event occurs. Similar to other quality-tracking processes, tracking patient satisfaction is improved in an electronic environment. From the time the patient enters the system—at the preoperative visit, for example—it is possible to track waiting times, times receiving care, and patient satisfaction via electronic means and surveys. Satisfaction data can be obtained from the patient by a care team member during a postoperative hospital visit or postdischarge telephone call and subsequently entered into the perioperative database.

Novel Approaches to Patient Safety

Current practice in a typical OR suite is for each OR to be equipped with a dry-erase board, the purpose of which is to convey relevant case information to multidisciplinary staff members who are present in the OR at various times during the procedure. Fields such as patient name, procedure, surgical side and position, allergies, and blood availability are often selected for presentation in this format. Typically, this information is handwritten by a staff member (e.g., a circulating nurse) between OR cases. However, such manual processes are frequently completed inaccurately due to transcription errors, lack of availability of a complete data set, lack of enough time, or someone forgetting to complete the task. Thus, incomplete or inaccurate data may serve as a risk to patients and defeat the purpose of the dry-erase board.

An AIMS can improve this process while simultaneously reducing the workload of the staff in the OR. Patient case data are already present in the information system and thus can be presented to the OR staff in the format of an electronic display such as an LCD screen (Fig. 16.2).[17] Due to the rapidly decreasing acquisition cost of large flat-panel displays, it is increasingly more cost effective to implement this solution as an add-on feature to an existing AIMS. Information presented on this board then becomes a focal point for crew-management initiatives such as the surgical timeout.[18] All OR staff can simultaneously view the same information at the same source and confirm its accuracy. Additionally, beyond the typical fields present on a handwritten board, the electronic board can be significantly more feature rich. It can display context-sensitive information, depending on the stage of the procedure. Staff names can be displayed (a crew-management feature) as staff log into and out of documentation, enabling improved communication in the OR by encouraging staff members to address each other by name. Patient-specific data such as medical-history synopses, medication lists, lab data, and vital signs can also be displayed to encourage situational awareness among OR staff members. When displayed on a large computer display such as an LCD panel, this information serves as a focal point during presurgical timeout procedures and as a general reference for the remainder of the procedure.

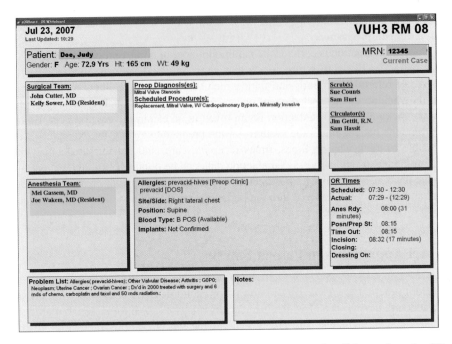

Fig. 16.2 A data display that shows surgery-related patient, case, and staff data to the entire OR team. When displayed on a large computer display such as an LCD panel, this information serves as a focal point during presurgical timeout procedures and as a general reference for the remainder of the procedure (screen shot courtesy of Acuitec, LLC, Birmingham AL)

Mobile Handheld Computers

Once implemented, electronic data systems produce a prodigious amount of data. While most of these data are held for offline review, they can also be immediately utilized. As with offline data analysis, the goals are to increase patient safety and surgical suite efficiency. Unlike offline analysis, during the normal course of care and in the background, computer systems can intelligently analyze data and send alerts to clinicians. Additionally, alerts can be sent to groups of clinicians or escalated from one clinician to another, depending upon the length and severity of the alert indicator. Alerts can be multifaceted and intelligent, based on logic involving physiologic (such as vital-sign data), process (such as patient location transfer), or other data. Integrated with these alerts is additional information based on case progress, historical context, or future prediction of state. By delivering these alerts to the clinician in real time, the electronic data system becomes both a method for recording and analyzing care that has been delivered and a system by which current and future care is guided and enhanced, maximizing efficiency and safety. Preliminary studies have shown that an intelligent alerting engine has the capability of providing a decreased percentage of false alarms, compared to a traditional limit-based monitor alarm system. Additionally, the creation of novel alarms and delivering them remotely to a clinician not present in the OR may increase the amount of new knowledge delivered to the distant clinician in terms of physiologic- or process-based changes.

With the advent of new hardware technology, this information/alert-delivery system can be extended to a portable computer. A pocket-sized, fully functional PC running the full version of an operating system puts an AIMS into the hands of a physician in an OR suite. Receiving the ASA first-place award for a scientific and education exhibit, the Vigilance System developed at Vanderbilt University Medical Center allows the clinician access to the full medical record, charting applications, and custom software applications that can access real-time waveforms from bedside monitors, live video from integrated camera systems, and process- and care-related information (Fig. 16.3). A handheld computer can provide a mobile clinician with a constant window to multiple sources of patient data, including bedside-monitor waveform displays, charting abstracts, live video feeds, and data from perioperative and central EMR repositories. This computerized physician's assistant also provides simultaneous views of several patients and increases situational awareness through the provision of data that are otherwise not known or not delivered in a timely fashion. Such technologies may lead to increased productivity while maintaining or improving safety and efficiency.

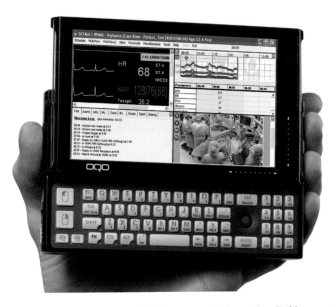

Fig. 16.3 Mobile data delivery on a handheld computer device. A handheld computer can provide a mobile clinician with a constant window to multiple sources of patient data, including bedside-monitor waveform displays, charting abstracts, live video feeds, and data from perioperative and central EMR repositories (photo courtesy of Acuitec, LLC, Birmingham AL)

Conclusion

Perioperative information management systems provide numerous mechanisms that facilitate process improvement in the OR. Data collection and analysis capabilities are paramount to designing systems that are able to rapidly respond to changes in the OR environment. Safety and efficiency initiatives, such as compliance with the Secure Communications Interoperability Protocol (SCIP, which is the US government's standard for secure voice and data communication) and analysis of block-time allocation, are enhanced by rapid and easy access to data. Likewise, access to EMR information can make the day of surgery both safer (by providing the right information to the right clinician at the right time) and more efficient (by decreasing delays and cancellations due to missing medical records). Beyond traditional electronic databases or medical records, information technologies hold several new areas for development. Technologies such as RFID can be integrated to provide distributed knowledge of location information for patients, clinicians, or equipment. Handheld computer technology holds the promise of increasing the situation awareness of clinicians in the OR suite through the integration and presentation of data from several sources to a single application screen delivered to a pocket-sized computer. The advantages of the information-enabled OR suite extend beyond the day of surgery. Quality-improvement programs, pay-for-performance programs, and financial efficiency all benefit from informatics systems. It is imperative that the paper-based systems of the past be treated as the dinosaurs they are. The advent of perioperative information systems provides a revolutionary opportunity in surgical care.

Key Points

- Process improvement requires significant data collection and analysis to be effective. Ideally, process improvement will enhance efficiency and patient and provider satisfaction, as well as facilitate improved patient safety and care.
- Data collection and analysis empower process-improvement initiatives.
- Access to electronic medical information improves efficiency and safety on the day of surgery.
- New technologies such as RFID and barcoding will advance existing information systems.
- Multisource data integration and delivery to clinicians using handheld computers will improve situational awareness in the OR suite.

References

1. Benson M, Junger A, Michel A, et al. Comparison of manual and automated documentation of adverse events with an anesthesia information management system (AIMS). Stud Health Technol Inform 2000; 77:925–9
2. Committee on Quality of Health Care in America, Institute of Medicine. Kohn LT, Donaldson MS, eds. *To Err Is Human: Building a Safer Health System.* Washington, DC: The National Academies, 2000
3. Committee on Quality of Health Care in America, Institute of Medicine. *Crossing the Quality Chasm: A New Health System for the 21st Century.* Washington, DC: The National Academies, 2001
4. Brailer DJ. Health information technology is a vehicle, not a destination: A conversation with David J. Brailer. Interview by Arnold Milstein. Health Affairs (Project Hope) 2007; 26:w236–41
5. Lee J. The anaesthetic outpatient clinic. Anaesthesia 1949; 4:169–74
6. St. Jacques PJ, Higgins MS. Beyond cancellations: Decreased day of surgery delays from a dedicated preoperative clinic may provide cost savings. J Clin Anesth 2004; 16:478–9
7. Pollard JB, Zboray AL, Mazze RI. Economic benefits attributed to opening a preoperative evaluation clinic for outpatients. Anesth Analg 1996; 83:407–10
8. Brown DL, Warner ME, Schroeder DR, et al. Effect of intraoperative anesthetic events on postoperative patient satisfaction. Mayo Clin Proc 1997; 72:20–5
9. Hepner DL, Bader AM, Hurwitz S, et al. Patient satisfaction with preoperative assessment in a preoperative assessment testing clinic. Anesth Analg 2004; 98:1099–105
10. Ferschl MB, Tung A, Sweitzer B, et al. Preoperative clinic visits reduce operating room cancellations and delays. Anesthesiology 2005; 103:855–9
11. Sandberg WS, Hakkinen M, Egan M, et al. Automatic detection and notification of "wrong patient-wrong location" errors in the operating room. Surg Innov 2005; 12:253–60
12. Meyer M, Chueh H, Egan M, et al. Using location tracking data to assess efficiency in established clinical workflows. AMIA Annu Symp Proc 2006:1031
13. Mazzei WJ. Operating room start times and turnover times in a university hospital. J Clin Anesth 1994; 6:405–8
14. Dexter F, Coffin S, Tinker JH. Decreases in anesthesia-controlled time cannot permit one additional surgical operation to be reliably scheduled during the workday. Anesth Analg 1995; 81:1263–8
15. Overdyk FJ, Harvey SC, Fishman RL, et al. Successful strategies for improving operating room efficiency at academic institutions. Anesth Analg 1998; 86:896–906
16. Vigoda MM, Lubarsky DA. Failure to recognize loss of incoming data in an anesthesia record-keeping system may have increased medical liability. Anesth Analg 2006; 102:1798–802
17. Meyer M, Levine WC, Brzezinski P, et al. Integration of hospital information systems, operative and perioperative information systems, and operative equipment into a single information display. AMIA Annu Symp Proc 2005:1054
18. Levine WC, Meyer M, Brzezinski P, et al. Usability factors in the organization and display of disparate information sources in the operative environment. AMIA Annu Symp Proc 2005:1025

Part B
Operating Room Management System

ORMS Case Scenario

Community Hospital decided to facilitate collection of quality data and improve access to patient information by installing an EMR system. A secondary goal was to decrease calls to the lab for results. The original interest in electronic records began with physicians from the ED. An electronic record was perceived to improve access to labs and historic patient data to enhance throughput of patient admission. The most significant problem to be alleviated was the incomplete information in the charts that arrived from the ED to other areas in the hospital. Administration opted to install a stand-alone product in the ED that included Web access as the first step. The physicians in the group were actively involved in vendor selection and development of the graphical user interface. Vendor-standard printed reports were available as well as customized reports requested by the ED staff. Physicians outside of the ED group were not involved in the process but were assured that they would be able to access the information.

Once the system was installed, the anesthesiologists immediately noticed problems. At first, patients were arriving in the OR without any records other than the surgical consent and demographic information. Because there was no handoff between members of the nursing staff, OR nurses had little information regarding the patients. The ED staff told the OR staff to "look it up on the computer," but they did not realize that the OR suite had only two computers, neither of which was in an actual OR. To resolve this concern, the chart information was subsequently printed upon patient transfer to the OR (but not to the floors). This printout consisted of a dozen pages of information, with data sorted alphabetically by type of note. One patient arrived with her first "Assessment" note commenting on the "good response to Narcan," but the actual doses of naloxone and narcotic given were recorded eight pages later, under "Procedure." Although the event had occurred 30 min earlier—which explained why the patient was somnolent, hypoxic, and acidotic on arrival to the OR—no documentation was readily apparent as to why the patient had even received narcotics.

When the implementation team was first queried about the order of the notes, the physicians were told that "it couldn't be changed" by the vendor (although less than a month later the order was changed to the more appropriate time-sorted flow of information).

The endless notes of nonessential clinical information, indicating that the patient bed was at the lowest height, the siderails were up, and the call-light was within reach, buried relative patient information. Other physicians asked to be able to access the system and were given read-only privileges via a separate Web-access program. Consistent access to this Web application was problematic, and physicians frequently complained that they did not know how to find the information they needed.

This program also reportedly had the ability to link into the PACS and a subsequently installed clinical system in Labor & Delivery (L&D). However, many were unable to use this function because of incompatibilities between the operating system of the L&D application and the browser portion of the ED system (a potentiality that had never been considered by the implementation team). Therefore, calls to the ED and lab for information did not significantly decrease.

The L&D system, from a different vendor, was deployed approximately 1 year after the ED system. It had functionality that was particularly useful for the patient population. The implementation team for this project included obstetricians, neonatologists, and anesthesiologists. However, this system remained incompatible with the ED system. Because it was also unable to interface with the lab system (which had been in use for over 10 years), labs still had to be looked up separately. Custom forms were generated in an attempt to match the layout of the paper forms, but the one-page "Anesthesia H&P" was now six pages, and the "Nursing Assessment," previously two pages, was now six pages. Moreover, data pass-through failed for three major items—medications, allergies, and labs. Physicians reading the chart (either electronically or on paper) still could not find important information, such as height, weight, and vital signs. Because of the pass-through failure, one anesthesiologist was unable to find the patient's medication list and was not aware that the patient was taking warfarin for her prosthetic valve until after he had placed an epidural. Fortunately, the vendor of the L&D system was very responsive to the needs of the hospital and, within 1 month, fixed the pass-through for medications and allergies (although the lab pass-through took longer, requiring a custom interface that could not be quantified in terms of delivery date), and the paper printouts were revised to be closer to the original forms. Within 6 months of implementation, all of the physicians and nursing staff were pleased and hated having to go back to paper in the rare instances of downtime.

The Chief Medical Officer (CMO), a surgeon, was extremely enthusiastic about implementing an "anesthesia record system," claiming that it would make the lives of the anesthesiologists much easier. But what he really wanted was an Operating Room Management System (ORMS), intended to improve patient tracking and charge capture. The infrastructure necessary to make such a system viable was lacking, and it was unclear if the management team truly realized the type and amount of hardware that would first have to be installed. The anesthesiologists spent a fair amount of time educating the CMO about the differences between AIMS and ORMS. Compatibility with the existing systems was emphasized. A system was chosen by the administration, but prior to implementation, the Director of Nursing, who had been the primary champion for the process, left the facility and no one was assigned to assume his role in the implementation process. The ORMS was not compatible with the other hospital clinical systems. None of the staff or physicians liked the new system, and they felt that it was forced upon them by the administration. Without a champion, many of the features were not used and most of the expected advantages were lost.

Realizing that huge expenditures had been made without adequate return on investment or improvement in patient safety, the hospital board put a moratorium on all future purchases of information technology until all of the various implementation problems had been resolved. Unfortunately, shortly after the administration enacted the moratorium, Community Hospital experienced an unannounced Joint Commission visit and failed accreditation based on several facets of the National Patient Safety Goals, including appropriate documentation of handoff between providers, medication reconciliation, and appropriate recognition of adverse events.

Chapter 17
Components of an ORMS

Marisa L. Wilson

What Is an ORMS?

An OR management system (ORMS) comprises a suite of integrated software modules within an application that contains the functional and technical capability to schedule cases (and reschedule them as necessary), organize and bill the materials and supplies used, plan the clinical staff required, and document clinical data at the point of care in all the perioperative areas. These functions are essential, as ORs are especially cost intensive, and effective use and management of the resources such as rooms, time, and staff, requires valid and accessible data in real time.[1] The relationships between the functional modules in a basic ORMS are depicted in Fig. 17.1. Although some ORMS application suites also contain an AIMS (as depicted in Fig. 17.1), the key functionality of only the ORMS segment will be described in this chapter. Importantly, this chapter will present a generalized description of functionality that is currently present in most of the vendor-produced ORMS products. The ORMS functionality descriptions in this chapter are not representative of the functionality of any specific vendor-based system but are based on generalized capabilities of all systems currently available on the market.

Each vendor-based system uses multiple methods to capture data. All of the ORMS products utilize standard, keyboard-driven, manual data entry for the screens. Most of them will capture data from physiologic monitors and incorporate that data into the clinical modules. Some of them utilize barcode technology (particularly for the materials-management and billing functions), and some utilize radio-frequency identification (RFID) transponders, or tags, along with RFID readers as methods for data entry (particularly for staff, patient tracking, and equipment). The input technologies that are ultimately used when interacting with the ORMS will depend upon what is available for use within the selected product offering and what can be supported by the healthcare enterprise infrastructure.

J. Stonemetz, K. Ruskin (eds.) *Anesthesia Informatics*,
© Springer Science+Business Media, LLC 2008

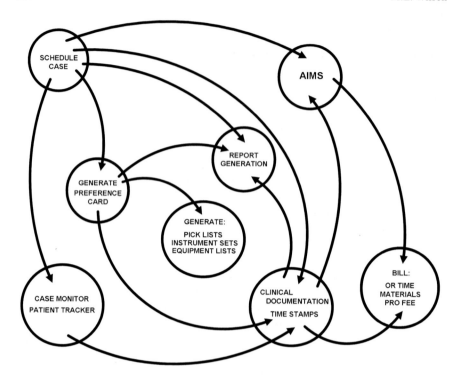

Fig. 17.1 Functional modules of an ORMS

The ORMS Functionality

Scheduling the Case

Scheduling the Surgeon, Case, Room, and Supplies

At the time it is decided that a patient needs to be scheduled for a surgical procedure (elective, emergent, or urgent), data are collected and entered to place the case onto the OR schedule. Usually, to schedule a case, the name of the surgeon, the name of the patient, the procedure(s) to be performed, the date, the time, the location, and the number of minutes required to complete the case are necessary. The minimum requirements will vary depending on how the institution chooses to establish the parameters of the ORMS. Some ORMS applications allow the calculation of an "average time" required for surgeons to complete specific procedures, based on historic data and various averaging calculations. Some ORMS applications will only allow the scheduling of cases into slots that contain a number of minutes that are equal to or greater than those required, on average, for a surgeon to complete a particular procedure based on the historic calculated average time. This averaging function is important, as it assists management to schedule cases into OR time slots to maximize efficiency. When cases go longer or shorter than scheduled on a consistent basis, nursing and anesthesiology departments incur excess labor costs because these departments must provide personnel either for more rooms or for longer intervals to complete all of the scheduled cases for that day.[2,3]

In addition to the data elements discussed, end users can enter a patient history number along with the name, which may bring forward patient-specific demographics, identifiers, and health data from a master patient index system. End users may also schedule the surgeon and the necessary clinical staff for the case. The types of scheduled clinical staff may include additional surgeons, surgical residents, assistants, circulating and scrub nurses, and additional monitoring personnel or technicians. The name of the anesthesiologist and the preferred method of anesthesia (from a surgical perspective) may also be placed into the scheduling module for a particular case during this process. Or, the ORMS may include a method by which an anesthesiologist and/or CRNA can be assigned to an OR for an entire day or part of a day and therefore be allocated to cases based on the room in which they are scheduled.

In some ORMS applications, the end user scheduling the case may be able to enter patient medical information that has direct relevance to anesthesiology, such as history of malignant hyperthermia, difficult airway, or allergies. Alternatively, upon correct identification of the patient, this medical information may be brought forward through the mechanism of an interface to the admitting system, a clinical data repository, an EMR, or whatever system may be considered a "source of truth."

Surgical equipment, surgical sets, instruments, and supplies needed for a case generally are accounted for by using an automatic process (described below) that occurs via the "pulling" of a preference card from the database when the case is being scheduled into a particular location. Specialty equipment, sets, instruments, implants, and supplies that are not part of the routine required items for the case being scheduled can also be added. In addition, it is possible to include equipment and supplies (including medications) needed by anesthesia through the same preference card mechanism (see below) or through the creation of various anesthesia equipment sets that may be added to a case.

Scheduling and the Block Model

Users of the ORMS who have the ability to schedule a case are generally limited to certain OR areas, if the facility has more than one. Users may also be limited to scheduling elective cases into certain ORs and on particular days and times for specific surgeons. These limitations can be set through the mechanism of the surgical block model. The block model allows facilities to designate ORs for priority use by individual surgeons, surgical groups, entire surgical departments, or specified procedures on specific days and at specific times, freeing the rooms for use by others at only designated times just before the day of surgery. The block model is designed to maximize efficiency, minimize staffing issues, and ensure profitable operations of the surgical suite. The ORMS block model functionality and database should assist managers in this process by supplying the historic data that will allow allocation of time based on maximum efficiency and thus avoid overutilization and/or underutilization of rooms.[4] ORMS applications must allow for input of the specific block models as designed by the surgical department for the various configurations (surgeon, surgical group, department, procedure, etc.). The ORMS must also allow the blocks to be edited, closed, and opened with ease, as well as released at various times, depending upon specialty or surgeon. The ORMS must be able to maintain a record of these changes to the schedule and the block model so that patterns can be discerned.

The ability to accommodate a fluid block model is vital, as salaries of the OR staff, specifically anesthesiology and nursing, account for most of the OR costs.[5] To have a significant impact on costs of patient care in the surgical suite, OR managers attempt to maximize labor productivity and decrease inefficiency by employing the fewest full-time nurses and anesthesiologists necessary to care for patients in fully utilized ORs. In this setting, the day on which to perform each elective case must be selected optimally to match the days on which full-time, trained OR personnel are scheduled to work.[6] This optimization is best accomplished through a customized block model.

The ORMS must have user profile variations that will allow some individuals to schedule cases anytime, anywhere, and in any location. These users may be scheduling urgent or emergent cases, or they may be responsible for coordinating the OR either the day before or the day of the case to optimize the room and space available. Scheduling and rescheduling of cases represent 78% of the communications that OR charge nurses have with surgeons just prior to case start.[7] The ORMS should allow these OR charge nurses and others (such as anesthesiology coordinators) to update the schedule with relative ease; it should also allow the ordering of equipment, supplies, and personnel, thereby reducing the risk of not having the necessary supplies on hand at the time of surgery. Other users should have a profile that only allows them access to the OR schedule for certain time periods, for example, no later than 72 hours in advance of the case time.

Scheduling Anesthesia

As stated, schedulers of OR cases are able to enter the name of a specific anesthesiologist on individual cases. Moreover, anesthesia managers should be able to schedule anesthesiologists and CRNAs to rooms for an entire day or part of a day. This action will incorporate the assigned anesthesia staff into the data for each case that occurs in that room for the day. Utilizing the capabilities of the ORMS to schedule anesthesia staff in addition to surgical staff will allow for, at a minimum, the generation of data to develop schedules for individual practitioners. Moreover, these data could then be interfaced to the AIMS, thereby maintaining synchronized schedules. Applying the names of scheduled anesthesia staff to cases or rooms and comparing that information to the names actually documented on the case in the clinical documentation function under the staff and their roles will also allow for an analysis of planned-versus-actual events. In addition to scheduling anesthesia personnel, users may enter data specifically relevant to anesthesia, such as type of preferred anesthesia, allergies, patient positioning, and significant health history and assessment information.

Scheduling an Intensive Care Bed

Some ORMS products have scheduling functions that allow for the designation of "Needs an ICU Bed" to specific procedures. With this capability, the bed requirement is automatically attached to the case each time the procedure is scheduled. In other ORMS products, this process is more complex, in that the need for an ICU bed is not tied to specific procedures but can be added as a request and sent as part of the admissions process so that an ICU bed will be "reserved." In this scenario, the request is then balanced against the current and estimated census figures for the date in question and the request is approved or disapproved for that date. With another method, ICU beds can be treated as equipment and a cap can be placed on the number that may be scheduled on any given day. When a request for an ICU bed is added to the case, as long as the cap on ICU beds has not been exceeded, the case can be scheduled for that date. If the cap on ICU beds has been reached, the case cannot be scheduled without permission and override from management. Generally, the ICU bed-reservation functionality of most ORMS products is rudimentary and only permits the sending of a request or the generation of a report of ICU bed requirements. Many facilities with high-surgical-acuity procedures may require a much more robust system than those available in current ORMS products to assist with the allocation of critical care bed resources.

Materials Management and Billing

Doctor Preference Cards

When a case is scheduled, data about the surgeon performing a procedure in a certain location are entered into the scheduling function of the ORMS. This process drives the selection of all equipment, surgical sets, supplies, instruments, and specifics related to procedures. Usually called the *doctor preference card* (DPC), the name of the function is a vestige from a time when the necessary items were actually listed on cards and kept in card boxes, which were pulled prior to the start of the case. In the ORMS of today, this "pulling of the DPC" occurs automatically. Fundamentally, each DPC lists all of the usual supplies, equipment, bed types, instrument sets, items, and patient specifics necessary to complete a case, along with the quantity of each typically used by the surgeon in a specific location or OR suite. As the DPC process is often onerous to manage, some ORMS applications allow for the creation of best-practice cards that are based on procedures, and not surgeons. With a best-practice card, multiple surgeons share the same card if they are performing the same procedure. Some ORMS applications allow for the creation of cards that contain the items needed for procedures that are not only the same, but are similar to each other. Each variation on this process is an attempt to control the number and variety of cards, which has a direct impact on the ultimate number of items that an enterprise must procure and manage and the sheer number of cards that must be kept accurate and current. Close management of DPC allows for standardization of inventory and has significant financial implications on inventory management.

Regardless of how the cards are created, each item listed on each card is processed during the shift before the case is scheduled to occur. Lists of equipment necessary for specific cases are sent to respective managers so that each item can be prepared and brought to the OR for use. Instrument requests are forwarded to the sterile processing areas to ensure that all will be ready for the day of surgery. Some ORMS applications contain instrument-tracking capabilities that are used to monitor instruments through the institution's sterile processing areas. All of the other items and supplies are processed onto pick lists or pick tickets that are then used by the surgical materials-management staff to stock the case carts from the storage shelves.

The materials-management processing functions of the ORMS usually work in conjunction with, and are interfaced to, the enterprise materials-management system so that item names, numbers, manufacturers, and stock levels are aligned, thus permitting a continuous loop of information to flow between both systems that informs users of new items, replacement items, and the need to send requisitions to manufacturers. The ORMS may also contain a native function that manages equipment, or it may interface with an equipment-management application. The equipment-management function allows the tracking of locations of each piece, as well as the manufacturer information. It may also include information on servicing schedules and may notify users or the biomedical engineering department when specific pieces are out for repair and when they are returned to the OR. Within the ORMS DPC and materials-management functions, cards can be built that contain the anesthesia supplies and medications necessary for procedures. Conversely, sets of supplies, equipment, and medications may also be built for the various types and recipients of anesthesia, which can then be added to the case and billed based on quantities used.

Surgical Billing

The materials-management function of the ORMS also serves to permit the billing of selected items. During the course of a procedure, the circulating nurse is responsible for documenting the quantity of items used against the quantity noted on the DPC. If the item is billable to the patient, the quantities are then sent to the enterprise billing system. All quantities used are sent to the larger enterprise materials-management systems to decrease quantities available and to trigger a reorder process. The quantities used during the case are also utilized within the ORMS application to monitor quantities on hand in local storage areas. The documentation of the supplies used within ORMS may be a totally manual process, with the circulating nurse manually changing each quantity listed by default on the DPC. Or, as an alternative mode of data entry, this process may be more automated and efficient with the use of barcode technology.

Professional-Fee Billing

Contained within the data elements to be documented in the clinical documentation function of ORMS is an accounting for each clinician who has a role in the case, the actual role performed, and the time on and the time off of the case while performing that role. Collecting these data in ORMS permits professional-fee billing (Profee) when required, as the roles and the time spent in those roles can be sent to the relevant department for processing. In addition, the times and the roles are attached to the case, which decreases missed opportunities for revenue generation. More generally, the collection of personnel names, roles, and time information will allow the generation of information related to the experience level of staff, which is very important in academic medical centers, where interns and residents keep logs of cases performed. Nursing staffs also utilize this information to determine the end of orientation periods or for certification purposes.

Clinical Documentation at the Point of Care

All ORMS applications contain mechanisms for documenting at the point of care. Most ORMS applications divide the perioperative process into phases of care: preoperative, intraoperative, and postoperative. The clinical documentation within the ORMS is generally nursing documentation. However, some ORMS applications contain a function that "grabs" particular data elements from among those documented and places them on a draft operative note that can be edited and signed by the surgeon. As stated previously, many ORMS applications also contain an AIMS. The AIMS functionality would then contain the clinical documentation elements relevant to anesthesiology staff.

The Preoperative or Preanesthesia Visit

Most ORMS applications contain functionality that allows for the documentation of the preoperative surgical and anesthesia H&Ps. Patient allergies can be verified. Laboratory and radiology results can be directly entered or interfaced from native hospital information systems. Current patient assessment data, including vital signs and current weight and respiratory, cardiovascular, and neurologic assessments, can be entered. Important details about the patient can be recorded for all care providers to view, such as mobility deficits, interpreters required, and current pain issues. History of malignant hyperthermia, difficult airway, and presence of pseudocholinesterase deficiency can be documented. Patient instruction and surgical preparation can be documented, as well as surgical procedures (as understood by the patient) and validation of surgical site.

The Preoperative Phase of Care

The preoperative/preanesthesia visit phase of care can be documented in the ORMS or AIMS, and which is chosen will depend on the product(s) that are selected and in use and on the amount of integration between the products; however, data are usually documented in the ORMS. At this point, the patient is imminently awaiting movement into the OR. If the data from the preoperative visit are placed into the ORMS, this information is available to the nursing and anesthesia staffs. During this phase, current patient physiologic assessment data are entered, which include vital signs, respiratory assessment, and pain and comfort levels. NPO status, medications taken (or held), allergies, postoperative plans, and surgical procedure and site are verified and documented. Point-of-care testing results are entered, such as blood glucose levels and pregnancy test results. IV access, fluids, and medications are documented once started or administered.

The Intraoperative Phase of Care

During the intraoperative phase of care, multiple data elements reflecting the procedure and patient condition are documented, typically by the circulating nurse. A list of the minimal data elements that are entered within the ORMS intraoperative documentation function can be found in Table 17.1.

Table 17.1 Minimal data elements entered in an ORMS intraoperative documentation function

Patient physical assessment
Patient position and positioning aids
Fluids in and out
Medications administered
Implant information (as required by the Food and Drug Administration)
Laser utilization, settings, on and off
Equipment used (including specific bed types)
Staff names, titles, and roles, along with times in and times out for each
Actual procedure(s) completed
Time stamps (set up and clean up, room start/stop, surgery start/stop, anesthesia start/stop, team time out, surgical incision time, etc.)
Tourniquets on and off, along with strength and location of tourniquets
Location of drains, tubes, and catheters, along with drainage

The Postoperative Phase of Care

Most ORMS applications continue the point-of-care documentation into the postoperative area using the same format as in the other phases of care. Documentation at this phase can be problematic because, often, sets of vital signs must be documented at very frequent intervals over specified periods of time. If the ORMS application can accept data from physiologic monitors, then this process becomes more efficient and accurate, as opposed to requiring the nursing staff to manually enter each value. However, the postoperative nursing staff should have the ability to designate the frequency of collection and to document conditions surrounding aberrations. In addition to the series of vital signs, the postoperative staff will document pain and comfort assessment, levels of consciousness, respiratory status, Aldrete scores, wound assessment, drains and tubes, and bowel and bladder functioning.

Case Monitors

Most ORMS applications come with some type of case monitoring functionality. Case monitors allow clinical staff within and outside of the OR to see the progress of the cases, usually projected on large, flat-panel screens. Data projected onto the case monitors come from the Scheduling and Clinical Documentation functions of the ORMS. Patient name or case number (to protect privacy), surgeon, and procedure are some of the data elements that can be projected onto the screens. The information projected can vary by location. The cases on the monitor can change color and pattern to indicate their phase and status based on the time stamps that are being documented. In other words, the case monitor provides a real-time reflection of what is happening during certain phases of care. Case monitors provide staff with the ability to plan care and to know what is happening around them in real time.

A more advanced type of case monitor is the Patient Tracker or the Day Manager. This type of monitor is interactive and is not merely a passive recipient of data from the Scheduling and Clinical Documentation functions. Cases can actually be moved from room to room on the monitor, thus allowing the Scheduling function to be a picture of the planned day and the Patient Tracker to be an image of what actually occurred. This information is vital to the study of efficiency and effectiveness in OR suites. These advanced monitors also usually contain a series of icons that can be activated during the case to signal that staff or supplies are needed. For example, if environmental services staff is needed, an icon can appear on the screen in the case area to signal the need. If an emergent case or trauma is arriving, a special icon can appear on the screen to signal that the staff should prepare to receive this patient.

Tracking the information provided automatically increases communications while decreasing interruptions, potential errors, and adverse events for the charge nurse and others who are coordinating the OR area on the day of surgery.[8] Therefore, the rigor, responsiveness, and facileness of the Case Monitor or Patient Tracker that comes with the ORMS must be seriously considered prior to selection. However, the Case Monitor or Patient Tracker must integrate and interface with the ORMS Scheduling and Clinical Documentation modules so that the power can be fully realized and another manual entry task is not created.

Report-Generation Capability

Most ORMS applications come with a supply of prebuilt reports that allow statistical, administrative, operational, and financial data to reveal knowledge to support safe and efficient care in the perioperative arena. A partial list of reports that may be available in an ORMS is provided in Table 17.2. Most surgical departments will require adjustments to the standard reports or will require reports not included in the set. Therefore, the ORMS database, which usually is created with a series of interrelated tables that are often in a complex arrangement of one to many, or many to many, and are joined by keys, will have to be "mined" by a report writer who fully understands the database structure and relationships. Most ORMS applications allow for the creation of custom reports using a standard report-writer application via Open Database Connectivity, which provides a way for client programs (e.g., report writers) to access a wide range of databases, including the ORMS database.

Table 17.2 Reports that may be available in an ORMS

OR schedules
Personnel schedules
Block utilization (one of the most difficult to create)
Equipment availability and utilization
Equipment out for repair
Procedures by surgeon
Procedures by location
Doctor preference cards and pick lists
Clinical documentation
Cost per procedure per surgeon

Conclusion

An ORMS is a large and complex application that allows end users to schedule OR procedures for specific surgeons in certain locations, on particular days, and for specified lengths of time. It also permits the requesting of materials, supplies, equipment, and other items necessary for the case, based on information related to the surgeon, location, and procedure. An ORMS will allow scheduling of anesthesia staff by case or by room and will permit the documentation of basic information with direct relevance to the safety of the anesthesia experience.

An ORMS also contains point-of-care clinical documentation to be completed by perioperative and perianesthesia nursing staff during all of the phases of care. These data include minimally: allergies, physiologic assessments, medications administered, fluids in and out, equipment, patient positioning, staff assigned to the case and staff roles, lasers and tourniquets used, wounds, drains, invasive lines, and catheters. These data should move forward through the phases of care to reduce the duplication of documentation and reduce risk to the patients in the process. Some ORMS applications will allow the creation of a draft operative note for the surgeon by pulling forward key data elements that are contained within the application and have been documented by other clinical staff at the point of care.

An ORMS allows all of the materials used during the operative process to be documented in the clinical functions module, which permits billing of supplies and the accumulation of usage data for equipment. An ORMS also contains a mechanism to track implants so that recall can occur if necessary. It should also come with a Case Monitor or Patient Tracker that integrates with the Scheduling and Clinical Documentation modules. This graphic depiction of the day of surgery assists managers and coordinators to provide a safe, efficient, and cost-effective experience for patients and staff.

An ORMS should contain a report-writing mechanism. The safe and efficient operation of the OR depends upon the ability to mine all of the data that are being gathered across the perioperative and perianesthesia experience in real or near-real time. ORMS may be configured with a suite of reports that can be altered somewhat (e.g., date ranges, locations, specific surgeons) or may provide the ability for an enterprise to develop its own custom reports based on need. Lastly, the ORMS must be tightly integrated with the AIMS. It may be preferential for both of the systems to be within the same application and same database platform. Integration, interface, and sharing of data between clinicians are paramount to safe and efficient care. Each collected data element must be assessed to reduce actual and potential redundancy in collection.

Key Points

- Most ORMS applications contain scheduling, clinical documentation, doctor preference cards, materials management, billing, and reporting functionality.
- The clinical documentation of the ORMS consists of point-of-care data from the preoperative, intraoperative, and postoperative phases.
- To ensure safety and efficiency, certain data elements must be shared and transferred from one phase of care to another.
- ORMS may contain an integrated AIMS, but many do not.

References

1. Junger A, Benson M, Quinzio L, et al. An anesthesia information management system (AIMS) as a tool for controlling resource management of operating rooms. Methods Inf Med 2002; 41:81–5
2. Abouleish A, Dexter F, Epstein RH, et al. Labor costs incurred by anesthesiology groups because of operating rooms not being allocated and cases not being scheduled to maximize operating room efficiency. Anesth Analg 2003; 96:1109–13
3. Abouleish A, Dexter F, Whitten CW, et al. Quantifying net staffing costs due to longer-than-average surgical case durations. Anesthesiology 2004; 100:403–12
4. Dexter F, Macario A. When to release allocated operating room time to increase operating room efficiency. Anesth Analg 2004; 98:758–62
5. Macario A, Vitez TS, Dunn B, et al. Where are the costs in perioperative care? Analysis of hospital costs and charges for inpatient surgical care. Anesthesiology 1995; 83:1138–44
6. Dexter F, Macario A, Lubarsky DA, et al. Statistical method to evaluate management strategies to decrease variability in operating room utilization: Application of linear statistical modeling and Monte Carlo simulation to operating room management. Anesthesiology 1999; 91:262–74
7. Moss J, Xiao Y, Zubaidah S. The operating room charge nurse: Coordinator and communicator. J Am Med Inform Assoc 2002; 9:S70–4
8. Moss J, Xiao Y. Improving operating room coordination: Communication pattern assessment. J Nurs Admin 2004; 34:93–100

Chapter 18
Integration of ORMS and AIMS

Marisa L. Wilson and Christine Doyle

The safe, efficient, and coordinated passage of a patient through the surgical and anesthesia experience begins long before the patient arrives at the hospital on the day of surgery. The process actually begins at the time a patient's health concern is recognized and a medical professional concurs that surgery is needed. From that moment forward, hundreds of data elements will be collected by multiple healthcare providers and placed into a variety of systems—electronic or paper, integrated or not. Within this complex matrix of information systems, some of these data will be redundant, some will be contradictory, some will overlap, some will pass from system to system, and some will reside only within a single database. Healthcare providers engaged in the process of safe care will sort through and try to collate and organize these data to generate a profile of the patient that will subsequently inform the process of care and evaluate the outcomes of multiple interventions. Ultimately, these data (which could be located in a variety of disparate systems) may be the key to creating new knowledge and evidence for practice innovation for anesthesiologists, surgeons, and nurses. The goal of this chapter is to stimulate thinking on the topic of data interchange and interoperable systems for the purposes of safe and efficient anesthesia care. Although the process is thought of as a simple linear one, the data collection is far from linear and may include data exchange in both directions as well as from multiple sites (Fig. 18.1).

Clinical Systems

The process of safe care throughout the perioperative and perianesthesia phases can be made more efficient and more advanced with the installation of interoperable, coordinated, and encompassing information systems, including the following:

1. Anesthesia Information Management System (AIMS)
2. Operating Room Management System (ORMS)
3. Pathology Information System
4. Radiology Information System (PACS, Picture Archiving and Communication System)
5. Computerized Physician Order Entry System (CPOE)
6. Electronic Medical Record (EMR)

J. Stonemetz, K. Ruskin (eds.) *Anesthesia Informatics*,
© Springer Science+Business Media, LLC 2008

DATA FLOW in PERIOPERATIVE SETTING

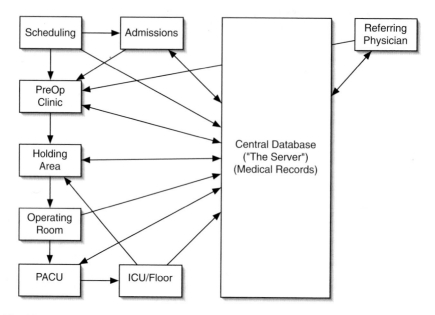

Fig. 18.1 Data exchange between ORMS and AIMS

Many healthcare enterprises have one or more of these systems in place now. The question is: Are these applications interoperable or do they exist as silos? *Coordinated* and *interoperable* are the key concepts to make this process work optimally, whether these systems are found within a uniform, enterprise-wide application or within separate "best of breed" applications.

The Institute of Medicine (IOM), in *Crossing the Quality Chasm*, recognized the need for automated clinical and administrative data to:

1. Enable health services research
2. Identify best practices
3. Permit the evaluation of the effects of various financing, organizing, and delivering methodologies[1]

The IOM promotes the use of IT systems in hospital-wide applications as a means of decreasing errors and costs. The IOM declared the implementation of IT systems to be of the highest priority. The Anesthesia Patient Safety Foundation has advocated for the implementation of automated documentation throughout the perioperative and anesthesia phases of care in order to improve safety.[2] Whether an institution is just beginning the process of acquiring an AIMS, ORMS, or EMR system, or it already has some or all the functionality of these systems in place, many issues are associated with their coordination, communication, and interoperability. Development of the appropriate requirements—and knowing what questions to ask—is critical. A framework that the reader can use to determine exact departmental needs will be provided in the sections that follow.

As with many endeavors, the better the plan, the better the final product, and the easier the transition. Although a discussion of database design and management is far beyond the scope of this chapter, some of the basic concepts are crucial to successful selection and deployment of these systems. The first and most important step is to identify and define the terms and data points in a consistent manner, which will allow relationships to be established between systems and the interchange of electronic data between them. The second step is to identify which data are actually going to be transferred between systems, along with identifying the system that will contain the source data.

Definition of Systems

For the purposes of this discussion, an AIMS is an IT system that allows for direct recording of intraoperative, anesthesia-sensitive, physiologic data, either manually or via interfaces with monitors. These anesthesia data would also include medications administered, quantities of fluids in and out, blood product administration, patient demographics, allergies, and commentary. The ORMS is a software system that allows for recording of information related to the perioperative phases of care around and within the OR environment. It allows for the collection of some of the same data as the AIMS. The specifics of the ORMS are fully described in Chap. 17. The preanesthesia or preoperative testing, preoperative preparation, and postanesthesia phases of care documentation can take place within either an AIMS or an ORMS. Healthcare providers within these phases of care gather and document data on patient demographics, allergies, vital signs, results of point-of-care testing, pain and comfort levels, levels of consciousness, relevant health history, current assessment, and other significant observations.

An EMR is a software system that accumulates information from a variety of information systems outside of the OR environment. It receives information from systems within the laboratory and radiology departments. It may receive and store summaries of the events that occurred during the perioperative and perianesthesia process. It may also be the medical record or a clinical repository. Minimally, the information sent out to the EMR takes the form of operative notes from the surgeon but could include anesthesia and nursing documentation summaries.

At this writing, the AIMS, ORMS, and EMR may be three individual systems or part of an integrated system in a variety of combinations. Data may be passed from system to system through interfaces, or various subsections of data within each system may be printed as necessary.

Data Elements

Data elements are single measurements or pieces of information that can be categorized into types: text, number, time, etc. Not every facility will need every one of these data elements for every procedure. Those that are considered crucial, along with associated follow-up or secondary items that may be important for the efficient use of the system and management of the OR, are listed in Table 18.1.

Consistency in naming and defining data elements between the systems is an important part of facilitating data exchange. Some data may be collected in more

Table 18.1 Data elements

Environment	Initial item	Follow-up or secondary item
Scheduling	Surgeon/provider	Assistant
	Case (procedure name)	Equipment requests
	Anesthesia type	Anesthesia requests
	Bed request (ICU)	
	Permanent risk issues	Allergies, isolation, difficult airway, etc.
Admitting	Demographics	
	Permanent risk issues	Allergies, isolation, difficult airway, etc.
Preop clinic	Pertinent history	
	Physical exam	
	Lab/EKG/x-ray	
	Permanent risk issues	Allergies, isolation, difficult airway, etc.
Preoperative	Consent	
	Preprocedure assessment	
	Physician's prep orders	Skin prep
		Labs (repeat K, PT, glucose)
		Breathing treatments
	Permanent risk issues	Allergies, difficult airway, isolation, etc.
Intraoperative		
Times	Room setup	Room clean up
	Room in	Room out
	Anesthesia start	Anesthesia stop
	Surgery start	Surgery stop
	Time out	
	Skin incision	
Clinical	Fluids in	Fluids out
	Medications administered	
	Transfusions	
	Positioning	
Materials	Supplies used	Number
	Implants	Number
		Location
		Manufacturer
	Equipment used	Number
		Type
		Specifics related to equipment
PACU	Vital signs	
	Aldrete score (or similar)	Respiratory status
		Level of consciousness
	Medications administered	
	Pain scale	
	Lines/tubes/drains	Placement
		Amount

than one location by multiple healthcare providers. Ideally, at each institution, a consensus should be reached regarding which system should be considered the "source of truth" for data related to "permanent risk factors" such as allergies, difficult airways, and malignant hyperthermia.

Time stamps comprise another group of important data elements. However, sometimes conflict arises as to definition, ownership, and which system should be accepted as the "source of truth." The American Association of Clinical Directors (AACD) has standardized and defined time stamps to promote the efficient use of resources, coordinate methods of data gathering, and develop standards for OR management. A partial list of selected time stamps and approved definitions is provided in Table 18.2.

Table 18.2 An abbreviated procedural times glossary

Time stamp	AACD definition
Room ready (RR)	Time when room is cleaned and supplies and equipment are ready for beginning of next case
Anesthesiologist of record in room (ARI)	Time of arrival in OR of anesthesiologist who is going to provide the service
Procedure physician (surgeon) of record in (PPRI) room	Arrival time of surgeon in the OR suite. The surgeon notifying the OR desk/manager about his entry into the hospital will expedite taking the patient to the OR.
Patient in room (PIR)/start time (ST)	Start time equals patient-in-room time
Anesthesia start (AS)	Time when anesthesiologist begins preparing the patient for an anesthetic
Anesthesia induction (AI)	Time when the anesthesiologist begins the administration of agents intended to provide a level of anesthesia required for the procedure
Anesthesia ready (AR)	Time at which the patient has sufficient level of anesthesia established to begin positioning/surgical preparation
Position/prep start (PS)	Time at which the nursing or surgical team begins positioning or prepping the patient for the procedure
Procedure/surgery start time (PST)	Time the procedure is begun (incision for surgery, scope for diagnostic procedure, beginning of exam under anesthesia, shooting for x-ray)
Procedure/surgery finish time (PF)	Time when all instrument and sponge counts are correct and verified as correct, all postop radiologic studies are complete; all dressings and drains are secured, and the surgeon(s) have completed all procedure-related activities on the patient
Anesthesia finish (AF)	Time at which the anesthesiologist turns over the care of the patient to a postanesthesia care team in the PACU/ICU. This is not to be confused with the time of arrival to the PACU/ICU.
Turnover time (TOT)	Time from prior patient-out-of-room to succeeding patient-in-room time for sequentially scheduled cases

From the American Association of Clinical Directors, http://www.aacdhq.org, with permission. Accessed August 10, 2007

Data Exchange

Data are collected in many locations in the system as a patient proceeds from the preoperative through postoperative phases, including Scheduling, Admitting, Preoperative or Preanesthesia Clinic (PEC, or PAT—Preanesthesia Testing), the Preoperative Prep or Holding Area, the Operating or Procedure Room, the PACU, and the Intensive or Surgical Care floor. For patients who are inpatients at the time of surgery, data may also have been collected within nursing Point-of-Care and Medication Administration Systems, in addition to the Order Entry, Laboratory, Radiology, and Pharmacy systems.

Location-Specific Functionality

Scheduling

In general, scheduling an operation will be one of the initial occurrences of data generation. The surgeon and surgical office staff will gather basic information related to the patient, the procedure, the clinical staff to be present, other tests required, the equipment required, and the preferred dates and times. Preliminary scheduling of the case may take place in the surgeon's office, with staff entering data directly into a computerized system, where the case remains as a request until validated. More commonly, the scheduling takes place upon receipt of the aforementioned data by a centralized scheduling staff after being transferred via telephone, fax, email, or by using specific functions within a computerized system. In any case, the data needed to actually schedule the case include information such as the surgeon's name; the procedure; the requested date, time, and room; any required equipment; the assistant (if any); the anesthesiologist (specific requests/needs); and inpatient bed request (including critical care unit requirements).

During the process of scheduling the surgical procedure, data pertinent to the patient's overall health should also be entered into the database, including allergies, patient weight, and known reportable infections. Other data may also include information from previous admissions and procedures, such as history of difficult airway or malignant hyperthermia. This information may come from the surgeon's office, old medical records, or the patient. Information provided during the scheduling process must be available not only to the OR staff, but also to the materials management, equipment, and instrument staffs (to ensure that necessary equipment and supplies are available), to the nursing supervisor or bed coordinator (to ensure appropriate bed assignment and nurse staffing), and ICU staff, if the patient is scheduled for admission to the ICU. Other departments (e.g., labor and delivery or neurophysiology) may also need access to the information if specialty monitoring is required.

Admissions

During the process of admitting the patient on the day of surgery, registrars or admitting clerks will enter and validate data on all of the patient demographic and insurance information. They may also be charged with gathering certain permanent information, such as ongoing infection-control issues (e.g., methicillin-resistant *Staphylococcus aureus*) and information about advance directives (Do Not Resuscitate/Do Not Intubate). The infection-control data may or may not be coming from a hospital-based epidemiologic or pathology information system if the patient has been admitted to the facility in the past, or it may be coming from the surgeon's office or the patient himself.

Preoperative or Preanesthesia Clinic

The Preoperative or Preanesthesia Clinic system may encompass a wide variety of functions and styles. It may include an actual clinic visit or merely be a place to collect information. Preoperative evaluation may be completed within the same healthcare facility in which the operation is to take place, making access to the data easier, or it may take place in a private-practice setting that includes printed, faxed, or phoned-in data from both the surgeon and other involved physicians. In general, such clinics collect data on each patient in the form of vital signs, weight, pertinent laboratory results, electrocardiographic results, and past medical history. The patient may complete the Preoperative Anesthesia Questionnaire at home, at the clinic, or in the surgeon's office and bring it in for review. The Preoperative Anesthesia H&P may be completed in the clinic by physicians or advanced practice nurses. In this clinical setting, significant patient teaching along with a thorough anesthesia H&P will be conducted and documented. It is here that the staff will review with the patient and/or the patient's family any ordered surgical preparations, fasts, and cleaning techniques that should occur prior to the patient's arrival on the day of surgery to ensure their understanding and compliance. The transmission of confirmation of this training and preparation to the Preoperative Clinic area of the system is essential in ensuring that the patient will be able to move forward with the surgery.

If the preoperative anesthesia H&P is completed within the same integrated healthcare system as the surgical procedure, then among the data collected should be "permanent items" such as history of allergies, difficult airway, malignant hyperthermia, and pseudocholinesterase deficiency. If this information is already in the patient's file, the system should flag these records in some manner. If the information is to be obtained from outside sources, such as a physician's office or another hospital, then a process must be developed to retrieve, validate, and incorporate the outside data into the larger hospital system.

Failed transmission of any of this information may contribute to delays on the day of surgery. In fact, a recent survey of practicing anesthesiologists revealed that nearly one-quarter of patients evaluated in such a clinic still encountered day-of-surgery delays. Proposed causes for these delays include failures of information transfer and lack of consensus on criteria for surgical readiness.[3]

Preoperative Holding Area

The Preoperative Holding Area encompasses both the outpatient prep area and the immediate preprocedure area. Information collected here includes validation of consent, allergies, and readiness for surgery (i.e., NPO status, medications, transport, and care for discharge). Identification bands with barcoded information coming from the admitting office may be placed, and the surgical site will be verified and marked. Nursing staff in this area will perform a head-to-toe assessment on the patient, which will include current vital signs, weight, level of consciousness, and current pain level. In addition, nursing may conduct point-of-care testing such as pregnancy tests and glucose finger sticks. The results of this testing will be entered into either an AIMS or ORMS. Additional lab work may be obtained, and results may or may not be automatically entered into an AIMS or ORMS. Nursing may start IV fluids or administer medications and will document such action in a Medication Administration Record that is often a function of the Order Entry application. Direct transmission of certain information gathered by reliable sources earlier in the perioperative process will greatly facilitate moving the patient through this area. In addition, advance knowledge of all patient health concerns reduces the risk of postponement or cancellation of cases. Moreover, it is reassuring to patients when they are not repeatedly asked the same questions at this highly stressful time. A summary of data collected in the Preop Clinic and the Preoperative Holding area that must be transmitted to the OR is provided in Table 18.3.[4]

Table 18.3 Preoperative area-to-operating room data transfer

Data elements	Specific details
Planned surgical procedure	Procedure name(s)
Surgical procedure verified	Site
	Side
	Verified: yes or no
Planned anesthesia type	General
	Epidural
	Spinal
	Local
	Monitored sedation
Allergies	Specific medication, food, or environmental substance
	No known drug allergy
	Unknown
	Unable to determine
Mental status	Level of consciousness
	Orientation
	Presence of cognitive deficits

(continued)

Table 18.3 (continued)

Data elements	Specific details
Language barriers	Yes or no Interpreter needed Specific language
Blood products/consent	Yes or no
Medications received in preop or taken at home	Medications Dosages
Antibiotics given	Routes Yes or no Specific antibiotic Time of administration Dosages Routes
Significant medical history	Blood pressure Asthma Cardiac history Renal history Neurologic history Liver history Infectious diseases Anesthesia history
Vital signs	Airway patency Respiratory status Breath sounds Artificial airway or ventilator Blood pressure (cuff or arterial) Pulse (apical or peripheral) Cardiac monitor rhythm Temperature Hemodynamic pressure reading
Equipment	Location Type
Catheters and drains	Location Type Amount
Musculoskeletal issues	Location Type
Skin integrity	Condition Color Dressing Incisions
Pain and comfort assessment	Location Descriptor Current level Goal level Comfort level

Adapted from American Society of Perianesthesia Nurses. *2006–2008 Standards of Perianethesia Nursing Practice*. Cherry Hill, NJ: American Society of Perianethesia Nurses, 2006, and Association of Operating Room Nurses. Sample Patient Hand-Off Tools, 2007. http://www.aorn.org/PracticeResources/ToolKits/PatientHandOffToolKit/.Accessed June 7, 2007

Operating Room

Multiple healthcare providers within the OR gather many data elements (see Table 18.1). Often, some of these data are duplicative and possibly contradictory or overlapping. Usually, this duplication is found within the nursing and anesthesia portions of the AIMS and ORMS. The most commonly duplicated data within the OR are allergies, surgical staff, procedure(s) name(s), room, patient positioning, time stamps, fluids in and out, blood product administration, medication administration, and vital signs.

If nursing and anesthesia are on separate systems, the systems may not be able to share these data. If they are documenting within specific modules of the same system, they still may not be able to share information if the functions of the application are not truly integrated. Two very important evaluation criteria that must be addressed when purchasing a system with an AIMS and ORMS are (a) the degree of integration between these functions and (b) the database platform upon which they function. Often, the functionality of the AIMS and ORMS is not truly integrated and the data are not residing on the same platform, making data exchange difficult and costly. This problem is occurring as larger vendors buy from smaller "best of breed" vendors whose systems were designed differently and whose databases are disparate. Until these acquired systems become integrated with the host system, data may not be able to be interfaced and shared within what appears to be a uniform product. In addition, if multiple nonintegrated systems are used, time stamps are particularly troublesome, as even extremely accurate computer clocks will not remain fully synchronized.

Postanesthesia Care Unit

As the patient is being prepared to leave the OR and travel to the next care area (PACU or ICU), a vast array of data are gathered in preparation for the imminent and fast-paced handoff between practitioners. The receiving PACU nurse usually is given verbal information from the circulating nurse while the case is still ongoing pertaining to the actual procedure(s) performed, the type of anesthesia used, the location of all wounds, the location of IV lines, the number and location of any drains and tubes, and the estimated time out of the OR. The data that should be transferred between these providers is summarized in Table 18.4.[5]

To assist with this transition, some healthcare enterprises are implementing Patient Trackers, which can designate the status of the case (in the room, started, closing, etc.) and broadcast that information to selected areas, including the PACU, particularly if an operational and accurate method exists for synchronizing time stamps between the various areas. This information is often limited to the basic information necessary to identify the patient, the procedure, and the surgeon. Some healthcare enterprises incorporate stand-alone products that can take data/information from a variety of systems and display it in a format that suits the workflow and information needs of the area. This information may include physiologic data from monitoring devices, medications given, and even images.

Without an interoperable system between the OR and the PACU or a coordinating system, the transmission of this information must be accomplished by telephone or in person. In consideration of the critical nature of the data and the highly charged environment in which this handoff action occurs, The Joint Commission promulgated National Patient Safety Goal 2E in 2006, which states that healthcare institutions must implement a standardized approach to handoff communications, including an opportunity to ask and respond to questions in ambulatory centers, critical-access hospitals, hospitals, and office-based surgery centers.[6] This scenario would include the handoff of care between and among OR nurses, OR and PACU nurses, PACU and ICU nurses, or the anesthesia team in any combination. Although The Joint Commission makes no demand regarding exact data that must be transmitted or the specific methodology for the handoff, it is clear that the data in Tables 18.3 and 18.4 must be considered.

In addition to the exchange of patient- and procedure-centric information that is collected within ORMS and AIMS, an additional data exchange occurs in the PACU, which involves the data embedded within order-entry processes. The order processing may occur manually or as an electronic process within a computerized physician order entry (CPOE) application. Regardless of the method of transmission, whether handwritten or computerized, the PACU staff becomes the recipient of postoperative orders coming from both the surgeon and the anesthesiologist in one work space. With the proliferation of CPOE applications in healthcare systems, the coordination of these orders becomes paramount. Which provider is responsible for the patient at which phase of postanesthesia care must be developed within the system. If the electronic orders are not coordinated, sequenced, and passed from surgeon to anesthesiologist to the nursing staff, then that nursing staff must attempt to sort through the orders to determine the precedence while they are accepting the patient, receiving report, and conducting their own assessment and interventions.

ICU/Surgical Floor

From the information documented in the preoperative area, OR, and PACU, some key data must be communicated to the clinical staff of the ICU or surgical floor, although the focus of the information may be quite different. The data to be included in the handoff and exchange are summarized in Table 18.4. The clinical staff must be prepared to receive and care for the patient by having advanced access to information about the patient, the procedure, the medications given in the OR and the PACU, and the fluids in and out. It would be safer for the patient and most expedient for the staff to have most of these data transferred into an application that is accessible to the staff of the clinical floor prior to the arrival of the patient. These data may be appropriately located in an EMR in a summary-type format or may be required in a CPOE application.

Table 18.4 OR-to-PACU/ICU data transfer

Data element	Specific details
Name and age of patient	
Names of surgeon(s)	
Procedure(s) performed	Procedure
	Site
	Side
Anesthesia type	General
	Epidural
	Spinal
	Local
	Monitored sedation
	Length of time
	Reversal agents used
Allergies	Specific medication, food, or environmental substance
	No known drug allergy
	Unknown
	Unable to determine
Mental status	Level of consciousness
	Orientation
Language barriers	Yes or no
	Interpreter needed
	Specific language
Estimated blood loss	Amount
Estimated fluid loss	Amount
	Type
Estimated fluid replacement	Amount
	Type
	Credit
Medications received in the OR and/or PACU	Medications
	Dosages
	Routes
	Times given
Pain management intervention	Intervention
	Effect
	Present pain score
	Patient goal
Vital signs	Blood pressure
	Heart rate
	Respiratory rate and status
	Temperature
	Oxygen saturation
Status of dressings/surgical sites	Location
	Type
	Draining
Comfort status	Presence of nausea
	Presence of vomiting

(continued)

Table 18.4 (continued)

Data element	Specific details
Catheters and drains	Location
	Type
	Drainage
Tests and treatments performed in OR and/or PACU	Radiology
	Pathology
Skin integrity	Pressure areas
	Wounds
	Drainage
Gastrointestinal assessment	Abdominal distention
	Bowel sounds
	Elimination
Genitourinary assessment	Voiding
Neurovascular assessment	
Ambulation	
Review of postoperative orders	

Adapted from American Society of Perianesthesia Nurses. *2006–2008 Standards of Perianesthesia Nursing Practice.* Cherry Hill, NJ: American Society of Perianethesia Nurses, 2006

Staff of the ICU and surgical floors may also want access to the real-time event timing of cases through the functionality of a tracker, which would allow selected staff to see the progress of key perioperative and perianesthesia events as they unfold. This knowledge permits preparation for the arrival of the patient well before the patient physically enters the unit or the floor.

Interoperability, Upgradeability, and Compatibility

Modern medicine uses various technologies in the care of patients, including communications and assessment devices. Several terms that are used in discussing these technologies require definition, as lack of understanding and incorrect usage of these terms may contribute to implementation failure. Reliable data, semantically and conceptually interoperable between systems, will support complete and accurate EMRs, the integration of niche applications (such as ORMS and AIMS), and complete and robust databases for continued quality improvement. The integration of these data across the perioperative and perianesthesia phases of care will facilitate true interdisciplinary evidence-based research. The ability of a system to be upgraded as technology and functionality improve and to be compatible with the variety of applications within a healthcare enterprise is fundamental to its long-term success as an application, as a data-collection tool, and as a source of information and knowledge for the professional practice.

What do the terms *interoperability*, *upgradeability*, and *compatibility* mean? They are all different aspects by which to assess how well a system will function at a facility, both on initial installation and over a period of time with and among other information systems.

The Institute of Electrical and Electronics Engineers defines *interoperability* as the ability of two or more systems or components to exchange information and to use the information that has been exchanged.[7] The lack of interoperability strongly implies that the described product or products were not designed with standardization in mind. Interoperability cannot be taken for granted, nor can it be assumed that it merely applies to the technical issues. Interoperability is also an organizational issue.

Medical-device interoperability has two major facets:

1. Data communication standards that support accurate data acquisition from monitors, infusion pumps, ventilators, portable imaging systems, and other hospital and home-based medical devices
2. Medical-device control standards that permit control of medical devices to create error-resistant systems, which may include safety interlocks between devices, closed-loop systems to regulate infusion devices, and remote access[8]

Some devices are well designed to be interoperable, known as "plug and play" (e.g., modular components in many ICU monitors). Others are not and, if they can be used with other systems at all, may require significant hardware and software adaptations. Furthermore, what is interoperable today may not be interoperable in 5 years; therefore, looking ahead is critical toward avoiding the necessity for continual system updates and instability. As mentioned, some large vendor products are not actually integrated (not internally interoperable) and may not be for some time. The cost and complexity of such seamless connectivity interferes with widespread deployment of these systems.[8]

Upgradeability may refer to hardware, software, or firmware. Common hardware upgrades include installing additional memory or storage space. Common software upgrades include installing a new version of an operating system, office suite, or proprietary database system. Firmware upgrades are less common and will rarely be seen in the arena discussed in this chapter.

Overall compatibility includes compliance with standards, either defined or de facto. Backward compatibility is critical in most facilities, as some piece of old equipment is always still in use (and generally not easily replaceable). *Generational compatibility* deals with older versions of software and is a specific variant on backward compatibility. The key here is the ability to read the data previously stored and archived.[9]

The product's *life span* must be distinguished from its *useful life*. Computers and similar equipment may have a product lifespan of 6 months (the time to the next generation of hardware or software), yet it may have a useful life of 2–5 years (or more). Furthermore, systems are not constantly upgradable; at some point, a new system will have to be acquired, just as versions of computer software must be regularly upgraded (from 1.0 to 1.1 vs. from 1.0 to 2.0).

Conclusion

The patient-care environment is rapidly becoming a vast information-technology system. Problems in information transfer can and will affect patient experience and outcomes. Communication failures are systematic and must be prevented or managed on the system level.

To ensure quality of care, an organization must:

1. Evaluate information flow within the organization to ensure that all possible cases are present in the database.
2. Investigate current hardware and software infrastructure to identify points of incompatibility and current capabilities.
3. Discourage duplication of data entry by multiple healthcare providers.
4. Determine which information systems are to contain the "source of truth."
5. Audit planned purchases to ensure forward compatibility and upgradeability.

Installation of any of the information-technology systems discussed above is only the starting point in the process. Every system will require continued attention to both software and hardware. Expect the unexpected—enterprises should not presume that errors cannot occur and should have a process in place to analyze errors and make improvements based upon the analysis.

Key Points

- AIMS typically consist of functionality that covers the preoperative, intraoperative, and postoperative phases of care.
- For patient safety, perioperative efficiencies, and staff effectiveness, data must be shared between the phases of care, regardless of whether the data are collected in an ORMS or an AIMS.
- Many healthcare institutions will choose an AIMS and an ORMS from different vendors in order to meet functional requirements. If this is the case, careful consideration must be given to the interoperability of the systems.
- Ownership of data elements that are carried over the phases of care will often change. Consideration must be given to which end user is the source of truth at any point in time.

References

1. Committee on Quality of Heath Care in America, Institute of Medicine. *Crossing the Quality Chasm*. Washington, DC: National Academy, 2001
2. Thys DM. The role of information systems in anesthesia. APSF Newsletter 2001 (Summer); 16(2). http://www.apsf.org/resource_center/newsletter/2001/summer/03Infosys.htm. Accessed June 5, 2007

3. Holt NF, Silverman DG, Prasad R, et al. Preanesthesia clinics, information management, and operating room delays: Results of a survey of practicing anesthesiologists. Anesth Analg 2007; 104(3):615–8

4. Association of Operating Room Nurses. Sample Patient Hand-Off Tools, 2007. http://www.aorn.org/PracticeResources/ToolKits/PatientHandOffToolKit/. Accessed June 7, 2007

5. American Society of Perianesthesia Nurses. *2006–2008 Standards of Perianesthesia Nursing Practice.* Cherry Hill, NJ: American Society of Perianethesia Nurses, 2006

6. The Joint Commission. National Patient Safety Goals, 2007. http://www.jointcommission.org/PatientSafety/NationalPatientSafetyGoals/07_hap_cah_npsgs.htm. Accessed June 7, 2007

7. *IEEE Standard Computer Dictionary: A Compilation of IEEE Standard Computer Glossaries.* New York: Institute of Electrical and Electronics Engineers, 1990

8. Goldman JM. Medical device connectivity for improving safety and efficiency. ASA Newsletter 2006 (May); 70(5). http://www.asahq.org/Newsletters/2006/05–06/goldman05_06.html. Accessed May 31, 2007

9. Doyle CA. Choosing an automated medical records system. American Society of Anesthesiologists Clinical Resources, 2005. http://www.asahq.org/clinical/ChoosinganAutomatedMedicalRecordsSystem.pdf. Accessed June 5, 2007

Chapter 19
Operating Room Scheduling and Capacity Planning

Luis G. Vargas, Jerrold H. May, William Spangler, Alia Stanciu, and David P. Strum

Managed care is placing severe financial and organizational pressures on health-care institutions, while at the same time capitation and competition are limiting resources. In response, institutions are beginning to re-engineer themselves from revenue to cost centers.[1,2] Research indicates that of the three major clinical service components that comprise the healthcare system (surgical, medical, and mental health), surgical services are among the most amenable to cost control by a systematic process of utilization review.[3] According to the National Heart, Lung, and Blood Institute, more than 33 million US residents undergo surgery annually, incurring charges of more than $450 billion, or nearly 10% of the entire healthcare budget.[4]

In the future, physicians will most likely be affiliated with centers of medical excellence, which are those facilities, hospital-based or free-standing, that deliver high-quality and reasonably priced care. In this respect, integrated scheduling systems are critical to cost containment and collaboration, particularly with regard to hospital expenditures. The total expenditures of hospitals in the US in 2002 are shown in Tables 19.1 and 19.2.[5] Approximately 86.9% of the hospitals in the US have ORs (Table 19.2). While the actual expenditure of different sized hospitals for running their ORs is not known with certainty, some estimates suggest that ORs account for ~10%–30% of total hospital expenditures. Thus, hospitals in the US spend between $30 and 90 billion on ORs annually, indicating that surgical facilities within hospitals and surgical centers are one of the most costly functional areas in the hospital.

As cost centers, ORs must be scheduled and run efficiently because they reflect on the financial health of the institution as a whole. Admission rates, OR utilization, and hospital census depend on a mix of surgical specialties and unimpeded access to surgical facilities.[6] Utilization problems occur when a hospital begins to run at or near capacity. If scheduling is inefficient, highly elective surgeries may occupy available beds to the detriment of less-elective surgeries, resulting in a decrease in the hospital's emergency capabilities. Conversely, if the institution preferentially allocates OR time for emergency services, elective surgeries, patient satisfaction, and access to surgical facilities may decrease.

Surgical facilities are similar to other competitive business enterprises—they must be able to deliver services at a competitive advantage.[7] That said, how does

J. Stonemetz, K. Ruskin (eds.) *Anesthesia Informatics*,
© Springer Science+Business Media, LLC 2008

Table 19.1 2002 US hospital expenditures

Bed-size category	Number of hospitals	Distribution of hospitals by bed category (%)	Expense per hospital ($ per year)[a]	Total expenses ($ per year)[b]
6–24	288	5.86	5.4	1.5
25–49	910	18.51	11.4	10.3
50–99	1055	21.46	20.8	22.1
100–199	1236	25.15	50.6	63.1
200–299	656	13.35	101.2	66.4
300–399	341	6.94	158.1	53.9
400–499	182	3.70	225.6	41.1
500+	247	5.03	386.3	95.4
Total	4915	1		353.1

[a]Dollar amounts are in millions
[b]Dollar amounts are in trillions
Data from *Hospital Statistics: The Comprehensive Reference Source for Analysis and Comparison of Hospital Trends*. Health Forum, ed. Chicago, IL: American Hospital Association, 2002

Table 19.2 2002 US hospital regional demographic distribution

Demographic areas	No. of hospitals	Hospitals with surgical units	Pop.[a]	Total hospital exp. ($ per year)[b]	Exp. per person ($ per person)	Inpatient surg. (per 1000 people)	Outpatient surg. (per 1000 people)
New England	228	180	13.3	20.8	1492	32.18	68.71
Middle Atlantic	472	406	39.7	61.0	1538	39.59	67.40
South Atlantic	806	692	51.8	61.4	1187	36.52	58.69
East North Central	759	685	45.2	60.2	1334	34.03	63.70
East South Central	384	345	17.2	21.4	1241	41.96	69.09
West North Central	706	649	19.2	26.4	1374	35.71	68.08
West South Central	811	635	31.4	36.1	1148	35.80	52.77
Mountain	339	299	18.1	17.5	960	30.33	46.14
Pacific	411	381	45.0	48.9	1085	26.60	40.90
Total	4915	4271					

[a]Dollar amounts are in millions
[b]Dollar amounts are in trillions
Data from *Hospital Statistics: The Comprehensive Reference Source for Analysis and Comparison of Hospital Trends*. Health Forum, ed. Chicago, IL: American Hospital Association, 2002

one know that a surgical facility is not competitive, and if so, what can one do to make it competitive? Answering the former question requires the assessment of the current performance of the OR suites. Answering the latter requires the use of scheduling methods to efficiently manage the resources available. To be competitive, surgical facilities must address two problems (a) how to select patients to be scheduled for surgery on a given day and (b) how to schedule patients according to certain criteria, such as minimizing the number of ORs used. Both problems require knowledge of the length of the procedure. The estimate of procedure duration is a critical step in the development of accurate and efficient schedules, as inaccuracies may lead to overtime and possibly inefficient use of scarce resources.

To allocate a specific starting time and duration for surgery, a surgeon's office typically contacts the admitting office and requests a reservation within an allotted time block. Requests are recorded in the admitting office and, with information on surgical teams and OR availability, are used to generate a prospective surgical schedule. The preliminary schedule is published and subsequently modified by the nursing and anesthesia departments. Patients are informed of their scheduled date of admission, and preoperative consultation and laboratory studies are arranged. When the patient is admitted, patient-specific information stored in the admitting office is transferred to the same-day surgery suite, where it is combined with new information generated at that location.

The major geographic locations through which patients traverse while receiving surgical services are illustrated with respect to a typical medical center in Fig. 19.1. Maximum throughput depends on efficient movement from location to location. Most patients arrive early on the day of surgery, accompanied by their families. A nursing history is obtained, the laboratory data are checked, and the patient is

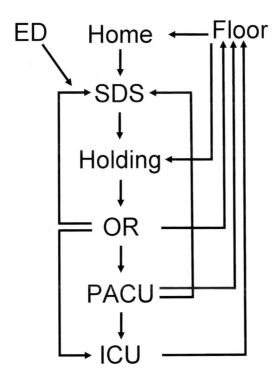

Fig. 19.1 Flow chart indicating patient flow and geographic locations in a typical surgical service. *SDS* same-day surgery

dressed for the OR. When ready, patients are sent to a holding area near the ORs, where they are interviewed by an anesthesiologist and the consent for surgery is obtained by a member of the surgical team. Inpatients move directly to the holding area from the inpatient wards. In the holding area, patients often request to speak with their family or surgeons before entering surgery. IV infusions are initiated, surgical preps are performed, and occasionally, casts are removed. If indicated, regional anesthesia is initiated in the holding area, using special equipment and monitoring.

When anesthesia, nursing, and surgical teams are ready, the patient is transported to the scheduled OR and is moved to the operating table, where monitors are applied, the patient is anesthetized, and surgery begins. Following surgery, the patient is transported to the PACU to recover before being returned to the same-day surgery unit or being moved to a ward bed. Same-day admission patients who are moved to a ward stay until their recovery can be managed at home. Outpatients who return to same-day surgery are reunited with their families, ambulated, instructed on follow-up care, and discharged home.

A few patients are sufficiently ill to require admission to an ICU following surgery. The surgery and anesthesia teams make such admission decisions together and are responsible for arranging reservations and admissions. The ICUs are remote from the operating suite, and communications typically occur by phone. Anesthesia must notify the ICU and arrange for beds, equipment, and personnel prior to the move. In some instances, the patient is taken to the PACU and later moved to the ICU.

Several problems may prevent the smooth progression of patients through the surgical services suites. These include, but are not limited to, late arrivals of patients or medical records, delays in support services, acute onset of abnormal medical conditions (infections, chest pain, etc.) that require delay or cancellation, inaccurate or inappropriate reservations, lack of a mechanism to enable dynamic scheduling, and delays that result in lost professional time. These and other problems lead to peaks and troughs in the demand for services, adding to inefficiency and dissatisfaction among patients, their families, and healthcare providers.

Scheduling in industrial environments requires taking into account three time horizons, expanding from short-term (daily), medium-term (several weeks), and long-term (6 months or more). Scheduling surgical facilities seems to have a similar structure. While the medium- and long-term horizons are usually determined by population demographics and medical practices, which generate emergencies and elective surgeries, daily scheduling must deal with the flow of people into and around the operating suite. The OR schedule is the point of departure for the daily flow. Once the day starts, it is rare that the schedule remains unchanged (Fig. 19.2). In fact, deviations from the schedule occur frequently, and people expect them to happen.

According to Gabel, an efficient and busy OR suite can process between 800 and 1000 cases per OR per year, depending on the case duration and mix.[7] In general, ~85% of the cases are elective (scheduled 2 or more days before surgery), and the remaining cases are emergencies or urgent. An *emergency* is a case in which the patient is in danger of losing life or a limb if surgery is not performed within some

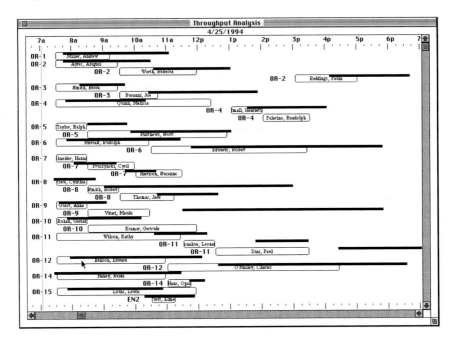

Fig. 19.2 Gantt chart of scheduled (*box*) and actual (*line*) procedure duration (patients' names are fictitious)

specified period of time. An *urgent* case is a case that requires attention within 24 hours. It is generally agreed within the medical community that the task of an OR scheduling system is to process elective cases, although ideally, all surgical cases are posted into the schedule.

Several competing goals are involved with the process of implementing an OR schedule, including (a) to meet the demands of surgeons for access to the ORs at suitable times and (b) to serve the institution's need for conserving resources such as people and space; i.e., the schedule should be able to fit as many cases as possible in busy days and open only as many ORs as necessary. The problems that may arise from these two contrasting objectives are exacerbated by the type of insurance patients may have. Managed care organizations require efficient and tightly packed schedules with little flexibility, while organizations that insure patients on a fee-for-service payment system require less efficiency and more convenience for their clients.

In summary, the goal of OR scheduling is predictable workload with adequate time for emergencies. Among other things, this means the joint and timely meeting of the surgeon, anesthesiologist, nursing staff, surgical suite, supplies, and special equipment. When a time slot in a particular surgical suite is selected, the availability of resources necessary to perform the procedure may be seriously affected by the use of a scheduling methodology that does not permit the timely performance of the procedure.[8]

A surgical schedule consists of a set of procedures (the durations of which are not known with certainty) and a set of ORs to which the procedures need to be assigned, satisfying some constraints with respect to the surgeon's availability, room preference (if any), and the type of OR in which the procedure can be performed. Thus, before surgical procedures can be assigned to ORs, their duration must be estimated. As the authors have reported,[9–11] we studied factors that influence the duration of surgical procedures and provided a model to statistically estimate their duration.[9] Our findings are summarized below.

Strategies that produce better estimates of surgical procedure times lead naturally to better utilization of surgical suites, higher productivity, and lower labor costs.[12–15] To this end, a number of management science methods and approaches have been applied to the problem of scheduling surgical suites. They include the use of mathematical programming and optimization techniques,[12–14] rule-based heuristic approaches,[15] statistical decision theory,[13] and computer-based simulation and algorithm evaluation.[12,16] These studies have shown significant success in improving overall utilization—and have shed light on the factors that impact efficient scheduling.

Estimating the Duration of Surgical Procedures

Efficient scheduling in a hospital is complicated by the variability inherent in surgical procedures, so that accurately modeling time distributions is the essential first step in constructing a planning and scheduling system. Modeling the nature of that variability has been of interest for the past 35 years. Rossiter,[17] e.g., notes that the two-parameter lognormal distribution visually appears to fit a waiting time distribution. In the literature, both the normal[18,19] and the two-parameter lognormal[20,21] distributions have been proposed for describing surgical times.

The authors showed a way to find the best distribution for each procedure and type of anesthesia using a large set of patient data from a larger project.[9] Our criterion for "best distribution" is the one that gives the best overall fit, using an appropriate statistical test. The literature suggested that the normal and lognormal distributions were two viable candidate distributions to consider; however, scatterplots of our data suggested that the lognormal would be the superior choice. A caveat to this statement is that minimum surgical procedure times, even for the simplest procedures, are strictly positive. Very common procedures (e.g., cardiac bypass) require at least several hours in the OR. *A lognormal distribution with a nonzero minimum* (also called the *origin*, *threshold*, or *location parameter*) had to be considered in addition to the usual two-parameter lognormal. The density function of a three-parameter lognormal is given by

$$f(x) = \frac{1}{\sigma(x-\theta)\sqrt{2\pi}} e^{-\left(\frac{1}{2\sigma^2}\right)(\ln(x-\theta)-\mu)^2}$$

where θ is the location parameter, and μ and σ are the mean and standard deviation of ln x, respectively.

A two-parameter lognormal obtains if $\theta = 0$. Estimating μ and σ is straightforward, but not so for the location parameter.

At least three methods to estimate the location parameter have been proposed in the literature. Assuming that our data set is typical of that which appears in at least other medical contexts, we recognized that a thorough analysis of the information could be used to derive rules about when to use a location parameter as part of the modeling process and, if so, which one to use. Consequently, we developed decision rules using data-mining techniques to select the most appropriate method to estimate the location parameter.[22]

Accurate estimation of the duration of a surgical procedure is the first step toward successful scheduling, but because of its randomness, the makespan or duration of the entire schedule is difficult to predict. The duration of surgical procedures impacts not only the schedule makespan, but also the revenue of the hospital. *Revenue management* (RM), also known as *demand management*, is an extension of inventory theory, as it grew out of the airline industry's attempt to maximize revenues. While healthcare and surgical management clearly are different from airline management, certain parallels can be drawn. For example, when a flight departs and a seat in the airplane is empty, the seat becomes worthless, just as an OR becomes worthless when it is not in use. Although the complete time cycle from flight offering to flight departure is longer than the time cycle in OR scheduling, the effect is the same; i.e., at the end of the day, the clock is reset and the resources become available again. In the airline industry, the price of a ticket is deterministic—a passenger usually pays for a seat in the airplane regardless of how tall or heavy he might be. In healthcare, the cost of a surgical procedure may be the same in two different institutions, but because the duration of the procedure varies, the revenue per unit of time is best modeled by a random variable. This method is equivalent to managing an airline in which the airplanes have benches rather than seats. Although all passengers would pay the same amount, the airline would prefer to include smaller people because it is seeking to maximize the number of passengers.

Consider the example of a helicopter tour in Hawaii. To balance the weight of the aircraft, the passengers are required to provide their body weight, which in turn introduces the possibility that someone could be denied a seat. Because the revenue of the tour company is a function of the weights of the individuals and because the tour company charges per individual, it would be to their advantage to maximize their revenue using the revenue per unit of weight, where weight is the random variable. Note that this problem is quite different from the one addressed in the RM literature.

Variability inherent in the duration of surgical procedures also complicates scheduling of surgeries composed of two or more procedures. Modeling the duration of these multiple-procedure surgeries is important operationally to produce accurate time estimates, improve utilization, reduce costs, and identify surgeries that might be considered outliers. Surgeries with multiple procedures are difficult to model because they are more difficult to segment and model in homogenous groups and because they are performed less frequently than single-procedure surgeries; therefore, relatively less data exist on which to base predictive models.

Investigating dual-procedure surgeries rather than making assumptions extrapolated from studies of single-procedure surgeries, we studied 10,740 surgeries each with exactly two CPTs and 46,322 surgical cases with only one CPT from a large teaching hospital to determine if the distribution of dual-procedure surgery times more closely fits a lognormal or a normal model. We tested model goodness-of-fit to our data using Shapiro-Wilk tests, studied factors affecting the variability of time estimates, and examined the impact of coding permutations (ordered combinations of CPT codes) on modeling.[23] Our analyses indicated that the lognormal model was statistically superior to the normal for modeling dual-procedure surgeries. Furthermore, permutations of component codes did not appear to differ significantly with respect to total procedure time or surgical time. To improve individual models for infrequent dual-procedure surgeries, permutations may be reduced and estimates may be based on the longest component procedure and type of anesthesia.

We recommend use of the lognormal model for estimating surgical times for surgeries with two-component procedures and believe it is reasonable to extrapolate similar principles to model three-component procedures. Our results also legitimized the use of log transforms to normalize surgical procedure times prior to hypothesis testing using linear statistical models. Multiple-procedure surgeries may be modeled using the longest (statistically most important) component procedure and type of anesthesia. In some data series, multiple-procedure surgeries account for up to a third of all surgeries and consequently have a large potential to impact surgical schedules.

Revenue Management and Patient Selection

RM is the process of generating incremental revenues from existing inventory or capacity through a better administration of the sale of the good or service. An organization that practices RM pays attention to customer segmentation, forecasting, pricing, and reacting actively to customer demand. Successful implementations of RM techniques have resulted in increased revenues for many organizations across various industries, most notably airline, hotel, restaurant, and car-rental businesses. The healthcare area, in comparison, has not made extensive use of RM, most likely because most segments within this industry are working on a nonprofit basis and because RM might raise ethical issues. Nevertheless, while any implementation of RM should be respectful of ethical concerns, the notion of hospitals as nonprofit organizations rather than revenue-maximizing units is not necessarily true. Hospitals will continue to survive and provide quality services only if they recover and/or reinvest the revenue generated by the wide range of services they provide to patients. Because waiting times for elective surgeries are increasing and waiting queues are piling up, solutions are sought to decrease the waiting times while maintaining an acceptable quality of service.

Businesses that sell perishable goods or services often must manage a fixed capacity of a product over a finite horizon. If in the market for these companies, customers are willing to pay different prices for the product, an opportunity is created to sell the product to different customer segments at different prices, e.g., charging different prices at different points in time or limiting the availability of products to price-sensitive customers. RM entails making decisions about which prices to charge and how to distribute products or services across each market segment, with the goal of increasing expected revenue. Thus, RM can be referred to as the art of maximizing the revenue that is generated from managing the limited capacity of a product over a finite horizon by selling each product to the right customer, at the right time, for the right price.[24]

An important concept underlying RM is market segmentation into multiple classes (e.g., leisure vs. business travelers), where different types of products (e.g., seats on an airline with restricted or fully refundable fares) are targeted to each class. Having its origins in research initiated by American Airlines, RM's main focus has been on the allocation of limited and perishable capacity to different demand classes. A resource is perishable if after a certain date it becomes either unavailable or ages at a significant cost. Examples of such perishable inventory include seats on a flight or in a theater, rooms in a hotel, and space on a cargo train. Thus, RM is primarily concerned with capacity allocation decisions. In the airline case, one of the tactical decisions is to determine the number of seats to make available to each fare class (protection levels) from a shared inventory and how many requests from each class to accept in order to maximize total expected revenues, taking into account the probabilistic nature of future demand for a flight.[25] In other words, given a booking request for a seat in an itinerary in a specific booking class, the fundamental RM decision is whether to accept or reject this booking, considering the past and future demands. In the hotel industry, the manager must decide at the operational level whether or not to rent a room to a customer who is requesting it for the target date, considering the reservations already made and potential walk-ins (customers who show up without a reservation). Therefore, it is not at all uncommon to deny an advanced booking (in either business) to price-sensitive customers for peak travel periods because it is anticipated that enough demand from higher-paying customers will develop. The analysis of capacity (seat) allocation (controlling the mix of discount fares and early booking restrictions) and overbooking (selling more seats than available when cancellations and no-shows are allowed) is supported by a thorough understanding of customer behavior and the capability to forecast future demand. The three most important RM interrelated aspects and areas of research are forecasting, seat allocation, and overbooking.

Surgical units within a hospital usually account for at least 60% of the total revenue generated by that hospital. The truth is that there will always be patients who need surgery, and it is also true that good management of scheduling the surgeries can lead to increased revenue for the hospital, which cannot be seen as at all detrimental to either the health of the patient or that of the institution. Additional revenue generated by an effective surgery-scheduling policy can be reinvested so that capacity will increase and more patients can be offered service and/or waiting times can be decreased. These developments can only occur by virtue of good management and revenue-generating strategies through a paradigm shift from the OR as a cost center to the OR as a revenue center.

Because healthcare-related costs are ever increasing, more attention must be given to controlling costs and revenues and to finding and implementing more efficient ways of using health resources. The competing demand in healthcare is more transparent than in the airline or hotel industries, but the costs involved are not; i.e., costs are known only with some degree of certainty before the actual service/intervention occurs. These characteristics, in turn, add more complexity to the efficient allocation and use of health resources. The "first-come, first-served" model of scheduling patients may concede to a higher-revenue method of scheduling and prioritizing patients. RM provides a fresh perspective with regard to patient scheduling. While the main objective of capacity allocation in the airline industry is to determine the number of units (seats) to sell at lower prices and the number to reserve for sale at higher prices, the analogy in healthcare is to determine the number of units of time the scheduling department should save for different classes of patients, with "class" defined as a combination of the patient's reimbursement category (e.g., the type of insurance that the patient possesses) and the type of surgery requested.

A few studies in the healthcare area have analyzed the implementation of such RM concepts. Chapman and Carmel used threshold curves, which are historic demand models used to predict and monitor future demand, to determine whether and when to apply discounts in order to increase the capacity utilization and revenue yield within Duke University's diet and fitness center.[26] In a more recent article, Green et al. analyzed the patient-scheduling problem faced by an MRI diagnostic service and identified threshold policies to manage patient demand and the capacity allocation (appointment scheduling and dynamic priority) by using a finite-horizon dynamic program.[27] The optimal (or near-optimal) policy determines at each point, based on a switching index, which patient class should be serviced next: inpatients, outpatients, or emergencies. While their assumption is that examination times are fixed and equal to the allotted time slot, here, we are attempting to incorporate the service-time randomness from the beginning in our analysis. Gerchak et al. developed an advanced reservation planning policy for elective surgery patients when the OR capacity is common for both elective and emergency surgeries.[28] In 2004, the PROS RM team along with Born et al. worked on optimizing the performance of contracts with insurers at Texas Children's Hospital.[29]

As the awareness of unacceptably long waiting times for elective surgeries within the public hospital system has become heightened in the past decade, dealing with this issue should be a focus at both the hospital and the national/governmental levels. An increase in admission rates to the hospital should be coupled with an increase of the available hospital resources (doctors, nurses, beds, etc.). One source of funding this capacity increase can be the internal financial resources (reinvesting the revenues), and the follow-up conclusion is that hospitals (and surgery units in particular) must undergo a paradigm shift in patient scheduling from a cost-driven approach to a net contribution-driven approach. Toward this end, RM methodology can become a new and important alternative worth considering.

The classical stream of research that explores multiple-class patient scheduling takes the form of priority queues. Solution approaches are (a) simulation and (b) (stochastic) linear and multiobjective mathematical programming. Various decision-support models for tactical decisions in the day-to-day hospital admission and surgical scheduling of the waiting lists have been proposed. For example, Everett, Lowery, and Ivaldi et al. have all described decision models that simulate elements of hospital operations, including patient arrivals and waiting lists, various types of surgical procedures, and overall throughput.[30, 31, 32] The simulation models are usually used as an operational tool to balance hospital availability and patient need while comparing the effectiveness of various alternative policies in this usually multicriteria decision setting. A first-come, first-served rule within a class of urgency is usually adopted, and no considerations are given to the various classes of financial characteristics.

Even if the first-come, first-served rule is most accepted in terms of fairness, hospitals must recognize the need for improved revenues, with the ultimate goal of self-preservation. As some patients may defer payment to the hospital, the only revenue of which the hospital can be certain is the fraction of the surgery cost covered by the patient's insurance company under the insurance agreement. From this perspective, patients with full insurance coverage have priority over those with partial insurance in the scheduling of a type of surgery. All categories of patients will be serviced within some limited time frame, but some purely elective patients may be postponed longer than others.

Assignment of Protection Levels

To help explain the parallelism between basic results in the airline industry and healthcare, we will first explain the former. Assume that a system has total capacity of C and that it must service two groups of customers, with each customer requesting exactly one unit (e.g., one seat on a flight) of total capacity. Each customer from Group 1 pays p_1 and each customer from Group 2 pays p_2, with $p_1 > p_2$. Let the probability density function for Group i's demand be f_i, its realized value, D_i, and its cumulative distribution, F_i. For simplicity, assume that the f_i values are continuous. Group 2 customers arrive before Group 1 customers, there are no cancellations, and overbooking is not permitted. Let x denote the protection level, i.e., the number of units of capacity reserved for Group 1 customers. Two cases are to be considered:

Case 1. Neither Group 1 nor Group 2 demand would exhaust the system capacity, but total demand would, so that the capacity allocation problem is nontrivial. That is, the probability that either group exceeds capacity is zero, $P[D_1 < C] = 1$ and $P[D_2 < C] = 1$, but together, the demand of both groups exceeds capacity, $P[D_1 + D_2 > C] = 1$. In this case, the return for a protection level x is rendered by

$$R(x) = p_2 \min\{D_2, C - x\} + p_1 \min\{D_1, x\}$$

and the value of x, x^*, that maximizes $ER(x)$ must satisfy the condition

$$P[D_1 > x^*] - \frac{p_2}{p_1} P[D_2 > C - x^*] = 0 \tag{19.1}$$

The expected loss from Group 1 brought about by setting the protection level at x^* is $p_1 P[D_1 > x^*]$, and the expected loss from Group 2 is $p_2 P[D_2 > C - x^*] = 0$. Equation (19.1) thus dictates that the protection level x^* should be set so as to exactly balance the expected revenue losses from the two groups of customers. This example could be applied to a clinic that serves people with private insurance and without insurance. For the people without insurance, the clinic is reimbursed by the government. It would not be unreasonable to assume that the demand from the uninsured would be larger than that of the group with private insurance, as the members of the latter group could have other choices of clinics.

Case 2. The demand D_1 of Group 1, the class that contributes more per unit of resource, would not exhaust system capacity, but the demand D_2 of Group 2, the class that contributes less per unit of resource, would exhaust system capacity, i.e., $P[D_1 < C] = 1$ and $P[D_2 > C] = 1$. This case is the situation considered by Littlewood[33]: $P[D_2 > C - x^*] = 1$, so that (19.1) reduces to

$$P[D_1 > x^*] - \frac{p_2}{p_1} = 0 \tag{19.2}$$

hence, we have

$$x^* = F_1^{-1} \left(1 - \frac{p_2}{p_1} \right)$$

Littlewood's formula (19.2) is a fundamental result for RM and is a critical component of later, more general, methodologies such as Belobaba's.[25] An example of this situation would be a clinic in which two groups of people with different private insurance coverages need different types of surgery. Together, they may exceed the capacity of the clinic, but individually they may not.

Now consider a situation in which the amount of the scarce resource (space, time, etc.) required by each customer is random. For example, consider a flat-fee legal clinic that serves both walk-in customers and those covered by employer-sponsored legal insurance. Consultation times are random, but historical data permit estimation of the distribution of time required to service a customer of either type. Professional ethics require the clinic to take customers on a first-come, first-served basis and to complete a consultation, regardless of the amount of time required. Customers covered by insurance pay less for a consultation than do walk-ins. How much of the fixed opening hours of the clinic should the clinic reserve for walk-in customers?

As before, assume that the system has total capacity of C and that there are two groups of customers. Each customer from Group i pays p_i regardless of the amount of capacity used, with $p_1 > p_2$. The density for the total number of units of capacity demanded by Group i is f_i. Let t_{ij} represent the amount of resource used by customer j of Group i. Assume that each value of t_{ij} is small enough relative to C so that it is possible to exactly schedule any desired level of capacity. Let

$$D_i = \sum_{j=1}^{N_i} t_{ij}, i = 1, 2$$

, where N_i is a random variable representing the number of customers of Group i requesting service.

For convenience, let $Q_i = p_i/T_i$, where the random variable T_i denotes the amount of the resource used by a customer from Group i. Q_i may be interpreted as the contribution per unit of resource by a customer of Group i. Q_1 and Q_2 are random variables because the t_{ij} are random. For the customers in Group i, the observed values of Q_i are $\dfrac{p_i}{t_{i1}}, \dfrac{p_i}{t_{i2}}, \dots, \dfrac{p_i}{t_{iN_i}}$. Let $E[Q_i] = \mu_i$, $i = 1,2$. It is also helpful to have notation for the conditional expectations $\mu_{i|Q_1 > Q_2} = E[Q_i \mid Q_1 > Q_2], i = 1,2$, and $\mu_{i|Q_1 < Q_2} = E[Q_i \mid Q_1 < Q_2], i = 1,2$. Although $p_1 > p_2$, because Q_1 and Q_2 are random, it is not certain that $Q_1 > Q_2$. Let θ denote the probability that Q_1 is greater than Q_2, i.e.,

$$\theta = P[Q_2 < Q_1] = P\left[\frac{Q_2}{Q_1} = \frac{p_2/T_2}{p_1/T_1} < 1\right] = P\left[\frac{T_1}{T_2} < \frac{p_1}{p_2}\right].$$

Note that $E[Q_i] \equiv \mu_i = \theta\mu_{i|Q_1 > Q_2} + (1-\theta)\mu_{i|Q_1 < Q_2}$, $i = 1,$ 2, so that $\mu_i \to \mu_{i|Q_1 > Q_2}$ as $\theta \to 1$; $\mu_i \to \mu_{i|Q_1 > Q_2}$ as $\theta \to 0$; $\mu_{2|Q_1 > Q_2} < \mu_{1|Q_1 > Q_2}$; and $\mu_{2|Q_1 < Q_2} > \mu_{1|Q_1 < Q_2}$.

With probability $(1 - \theta)$, Group 1 customers generate less revenue on a per-unit basis than do Group 2 customers. In that situation, allocating x resource units to Group 1 is an allocation decision, as opposed to a way to "protect" part of a scarce resource for the more financially desirable customer group. To keep the terminology consistent, however, we continue to refer to x as the protection level even when individual utilizations are random. The next result shows that when utilizations are random, a unique protection level exists for Case 1, with the prices of (19.1) replaced by the contributions per unit in (19.3). We give without proofs the following results, given in detail in the work of Vargas et al.[34]

Theorem 1. *Under the conditions of Case 1, when customer resource utilization is random, the unique optimal protection level for Group 1, x^*, satisfies the condition*

$$P[D_1 > x^*] - \frac{\mu_2}{\mu_1} P[D_2 > C - x^*] = 0 \tag{19.3}$$

When individual resource utilizations are deterministic, Case 2 simplifies Case 1 by assuming that, relative to total system capacity C, the demand for the lower-revenue Group 2 is unbounded. The analogous assumption when individual resource utilizations are random is that the total demand of the group with lower contribution per unit is (relatively speaking) unbounded. That is, instead of Case 2, we have:

Case 2'. The demand of the class that contributes more per unit of resource would not exhaust system capacity, but the demand of the class that contributes less per unit of resource would exhaust system capacity. That is, with probability θ, $Q_1 > Q_2$, so that $P[D_1 < C] = 1$ and $P[D_2 > C] = 1$, and with probability $(1 - \theta)$, $Q_2 > Q_1$, so that $P[D_2 < C] = 1$ and $P[D_1 > C] = 1$.

When individual resource utilizations are deterministic, one group that has (relatively speaking) unlimited demand simplifies the calculation of the protection level; (19.2) is a specialization of (19.1). The next result shows that when individual resource utilizations are random, a protection level can still be determined when the less financially desirable group has unlimited demand, but the formula in such a situation is more complicated than the one that applied in Case 1. After the proof, we show that Littlewood's rule (19.2) is the limiting case of (19.4) in Theorem 2 as $\theta \to 1$ or as $\theta \to 0$.

Theorem 2. *Under the conditions of Case 2', when customer resource utilization is random, the unique optimal protection level for Group 1, x*, satisfies the condition*

$$P[D_1 > x^*] - \left(\frac{1-\theta}{\theta}\right)\frac{\mu_{2|Q_1 < Q_2}}{\mu_{1|Q_1 > Q_2}} P[D_2 > C - x^*] = \frac{\mu_{2|Q_1 > Q_2}}{\mu_{1|Q_1 > Q_2}} - \left(\frac{1-\theta}{\theta}\right)\frac{\mu_{1|Q_1 < Q_2}}{\mu_{1|Q_1 > Q_2}} \quad (19.4)$$

Corollary. *Under the conditions of Case 2', when customer resource utilization is random, but it is known with certainty if $Q_1 > Q_2$ or $Q_1 < Q_2$, the unique optimal protection level for Group 1, x*, satisfies the condition* $P[D_1 > x^*] = \mu_2 / \mu_1$, *or equivalently* $x^* = F_1^{-1}(1 - \mu_2 / \mu_1)$ *if* $Q_1 > Q_2$ *and* $P[D_2 > C - x^*] = \mu_1 / \mu_2$, *or equivalently,* $x^* = C - F_2^{-1}(1 - \mu_1 / \mu_2)$ *if* $Q_1 < Q_2$.

These simple results show that the protection levels are not deterministic but random variables and that the expected revenue can be maximized by selecting appropriate levels based on the average contribution per unit of resource.

In the case of surgical services, the number of classes is a function of the total number of procedures considered and the levels of funding. For example, if we consider 100 CPT categories and three levels of funding, there are 300 possible classes from which patients will have to be selected to form the portfolio of procedures for a given day.

In general terms, the problem is as follows. Given N surgeries (CPTs) and M reimbursement categories, a patient's class is determined by the type of surgery requested and the reimbursement category under which he falls. The class to which the request belongs is defined by j, with $j = 1, ..., n$ and $n = M \times N$, as a combination of patient's insurance type and surgery requested. The ranking within the j classes of patients will change based on some random realization of surgery time, which is assumed to be lognormally distributed as shown in the previous section. Thus, although the price per surgery (p_j) is fixed, by considering that the actual surgery time follows some probability distribution, the revenue/ unit of time obtained (q_j) will also be a random variable, with some finite mean and standard deviation. The problem then is: How many time units (min, 5-min periods, etc.) should be protected, in a nested fashion, for class j and higher, in order to maximize expected revenue?

Once nested protection levels are selected for the different classes of patients (a class is defined by the subspecialty CPT and the level of funding), it can be decided which patients should be scheduled on a given day. The protection levels determine the number of patients of a given class that are selected. The next step is to schedule them in the appropriate ORs.

Surgical Scheduling

Two methods are used to allocate surgical procedures to ORs: on a first-come, first-served basis and block scheduling. In the latter, time is reserved in ORs for a surgeon, a surgical group, or a particular type of surgical service. The size of the blocks is based on demonstrated use. As a rule of thumb, block time is increased if utilization is >80%–85% and decreased if utilization is >70%–75%. Block scheduling is advantageous to surgeons who serve patients for elective surgeries because it improves utilization of the OR. Block scheduling is not advantageous for surgeons who serve patients for urgent and emergent surgeries because lack of flexibility impairs access to the needed OR. Voss recommends a combined block and first-come, first-served approach to scheduling, as well as practical guidelines for constraining the times of day for particular types of patients and procedures.[35] Retaining surgical blocks is important because of the political constraints involved in allocating OR time. The first-come, first-served scheduling mechanism increases utilization by filling in unused time between blocks, as well as time that might be released within blocks. Blocks are typically reserved in advance and are amenable to offline packing approaches, in which all of the items that must be scheduled are known in advance and may be sorted before being scheduled. First-come, first-served procedures may need to be reserved online, meaning that times must be committed to them as they are called in, and they cannot be later moved solely for the convenience of the scheduler.

Notation

An *operating suite* is a room in which surgery is performed, and a subspecialty surgical *block* is a group of operating suites the equipment and personnel of which are interchangeable with each other but not necessarily with suites outside the block. Let

s_i Starting time of the ith procedure

t_i Ending time of the ith procedure, and $s_i < t_i$

a_i Duration of the ith procedure, and $t_i = si + a_i$

x_{ij} Binary assignment variable ($x_{ij} = 1$ if the ith procedure is assigned to the jth OR, and $x_{ij} = 0$, otherwise)

T_j Time at which the budget for the jth operating suite ends. We assume without loss of generality that the budgeted day starts at time 0 for all ORs and that all ORs are budgeted the same amount of time, i.e., $T_j = T$ for all j.

y_j Binary assignment variable ($y_j = 1$ if the jth OR is used, and $y_j = 0$, otherwise)

z_j Amount of time (overtime) an OR is used beyond the budgeted time T_j

c Fixed cost of opening an OR for a period of time $[0, T_j]$

d Cost of a unit of overtime

C_o^i Cost of overutilizing an OR assigned to the ith surgical block

C_u^i Cost of underutilizing an OR assigned to the ith surgical block

B_i Amount of time budgeted for the ith surgical block

B_i^* Amount of time budgeted for the ith surgical block that minimizes the expected cost

x_i Amount of time used by the ith surgical block

w_j Binary variable ($w_j = 1$ if the jth OR is used beyond the budgeted time; $w_j = 0$, otherwise)

Block Scheduling: Minimal Cost Analysis Model

To analyze utilization of surgical subspecialty operating theaters, it is necessary to define several important terms. *Usage* is the total time an operating suite is used, i.e., the surgical demand, to be distinguished from *utilization*, which is the ratio of operating suite time used to that of the available time. Utilization is a relative term without units, while usage is an absolute measure defined in minutes or hours. *Classical utilization* is the ratio of total time used to budgeted OR time. *Budgeted utilization* is the ratio of budgeted time used for surgery to total budgeted OR time. Budgeted OR time not used is defined as *underutilization*, while surgical cases beginning/ending outside budgeted OR time are categorized as *overutilization*. Surgical cases that overlap budgeted and nonbudgeted OR time are parsed, and the portions assigned appropriately.

To minimize costs, we developed a model applicable to capacity planning for surgical subspecialty block times.[35] The minimum cost solution can be determined by knowing only the distribution of the X_i, the total time used in ith block, and the relative hourly cost of under and overutilization; this is true regardless of how the distribution of the X_i is determined. As these blocks can be independently budgeted, they can be optimized separately or together. Let us assume that there are n noninterchangeable blocks of operating suites and that the operating suites within each block are interchangeable. For each of these blocks, we can determine the optimum amount of time (Bi) that they should be budgeted to minimize the total expected cost.

Let $C(x_i)$ be the total cost associated with utilizing the blocks of operating suites $1, 2, \ldots, n$, $x_1, x_2, \ldots, x_n$ time units, respectively. This cost can be written as the sum of the costs of overutilization given by $\sum_i C_o^i [\max\{x_i - B_i, 0\}]$, and the costs of underutilization given by $\sum_i C_u^i [\max\{B_i - x_i, 0\}]$.

The total cost is given by

$$C(x_i) = C_o^i [\max\{x_i - B_i, 0\}] + C_u^i [\max\{B_i - x_i, 0\}]. \qquad (19.5)$$

The amount of time that the ith block of operating suites must be allocated to minimize the expected cost is the value of $B_i = B_i^*$ such that

$$P[X_i \le B_i^*] = \frac{C_o^i}{C_o^i + C_u^i} \quad \text{or} \quad P[X_i \le B_i^*] = \frac{C_o^i / C_u^i}{1 + C_o^i / C_u^i}. \qquad (19.6)$$

Simply stated, $B_i = B_i^*$ is the $100(C_o^i / C_u^i)(1 + C_o^i / C_u^i)^{-1}$ percentile of the probability distribution of X_i. Thus, if, e.g., the cost of overutilization exceeds underutilization by ratios of 1, 2, or 3 ($C_o^i / C_u^i = 1, 2,$ or 3), then $B_i = B_i^*$ is the 50th, 67th, and 75th percentile, respectively. Note, that to perform the analysis, it is not necessary to know the actual cost of overutilization and underutilization—only their relative cost, i.e., C_o^i / C_u^i. The amount of time that this model allocates to each block, $B_i = B_i^*$, depends on the distribution of surgical demand.

Application

To illustrate the minimal cost analysis model, we borrowed results from our previous work in which we used data from 58,251 computerized records of surgical cases that consisted of 5122 different CPT-coded procedures of which 3166 procedures occurred two or more times.[36] Each CPT code had 1–1746 cases assigned to it, with analyzed data for ten subspecialty surgical blocks for 1591 weekdays or 328 weeks using from 9 to 18 operating suites daily. Block-specific daily surgical demand was modeled by one of four probability distributions. Aggregate usage (surgical demand) from each of the ten subspecialty blocks was fit to each of the models (normal, Weibull, gamma, or lognormal) for each day of the week. We tested each fitted distribution with a Kolmogorov-Smirnov test for goodness of fit and retained the best-fit model for each surgical subspecialty block day. By solving the block-specific best-fit model for the appropriate ratio of costs, we predicted the level of surgical demand most likely to minimize the costs of underutilization and overutilization. Thus, we predicted the block-specific surgical time allotment most likely to cater to the expected surgical demand while minimizing the cost of operating the block. The fitted probability distributions of the amount of time used by cardiothoracic procedures are shown in Table 19.3, and estimates of savings for the cardiothoracic block under three different cost scenarios are provided in Table 19.4.

Table 19.3 Probability distributions of weekday surgical usage and the minimal cost analysis block time allotment (hours) for cardiothoracic

Weekday	Monday	Tuesday	Wednesday	Thursday	Friday
Distribution	Normal	Normal	Normal	Normal	Normal
No. of days	311	328	328	325	327
No. of cases	1370	1603	1413	1573	1437
KS p value	0.40	0.59	0.99	0.77	0.90
Parameters	$\hat{\mu} = 24.6$ $\hat{\sigma} = 8.9$	$\hat{\mu} = 26.1$ $\hat{\sigma} = 8.4$	$\hat{\mu} = 24.9$ $\hat{\sigma} = 8.7$	$\hat{\mu} = 25.7$ $\hat{\sigma} = 8.2$	$\hat{\mu} = 24.0$ $\hat{\sigma} = 9.1$
Budget percentile	MCA block time (hours)				
50th	24.6	26.1	24.9	25.7	24.0
67th	28.5	29.7	28.7	29.3	27.9
75th	30.7	31.8	30.8	31.3	30.1

Three surgical suites in the block. *KS,* Kolmogorov-Smirnov test for goodness of fit. $\hat{\mu}$ and $\hat{\sigma}$ are the location and scale parameters respectively for the Normal distribution. *MCA,* minimal cost analysis. From Strum DP, Vargas LG, May JH. Surgical subspecialty block utilization and capacity planning: A minimal cost anlysis model. Anesthesiology 90(4); 1999: 1176–85, with permission.

Table 19.4 Minimal cost analysis (MCA) budget estimates, actual costs of operation, and potential savings to be realized if the MCA time allotments were to be implemented

Cardiothoracic		Co = Cu	Co = 2Cu	Co = 3Cu		Utilization (%)
Mondays	MCA budget	$17,997	$20,577	$21,776	Classic	105.4
	Actual cost	$19,524	$23,912	$28,300	Over	28.3
	Savings	7.8%	13.9%	23.1%	Under	22.9
Tuesdays	MCA budget	$18,786	$21,265	$22,578	Classic	107.1
	Actual cost	$19,911	$24,406	$28,901	Over	28.5
	Savings	5.6%	12.9%	21.9%	Under	21.4
Wednesdays	MCA budget	$18,432	$21,101	$22,487	Classic	103.9
	Actual cost	$20,559	$25,751	$30,942	Over	32.6
	Savings	10.3%	18.1%	27.3%	Under	28.7
Thursdays	MCA budget	$18,681	$21,049	$22,312	Classic	106.2
	Actual cost	$20,174	$24,863	$29,551	Over	29.8
	Savings	7.4%	15.3%	24.5%	Under	23.6
Fridays	MCA budget	$17,989	$20,828	$22,293	Classic	102.1
	Actual cost	$19,437	$23,679	$27,921	Over	26.9
	Savings	7.5%	12.0%	20.2%	Under	24.8

Values are daily averages for three surgical suites. Co cost of overutilization, Cu cost of underutilization. $n = 60.388$ surgeries. From Strum DP, Vargas LG, May JH. Surgical subspecialty block utilization and capacity planning: A minimal cost analysis model. Anesthesiology 1999; 90(4):1176–85, with permission

Block scheduling is similar to protection levels in RM, with the difference being that the criterion is not revenue per unit of resource, but cost. Both ways of selecting patients and scheduling them can coexist, provided that a tradeoff is made between the two objectives that, on occasion, may contradict each other.

Scheduling Individual Procedures

Assigning surgical procedures to ORs is analogous to a bin-packing problem (BPP) that has been studied in the operations research/management literature since at least 1974. The objective is to minimize the total number of ORs (bins) required to perform the surgical procedures. Surgical scheduling can be thought about in two ways: online and offline. The latter is performed to create the schedule with which the surgical day starts. The former is used as the schedule evolves because the procedure duration may be unknown and it is represented with a random variable or because the procedures are selected in a first-come, first-served basis without prior scheduling. Here, we deal with offline scheduling of procedures to ORs.

As indicated above, the duration of a surgical procedure is a random variable. To describe the problem, we assume that the duration of a procedure is known. We will estimate it using the model presented in the section above on "Estimating the Duration of Surgical Procedures." Thus, we deal with deterministic offline scheduling. Given a surgical schedule for a given day consisting of n procedures, each of them must be assigned to an OR (bin) from among m possible ORs. The traditional BPP is given by

$$\text{Minimize} \quad F(y) \equiv \sum_{j=1}^{m} y_j$$

$$\text{such that} \quad \sum_{i=1}^{n} a_i x_{ij} - T_{Yj} \leq 0, \; j = 1, 2, \ldots, m$$

$$(\text{BPP}): \quad \sum_{j=1}^{m} x_{ij} = 1, \; i = 1, 2, \ldots, n$$

$$x_{ij} = 0, 1, \; i = 1, 2, \ldots, n, \; j = 1, 2, \ldots, m$$

$$y_i = 0, 1, \; j = 1, 2, \ldots, m$$

An example of a surgical schedule formulated as a BPP is provided in Fig. 19.3.

The current state of knowledge in theoretical computer science supports the contention that an efficient algorithm to solve the BPP exactly does not exist. The BPP is considered to be NP-hard,[37,38] meaning that it is as difficult to solve as a large class of other problems, all of which are believed to not be solvable by efficient algorithms. Because an efficient exact solution method is unlikely, it is of interest to find efficient heuristics, i.e., approximate methods that provide near-optimal solutions[39] and to compute both the average-case and the worst-case performance ratios for those heuristics.[40,41] Coffman et al. provide a comprehensive review of various heuristic algorithms.[38] We have found only one reference that studies their use in a hospital environment.[42]

Operating Room Bin-packing Problem with Overtime Costs

Because the duration of surgical procedures is uncertain and varies due to surgeon experience, type of anesthesia, and other factors,[11] the use of an OR may extend beyond the budgeted time, which is usually 8 hours per day. Depending on the cost of overtime versus regular time, we need to find out when it is efficient to open a new OR or extend those already open into overtime. Allowing overtime is similar to a BPP with variable bin size.[43] A similar problem has been studied by Leung et al.[44] They consider what they call the open-end BPP, in which a bin is assigned an item if the bin has not yet reached a level C or above, but it is closed as soon as it reaches that level.

Our problem with variably sized bins is somewhat different from those mentioned above. Here, considering variable bin sizes leads to the question: Is the amount of

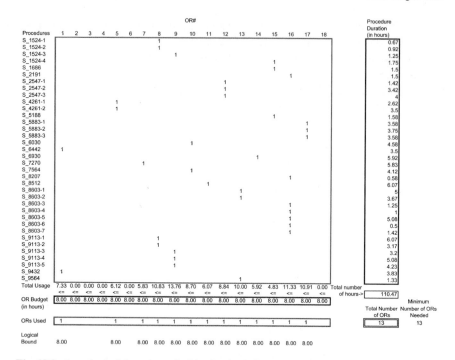

Fig. 19.3 Actual schedule at the end of the day for 01/07/1992. Surgeons' labels are formatted as S_xxxx-y, where S identifies a surgeon, xxxx represents an anonymous surgeon-specific identifier, and y is case specific

overtime cost greater than the cost of opening another OR (bin)? We refer to this new problem as the *BPP with overtime costs* (BPPwOC). The objective function represents the total cost of the bins with overtime:

$$\text{Minimize} \quad G(y,z) \equiv \sum_{j=1}^{m} \left(cy_j + dz_j \right)$$

$$\text{such that} \quad \sum_{i=1}^{n} a_i x_{ij} - z_j - T_j y_j \le 0, \ j = 1, 2, \ldots, m$$

$$(BPPwOC): \quad \sum_{j=1}^{m} x_{ij} = 1, \ i = 1, 2, \ldots, n$$

$$z_j \le [c/d] w_j, \ j = 1, 2, \ldots, m$$

$$y_j \ge w_j, \ j = 1, 2, \ldots, m$$

$$x_{ij} = 0, 1, \ i = 1, 2, \ldots, n, j = 1, 2, \ldots, m$$

$$y_j = 0, 1, \ j = 1, 2, \ldots, m$$

$$w_j = 0, 1, \ j = 1, 2, \ldots, m$$

$$z_j \ge 0, \ j = 1, 2, \ldots, m$$

Consider the OR schedule (see Fig. 19.3) that resulted at the end of the day at a large teaching hospital. It consists of 36 cases performed by 18 surgeons using 18 available ORs. For the purpose of discussion, we assume that all of the cases can be done in any of the 18 available rooms. The actual schedule in this example had 21.1 hours of overtime and 11.9 hours of unused regular time (underutilization). Figure 19.4 shows a Gantt chart of the schedule. This day, the ORs opened at 7:00 a.m. and theoretically would close at 3:00 p.m. Thus, any procedure that starts before 7:00 a.m. or goes beyond 3:00 p.m. is considered to be using overtime.

A solution to the classical BPP for this example, without considering overtime, is shown in Fig. 19.5. The minimal number of ORs without overtime is equal to 14 versus the 13 actually used. Of course, the actual schedule has overtime and inefficiencies, as shown by the amount of unused regular time (Fig. 19.6). To decide which heuristic we should use, we performed a simple experiment, which is detailed in the next section.

Bin-packing Heuristics for Offline Surgical Scheduling with Overtime Costs

It is known that the BPP is an NP-hard problem[37] and that no polynomial-time algorithms are known that produce an optimal packing in every case. However, algorithms are known that produce near-optimal packings.[38,45] They are divided into online and offline algorithms. The construction of a surgical schedule from a set of given surgical requests is done offline. The four well-known algorithms are: first-fit,

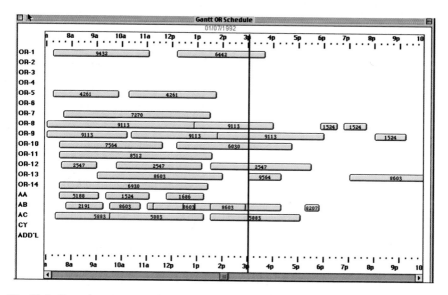

Fig. 19.4 Gantt chart representation of the actual schedule (end of the day, 3:00 p.m.). Numeric labels are anonymous surgeon-specific identifiers

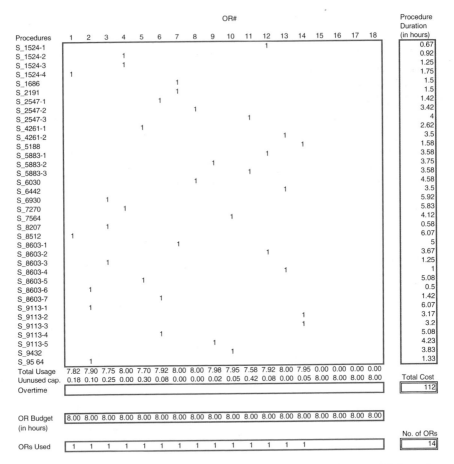

Fig. 19.5 An optimal solution for the classical BPP without overtime. Surgeons labels are formatted S_xxxx-y, where S identifies a surgeon, xxxx represents an anonymous surgeon-specific identifier, and y is case specific

best-fit, next-fit, and worst-fit. The items to be packed are usually ordered in increasing or decreasing size. For a given item:

- *First-fit decreasing/increasing* (FFD/FFI) assigns the item to the first bin in which it fits.
- *Best-fit decreasing/increasing* (BFD/BFI) assigns the item to the bin that leaves the least unused room in it after the assignment, i.e., the best-fit.
- *Worst-fit decreasing/increasing* (WFD/WFI) assigns the item to the bin with the largest capacity.
- *Next-fit decreasing/increasing* (NFD/NFI) only keeps one bin open at a time. It assigns the item to the bin being used at the moment, the opened bin, if there is room; otherwise, the bin is closed and the item is assigned to a newly opened bin.

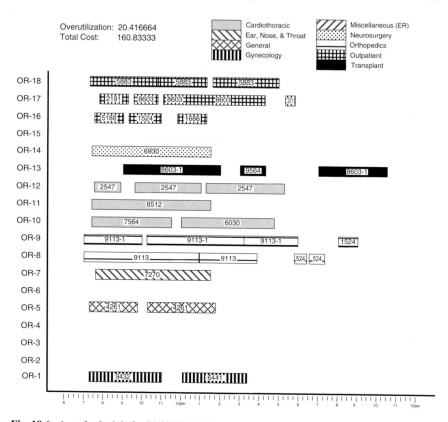

Fig. 19.6 Actual schedule for 01/07/1992. Block-specific surgeries are represented with the same colors. Numeric labels are anonymous surgeon-specific identifiers

The performance of these heuristics is measured by the *worst-case* and the *average-case performance ratios*. The former is given by the ratio of the objective function value that corresponds to the bin-packing heuristic and the objective function value of the optimal solution. The classical BPP has well-known worst-case performance ratio bounds. Johnson showed that the asymptotic worst-case for both FFD and BFD is 11/9.[41] However, performance ratios are not known for the BPP with overtime costs. To estimate the worst-case performance ratio for each of the heuristics mentioned, we sampled and solved BPPs with overtime for surgical schedules from a set of schedules from a large teaching hospital. The database contains daily schedules starting on July 1, 1989, and ending on November 1, 1995. We selected 1 day per month at random, ensuring that the day of the week was not always the same. Thus, for each month starting in July 1989, we selected a total of 76 schedules. Each day was then packed using the four heuristics mentioned, the optimal solution for the integer formulation, and the relaxed problems estimated. As the problem was formulated as an integer programming problem, we cannot be certain

Table 19.5 Heuristics for worst-case performance ratio statistics for the bin-packing problem with overtime costs

	BFD	FFD	NFD	WFD
n	76	76	76	76
Average	1.02113	1.03121	1.13938	1.2729
Standard deviation	0.0256016	0.0328689	0.092736	0.111009
Max	1.08048	1.12053	1.3989	1.68013

$n = 60{,}388$ surgeries. *BFD* best-fit decreasing, *FFD* first-fit decreasing, *NFD* next-fit decreasing, *WFD* worst-fit decreasing

that the optimal solution is the one that we obtained. However, because we also solved the relaxed linear programming problem, we have an idea of how close we could be to the integer optimal solution. The results of this sampling experiment (shown in Table 19.5) were that, on average, the heuristic best-fit decreasing algorithm provides estimates of the solution closest to the optimal integer solution. These heuristics provide an upper bound to BPPwOC.

Overtime is not the only constraint involved in surgical scheduling. In addition to the cost of extending the bins, the starting and the ending times of the procedures must be considered to take into account surgeons' constraints and preferences, including: the surgeons' procedure may not overlap (overlapping constraint), ORs may not be used for some procedures (resource constraint), some procedures must be performed in certain blocks of rooms at specified times (block constraint), some institutions prefer to start the schedule with the longest procedures (preference ordering), etc. Here, we consider only nonoverlapping and preference-ordering constraints.

The Bin-packing Problem with Preference Constraints and Overtime Costs (BP3)

A surgical procedure time is divided into four periods: from arrival until anesthesia ready (T1), positioning (T2), surgical time (T3), and anesthesia emergence time (T4), which implies that when a block of ORs belongs to a surgeon/practice, the surgeon may not be present for the entire surgery. Surgical procedures are allowed to overlap on periods T1 and/or T2 but not on period T3, in which the surgeon(s) are performing the procedure (Fig. 19.7). Thus, for any two procedures i_1 and i_2 either $s_{i_2} > t_{i_1}$ or $s_{i_1} > t_{i_2}$.

Until recently, bin-packing heuristics did not consider constraints on the order in which the items must be packed into the bins (e.g., see the work of Trumbo et al.[46,47]). In surgical scheduling, these constraints result from preference orderings on procedures imposed by surgeon availability. For example, surgeon 1524 in the schedule of Fig. 19.3 performed four procedures. Assuming that he performs the procedures himself, the procedures should take place sequentially. Let $w_{ii'} = 1$ if procedure i must be done before procedure i', and $w_{ii'} = 0$, otherwise. Clearly, $w_{ii'} + w_{i'i} = 1$, for all pairs of procedures i and i'. For any two procedures i and i' for which $w_{ii'} = 1$, we must have $t_i \leq s_{i'}$, i.e., the starting time of procedure i' must be greater than or equal to the ending time of procedure i. Let $xij = 1$ if the ith procedure is assigned

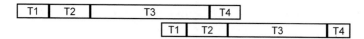

Fig. 19.7 Procedures with nonoverlapping surgical times. T1, time from arrival until anesthesia ready; T2, positioning time; T3, time from incision until surgical closure; T4, emergence time until patient is stable in recovery room

to the jth OR. Overtime is given by $z_j = \max\{\max_{1 \le i \le n}\{t_i x_{ij}\} - T_j, 0\}$. We assume without loss of generality that $a_1 \le a_2 \le \cdots \le a_n$. Incorporating preference and resource constraints to the problem, we have the formulation in (BP3), where the constraints in (1) are preference-ordering constraints; (2) ensures that $y_j = 1$ whenever the room is used; (3) ensures that a procedure is performed in one room only; (4) and (5) are binary conditions; and (6)–(8) are constraints on the overtime.

$$\textit{Minimize} \quad G(y,z) \equiv \sum_{j=1}^{m}\left(cy_j + dz_j\right)$$

$$\textit{such that}$$

$$(1) \quad t_i w_{ii'} \le S_{i'}, i, i' = 1, 2, \ldots, n$$

$$(2) \quad \max\{t_i x_{ij}\} - z_i \le T_j y_j, j = 1, 2, \ldots, m$$

$$(BP3):(3) \quad \sum_{j=1}^{m} x_{ij} = 1, i = 1, 2, \ldots, n$$

$$(4) \quad y_j = 0, 1, j = 1, 2, \ldots, m$$

$$(5) \quad x_{ij} = 0, 1, i = 1, 2, \ldots, n, j = 1, 2, \ldots, m$$

$$(6) \quad z_j \le [c/d] w_j, \quad j = 1, 2, \ldots, m$$

$$(7) \quad y_j \ge w_j, \quad j = 1, 2, \ldots, m$$

$$(8) \quad w_i = 0, 1, z \le 0, \quad j = 1, 2, \ldots, m .$$

Other types of constraints could also be imposed (two procedures i and i' must be performed in the same room, etc.). In that case, not only $w_{ii'} = 1$, but

$$x_i \equiv \sum_{j=1}^{m} j x_{ij} = x_{i'} \equiv \sum_{j=1}^{m} j x_{i'j}.$$

Constraint Programming Formulation

Problems with soft constraints have been the subject of attention in the operations research and computer science literature under the name *constraint programming* (CP).[48,49] Its commonalities with optimization (i.e., search and inference methods to accelerate the search) make CP a suitable methodology to solve this problem. One key distinction between CP and optimization is that CP formulates a problem within a programming language. CP exploits problem structure to direct the search. It relies on logic-based methods such as domain reduction and constraint propagation. Domain reduction uses restrictions on the domain of the variables to deduce that other variables can only take certain values. Constraint propagation is the act of passing the reduced domains of the variables to other constraints until each variable's domain is reduced to a single value and a feasible solution is identified. According to Hooker, "…constraint programming is more effective on 'tightly constrained' problems, and optimization more effective on 'loosely constrained' problems."[49] Following these principles, we formulated the modified BPP as follows. We assume without loss of generality that $T_j = T$ (see definition of T_j above). Let xi be the OR number to which the ith procedure is assigned. Let $z_j \equiv \max\{\max_{\{i|x_i=j\}}\{t_i\} - T, 0\}$ be the overtime created by the assignment of the ith procedure to OR xi. Let y_{x_i} be the variable representing that an OR is in use when a procedure is assigned to it.

$$\text{Minimize} \quad G(y,z) \text{''} \sum_{j=1}^{m}(cy_j + dz_j)$$

such that

(CP1):

(1) $\quad t_i w_{ii'} \le s_{i'}, \quad i, i' = 1, 2, \quad , n$

(2) $\quad t_i - z_{x_i} \le T y_{x_i}, \quad i = 1, 2, \quad , m$

(3) $\quad z_j \le [c/d] w_j, \quad j = 1, 2, \quad , m$

(4) $\quad w_j = 0, 1, \quad j = 1, 2, \quad , m$

(5) $\quad x_i \in \{1, 2, \quad , m\}, \quad i = 1, 2, \quad , n$

(6) $\quad y_j \not{\nmid} w_j, \quad j = 1, 2, \quad , m$

(7) $\quad w_j = 0, 1, \quad j = 1, 2, \quad , m$

(8) $\quad y_j = 0, 1, \quad j = 1, 2, \quad , m$

To implement the BPP with resource and preference constraints (CP1), we developed the following heuristic:

(S1) Determine which surgeons require more than one OR. Let S be the set of surgeons and let $S_{>1}$ be the set of surgeons who require more than one OR.

(S2) For every surgeon $i \in S_{>1}$, create a dummy surgeon i_D. Let S_D be the set of dummy surgeons.

(S3) Solve the following problem (CP2) for the procedures corresponding to the set of surgeons $\bar{S} = \{S - S_{>1}\} \cup S_{>1} \cup S_D$.

Problem CP1 is an NP-hard problem. Thus, a heuristic (HCP1) based on a bin-packing heuristic, taking into account preference and resource constraints, might provide an adequate solution.

HCP1

(S1) Determine which surgeons require more than one OR.

(S2) For every surgeon $i \in S_{>1}$, create a dummy surgeon i_D.

(S3) For each new surgeon, create procedures whose duration equals the sum of the durations of all of the procedures assigned to that surgeon.
(S4) Arrange the new procedures in decreasing order of duration.
(S5) Apply the heuristic best-fit decreasing with overtime costs.

The question remains: How does this heuristic perform?

Application of the Heuristics to Actual Surgical Schedules

As an illustration, consider the schedule shown in Fig. 19.6, which contains 36 procedures and 18 surgeons. Six of the surgeons performed 24 of the 36 surgeries. CP first creates dummy surgeons for those surgeons who could have overlaps and creates dummy procedures with all of those procedures of a given surgeon that need to be done sequentially without overlaps. Procedures are then bin-packed using the best-fit decreasing heuristic with overtime costs to minimize the total cost of the schedule. CP reduced the size of the feasible space by first satisfying resource and preference-ordering constraints, and then optimized the assignment of the remaining procedures. The CP solution is shown in Fig. 19.8.

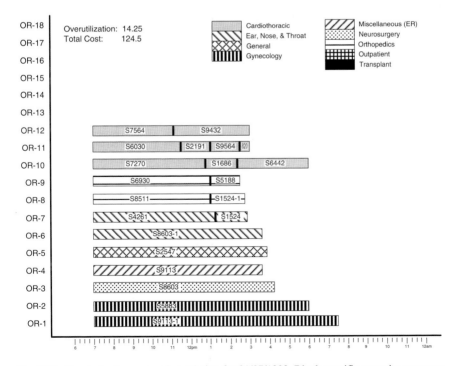

Fig. 19.8 Constrained programming solution for 01/07/1992. Block-specific surgeries are represented with the same patterns. Numeric labels are anonymous surgeon-specific identifiers

Note that even in the case of CP, the amount of overtime in a given OR may be larger than c/d (the ratio of the budgeted time value of an OR and the cost per unit of overtime); in our case, $c/d = 8/2 = 4$ units. This value is due to preference ordering and resource constraints, but when feasible, it will always be less than c/d.

Using the heuristics mentioned, we implemented the schedules in the database for the years 1989–1995. The total cost in hours and the percentage savings are shown in Tables 19.6 and 19.7, respectively.

Note that as constraints are added to the schedule (CP heuristic), the cost of the schedule increases (as would be expected). If rather than using the actual procedure times, the estimates computed in the model presented (in the section concerning "Estimating the Duration of Surgical Procedures") are used, the savings drop by ~5% across all heuristics. Nonetheless, the potential savings are still considerable, illustrating how important it is to accurately predict the length of procedure times. How the procedures are later scheduled has as great an impact on the total cost as does the accuracy of the predictions. Note that we have only depicted heuristics based on preordering the procedures prior to scheduling in decreasing order; i.e., we scheduled longest cases first. Scheduling shortest cases first increases the cost of the schedule (Tables 19.8 and 19.9). Based on these results, we could say that this hospital appears to schedule procedures according to a best-fit increasing

Table 19.6 Actual yearly total costs (h) for various packing heuristics

Year	BFD ($)	FFD ($)	NFD ($)	WFD ($)	CP ($)	Actual ($)
1989	14,146.17	14,154.17	16,560.17	19,606.17	15,152.25	18,759.86
1990	32,029.41	32,038.25	36,179.98	40,536.56	33,857.27	41,989.10
1991	40,830.57	40,839.13	38,426.27	46,901.44	36,366.61	57,299.86
1992	37,013.75	37,020.34	39,293.43	41,937.26	39,213.37	47,933.49
1993	37,809.43	37,812.00	39,132.41	42,166.41	39,869.61	49,150.54
1994	39,168.23	39,174.72	39,321.78	43,065.80	41,590.40	50,554.91
1995	35,006.14	35,010.77	33,688.04	37,484.68	37,218.58	45,326.05

$n = 60,388$ surgeries (1989 results are based on 6 months and not 12 months of data). *BFD* best-fit decreasing, *FFD* first-fit decreasing, *NFD* next-fit decreasing, *WFD* worst-fit decreasing

Table 19.7 Percentage savings with respect to the actual costs

Year	BFD (%)	FFD (%)	NFD (%)	WFD (%)	CP (%)
1989	24.59	24.55	11.73	−4.51	19.23
1990	23.72	23.70	13.83	3.46	19.37
1991	28.74	28.73	32.94	18.15	36.53
1992	22.78	22.77	18.03	12.51	18.19
1993	23.07	23.07	20.38	14.21	18.88
1994	22.52	22.51	22.22	14.81	17.73
1995	22.77	22.76	25.68	17.30	17.89

$n = 60,388$ surgeries. *BFD* best-fit decreasing, *FFD* first-fit decreasing, *NFD* next-fit decreasing, *WFD* worst-fit decreasing, *CP* constraint programming

Table 19.8 Costs for heuristics based on shortest cases first

Year	BFI ($)	FFI ($)	NFI ($)	WFI ($)	CP ($)	Actual ($)
1989	17,147.17	17,147.17	17,147.17	21,398.36	15,152.25	18,759.86
1990	38,907.59	38,907.59	38,907.59	45,846.08	33,857.27	41,989.10
1991	50,263.59	50,263.59	42,400.52	47,143.52	36,366.61	57,299.86
1992	46,947.86	46,947.86	46,947.86	50,494.10	39,213.37	47,933.49
1993	48,198.51	48,198.51	48,198.51	51,301.69	39,869.61	49,150.54
1994	50,438.83	50,438.83	50,438.83	52,795.17	41,590.40	50,554.91
1995	45,412.20	45,412.20	45,412.20	46,785.94	37,218.58	45,326.05

$n = 60{,}388$ surgeries. *BFI* best-fit increasing, *FFI* first-fit increasing, *NFI* next-fit increasing, *WFI* worst-fit increasing, *CP* constraint programming

Table 19.9 Percentage of savings for heuristics based on shortest cases first

Year	BFI (%)	FFI (%)	NFI (%)	WFI (%)	CP (%)
1989	8.60	8.60	8.60	−14.06	19.23
1990	7.34	7.34	7.34	−9.19	19.37
1991	12.28	12.28	26.00	17.72	36.53
1992	2.06	2.06	2.06	−5.34	18.19
1993	1.94	1.94	1.94	−4.38	18.88
1994	0.23	0.23	0.23	−4.43	17.73
1995	−0.19	−0.19	−0.19	−3.22	17.89

$n = 60{,}388$ surgeries. *BFI* best-fit increasing, *FFI* first-fit increasing, *NFI* next-fit increasing, *WFI* worst-fit increasing, *CP* constraint programming

methodology, which is more advantageous to patients, as scheduling shortest procedures first will minimize the average waiting time of the patients.

Conclusion

The classic definition of OR utilization is the ratio of the total OR time used to the total OR time allocated or budgeted.[4,5] While medical centers operate surgical services (excluding emergency patient care) at an estimated 50%–60% utilization rate, managers generally recognize that ORs could be at least 80% utilized in the care of elective surgical patients. They also agree that the additional 15%–20% gain in OR utilization will require a real-time communications and resource-coordination system (Fig. 19.9). The main objectives of such a system should be:

- Collect and make available site-specific information generated by the work process (e.g., the preoperative checklist from same-day services) to other units of surgical services. As a result, patient management decisions can be based on an appreciation of the overall hospital situation, which should improve the reactive coordination of personnel, space, and equipment.
- Seek an unobtrusive, reliable, and *accurate* method of recording surgical services *utilization* data for analysis and subsequent predictive scheduling of hospital resources, including personnel, space, and equipment.

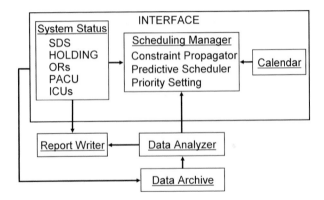

Fig. 19.9 Components of a surgical-scheduling and capacity-planning system

- Improve the quality and reliability of data by automating data collection.
- Empower healthcare providers by returning locally generated data to the healthcare providers who use it.
- Improve time management and operational efficiency of key healthcare professionals and administrators involved in the delivery of surgical services.
- Document surgical diagnosis and procedures perioperatively as an objective basis for total quality improvement procedures.
- Help to explore the impact of improved communications on the evolution and maintenance of surgical culture.

All of these objectives require an accurate prediction of the duration of surgical procedures, selection of patients to form part of a daily schedule, scheduling of the procedures, and measurement of the schedule outcomes.

References

1. AHA. Ambulatory Surgery. *Trendlines*. Society for Ambulatory Care Professionals, 1994
2. AHRQ. AHRQ data show rising hospital charges, falling hospital stays. AHRQ Res Activities 2002; 266(Oct):21–2
3. Wickizer TM. Effect of hospital utilization review on medical expenditures in selected diagnostic areas: An exploratory study. Am J Public Health 1991; 81:482–4
4. Mangano DT. Perioperative Medicine: NHLBI Working Group Deliberations and Recommendations. J Cardiothor Vasc Anesth 2004; 18(1):1–6
5. Hospital Statistics: The Comprehensive Reference Source for Analysis and Comparison of Hospital Trends. Health Forum, ed. Chicago, IL: American Hospital Association, 2002
6. Stewart JT. Surgical specialties affect scheduling. Hospitals 1971; 17:132–6
7. Gabel RA, Kulli JC, Lee BS, et al. *Operating Room Management*. Oxford, UK: Butterworth and Heinemann, 1999
8. Hancock WM, Isken MW. Patient-scheduling methodologies. J Soc Health Syst 1992; 3:1083–6
9. May JH, Strum DP, Vargas LG. Fitting the lognormal distribution to surgical procedure times. Decision Sci 2000; 31(1):129–48

10. Strum DP, May JH, Sampson AR, et al. Individual surgeon variability is a multiplicative function of surgical time. Anesth Analg 1999; 88(2S):Suppl: 48S
11. Strum DP, May JH, Sampson AR, et al. Surgeon and type of anesthesia predicts surgical variability and affects the scheduling of surgery. Anesthesiology 2000; 92(5):1454–66
12. Dexter F, Macario A, Traub RD, et al. An operating room scheduling strategy to maximize the use of operating room block time: Computer simulation of patient scheduling and survey of patients' preferences for surgical waiting time. Anesth Analg 1999; 89(1):7–20
13. Blake JT, Dexter F, Donald J. Operating room managers' use of integer programming for assigning block time to surgical groups: A case study. Anesth Analg 2002; 94(1):143–8
14. Blake JT, Donald J. Mount Sinai hospital uses integer programming to allocate operating room time. Interfaces 2002; 32(2):66–73
15. Dexter F, Macario A. Changing allocations of operating room time from a system based on historical utilization to one where the aim is to schedule as many surgical cases as possible. Anesth Analg 2002; 94(5):1272–9
16. Dexter F, Macario A, Traub RD. Which algorithm for scheduling add-on elective cases maximizes operating room utilization? Use of bin packing algorithms and fuzzy constraints in operating room management. Anesthesiology 1999; 91(5):1491–500
17. Rossiter CE, Reynolds JA. Automatic monitoring of the time waited in out-patient departments. Med Care 1963; 1:218–25
18. Barnoon S, Wolfe H. Scheduling a multiple operating room system: A simulation approach. Health Serv Res 1968; 3(4):272–85
19. Dexter F. Application of prediction levels to OR scheduling. AORN J 1996; 63(3):1–8
20. Hancock WM, Walter PF, More RA, et al. Operating room scheduling data base analysis for scheduling. J Med Syst 1988; 12:397–409
21. Robb DJ, Silver EA. Scheduling in a management context: Uncertain processing times and non-regular performance measures. Decision Sci 1996; 6(24):1085–106
22. Spangler WE, May JH, Strum DP, et al. A data mining approach to characterizing medical code usage patterns. J Med Syst 2002; 26(3):255–75
23. Strum DP, May JH, Sampson AR, et al. Estimating times of surgeries with two component procedures: Comparison of the lognormal and normal models. Anesthesiology 2003; 98(1):232–40
24. Talluri KT, Van Ryzin GJ. The Theory and Practice of Revenue Management. New York: Springer/Business Media, 2004
25. Belobaba PP. Application of a probabilistic decision model to airline seat inventory control. Oper Res 1989; 37(2):183–97
26. Chapman SN, Carmel JI. Demand/capacity management in health care: An application of yield management. Health Care Manage Rev 1992; 17(4):45–55
27. Green L, Savin S, Wang B. Managing patient service in a diagnostic medical facility. Oper Res 2006; 54(1):11–25
28. Gerchak Y, Gupta D, Henig M. Reservation planning for elective surgery under uncertain demand for emergency surgery. Manage Sci 1996; 42:321–34
29. Born C, Carbajal M, Smith P, et al. Contract optimization at Texas Children's Hospital. Interfaces 2004; 34(1):51–8
30. Everett JE. A decision support simulation model for the management of an elective surgery waiting system. Health Care Manage Sci 2002; 5:89–95
31. Lowery JC. Design of hospital admissions scheduling system using simulation. Proceedings of the 1996 Winter Simulation Conference 1996:1199–204
32. Ivaldi E, Tanfani E, Testi A. Simulation supporting the management of surgical waiting lists. Discussion Paper della Sezione di Economica Politica e Studi Economici Internazionali, 2003
33. Littlewood, K. Forecasting and control of passenger bookings. J Revenue Pricing Manage 2005; 4:111–23
34. Vargas LG, May JH, Stanciu A. Revenue management with random resource requirements. 2008 (in preparation)

35. Voss SJ. Ambulatory surgery scheduling: Assuring a smooth patient flow. AORN J 1986; 43(5):1009–12
36. Strum DP, Vargas LG, May JH, et al. Surgical suite utilization and capacity planning: A minimal cost analysis model. J Med Syst 1997; 21(5):309–22
37. Johnson DS. Fast algorithms for bin-packing. J Comput Syst Sci 1974; 8:272–314
38. Coffman EG, Garey MR, Johnson DS. Approximation algorithms for bin packing: A survey. In: Hochbaum D, ed. *Approximation Algorithms for NP-Hard Problems*. Boston, MA: PWS, 1997:46–93
39. Scholl A, Klein R, Jurgens C. BISON: A fast hybrid procedure for exactly solving the one-dimensional bin packing problem. Comput Oper Res 1997; 24(7):627–45
40. Johnson DS. Near-optimal bin-packing algorithms, in electrical engineering. Doctoral Dissertation. Massachusetts Institute of Technology, Cambridge, MA, 1974
41. Johnson DS, Demers AJ, Ullman JD, et al. Worst-case performance bounds for simple one-dimensional packing algorithms. SIAM J Comput 1974; 3:299–326
42. Kennedy MH. *Bin-Packing, Knapsack, and Chance-Constrained Approaches to Operating Room Scheduling*. Troy, NY: Rensselaer Polytechnic Institute, 1992
43. Dell'Olmo P, Kellerer H, Speranza MG, et al. A 13/12 approximation algorithm for bin-packing with extendable bins. Inform Process Lett 1998; 65(5):229–33
44. Leung JY-T, Dror M, Young GH. A note on an open-end bin packing problem. J Scheduling 2001; 4:201–7
45. Fleszar K, Hindi KS. New heuristics for one-dimensional bin-packing. Comput Oper Res 2002; 29:821–39
46. Trumbo M, Lee HS, Knoth B. *A Constrained Bin-Packing Problem*. Yorktown Heights, NY: IBM TJ Watson Research Center, 1996:13
47. Lee HS, Trumbo M. *An Approximate 0–1 Edge-labeling Algorithm for Constrained Bin-packing Problem*. Yorktown Heights, NY: IBM TJ Watson Research Center, 1997:6
48. Lustig IJ, Puget J-F. Program does not equal program: Constraint programming and its relationship to mathematical programming. Interfaces 2001; 31(6):29–53
49. Hooker JN. Logic, optimization and constraint programming. Informs J Comput 2002; 12(4):295–321

Part C
Mobile Computing, Education, and Simulation

Communication Case Scenario

Dr. Schwartz, the chair of the department of anesthesiology at Greater Metropolitan, a large community hospital, and president of the practice group, recently conducted an investigation of an incident that occurred at Greater Metropolitan. One of the partners was transporting a patient to the ICU while also supervising a CRNA in another OR. Although the CRNA in the room paged the anesthesiologist several times, he claimed that he never received the call. Over the course of this investigation, Dr. Schwartz identified lapses in communication to be the root cause of this and several anesthetic complications that had occurred over the preceding year. In response to this problem, the members of the group decided to purchase a new communication system that provides instantaneous contact between any two staff members.

The anesthesiologists identified the requirements for their new communication system, the most important of which were high reliability, continuous availability, ease of use, and confidentiality of protected health information. They also wanted automatic notification of abnormal laboratory values and, ideally, wanted to be notified if a monitor were to generate certain critical alarms. With no windows, the ORs were located in the interior of the building. As a result, cellular telephone service was nonexistent in the ORs; it was therefore necessary to install antennas throughout the area. As Greater Metropolitan was in a coastal city, it was also important that the system work during power or telephone outages that may occur during a hurricane. The group intended to evaluate voice-over-IP (VoIP) technology, handheld radios, text-messaging systems that use wireless Ethernet, and cellular telephones.

The group contacted several cellular telephone providers. Each company offered discounts if every member of the group became a subscriber and even larger discounts if the hospital agreed to use their services. One provider offered to set up a repeater with an antenna on the roof of the building that would point to a base station, an amplifier, and antennas throughout the OR and would provide seamless coverage.

Two other providers offered to put a dedicated cellular base station in the OR, a configuration that would also provide seamless coverage. As an added benefit, the base station could direct each user's mobile telephone to use the lowest power setting, saving battery power and minimizing the already low risk of interference with electronic patient-care equipment.

One provider developed mobile cellular stations that were powered by generators and could be brought into place by truck after a storm or other disaster. The same company offered a "walkie talkie" service that would allow any member of the group to contact any other member by pushing a button. The anesthesia group decided to choose this company to provide communication services. Greater Metropolitan already had an AIMS in place and was working with the developer of that system and an outside consultant to create an automatic paging system that would be activated by specific alarm conditions and that would allow the CRNA to page the supervising anesthesiologist by pressing a button on the AIMS.

The anesthesia group was proactive and brought the hospital administration into the negotiations with the cellular service provider. Physicians with privileges at the hospital were encouraged to use the hospital's cellular service provider in exchange for improved coverage inside the hospital and a significant discount. The anesthesiologists received immediate benefits from switching to cellular telephones: The partners could respond to situations almost immediately and were much more comfortable leaving the OR to attend to other duties. The nursing staff noticed that their calls were answered much more quickly, and the quality assurance department noticed fewer errors in patient care. Greater Metropolitan's IT department developed a module for their laboratory system that automatically sent text messages for abnormal laboratory results to responsible personnel. As a result of this improved communication system, the quality assurance department noticed that the time required to initiate treatment of abnormal laboratory values dropped significantly.

Shortly after the system was installed, high winds and a thunderstorm caused severe, widespread power outages that disrupted nearly every aspect of patient care at a hospital across town. However, the cellular service at Greater Metropolitan and among the community physicians continued without any problems, and business continued as usual.

Chapter 20
Information Technology in Anesthesia Education

Viji Kurup and Keith J.Ruskin

The changing face of healthcare, along with changing expectations from residents with respect to the quality of education that they receive, has challenged residency programs, to rethink the model that they use and develop new strategies with consideration of the new environment. Furthermore, the volume of information in the medical field is growing exponentially; every year, more than two million scientific papers are published in biomedical journals, and more than seven million pages of information are added to the World Wide Web everyday. Keeping pace with the volume demands the introduction of innovative methods in learning, teaching, and assessing medical professionals.[1,2]

The patient population of today is sicker than those of the past, and it is not sufficient for a healthcare professional to rely solely on textbooks to stay current with the field. Further, the focus on evidence-based medicine has highlighted the need for healthcare providers to keep current with the literature and have access to the latest trends in patient care. As information technology has touched almost every aspect of life at the turn of the millennium, the healthcare profession is no exception. This chapter will discuss the various aspects of technology that have been used in medicine, with particular emphasis on residency training in anesthesia.

As early as the 1980s, the drive to integrate computers into medical education was gaining momentum, and the disconnect between the use of technologic advances in the clinical versus the educational field was highlighted.[3] Numerous studies have shown that traditional lecture formats are ineffective teaching tools.[4] The report "Assessing Change in Medical Education: The Road to Implementation" emphasized that medical students must be given a strong grounding in the use of computer technology to manage information, support patient-care decisions, select treatments, and develop their abilities as lifelong learners.[5]

An essential component of facilitating learning is to understand the learners—a population that has changed over the years. The learners of today are exposed to computers from an early age; even young children can produce three-dimensional computer images with easy-to-use software. They have grown used to assimilating

J. Stonemetz, K. Ruskin (eds.) *Anesthesia Informatics*,
© Springer Science+Business Media, LLC 2008

knowledge with animation. A number of terms are used to describe the present generation, among which are "Generation X" for those born between 1965 and 1976 and "The Millennials" for those born between 1977 and 1998, although the dates change depending on the source. The Millennials have always had technology as part of their lives. They are described as being tech savvy and media saturated. A vast majority of them use the Internet for schoolwork, and email and instant messaging are natural communication and socialization mechanisms. Multitasking is a way of life, and staying connected is essential to them. They grew up facing time pressures that were traditionally reserved for adults. They are very family centered and do not typically regard their jobs with the same measure of loyalty historically shown by their parents. Instead, they are driven by goals and achievements. They work well in teams, but are focused on their own personal development. They have a strong desire for immediacy and zero tolerance for delays. They have little fear of authority. Understanding this generation and developing programs and curricula that suit their needs and values are key to attracting this group of students. Many teachers who did not use computers during their education are not as familiar with new technologies; therefore, a disconnect occurs between the teachers and learners. It is important for institutions to understand this issue if they want to attract the best and the brightest to their institution. Students actively compare programs at interviews and make decisions based on the values that they think are important to them. Many institutions now have online chat tools that respond to queries of students in real time. Furthermore, the profession has come a long way from the apprenticeship-based model for training physicians. Today, patient care is delivered by teams of specialized providers in a complex healthcare system, and training models must be adjusted to conform to this new reality.

E-Learning

E-learning refers to the use of Internet technologies to enhance knowledge. The term *e-learning* encompasses the use of computers and networks in education, providing online course administration, online course information, and online communication.[6] It is also referred to by other terms: *online learning*, *computer-assisted learning*, or *Web-based learning*. Simply conducting searches or reading literature on the Web does not constitute e-learning. E-learning involves a virtual classroom with students and a tutor(s), educational modules with rich multimedia teaching files, and some method of interaction and feedback between the tutors and students. This method puts the learner in charge of his own education. He can control the pace, timeliness, content, and sequence of learning.[7] By using rich multimedia content, the learner becomes an active participant in the learning. E-learners have demonstrated increased retention rates and better utilization of content.[8] Studies designed to assess the role of technology in academic achievement have shown that it has a positive effect in teaching complex problem-solving skills but a negative effect when used for low-order thinking skills.

The number of residency programs that use computer-aided instruction has grown over the past few years, and several methods have been tried and tested. Interactive tutorials using hypertext and links that allow students to customize their learning have become very popular. Proponents of computer-aided instruction believe that student learning is enhanced when complex information is presented in multiple formats. A meta-analysis demonstrated that students' achievements were positively influenced by visuals (pictures, illustrations, etc.) and that they facilitate superior recall of information.[9] Models that help the student manipulate variables and observe the outcomes of physiologic processes (e.g., drug kinetics and hormone regulation) are in use, as well as interactive simulations that present case-based scenarios or artificial environments. A meta-analysis of Continuing Medical Education (CME) programs that use traditional didactics versus interactive instruction versus mixed instruction showed that didactic sessions are not an effective method by which to change physician performance.[4] Italy is leading the way in e-learning, with the Italian Society for Anesthesia and ICU establishing a task force to promote the use of e-learning in anesthesia.[6]

In the US, a growing number of institutions use *course-management software* in training anesthesia residents. Most systems are Web based to facilitate "anytime, any place, any pace" access to learning content and administration. Educators can use course-management systems such as Blackboard for a wide variety of activities, including designing the curriculum and posting the syllabus, required reading, and interesting articles or videos. Periodic tests can be administered, and residents can be evaluated serially. These systems can be used to track resident activity, gear programs to resident interests, and generate statistics on the use of the various modules by residents. Because the curriculum is posted in electronic form, it can be adapted quickly and efficiently to reflect changes in current recommendations and guidelines on specific topics. The Web-based software can be accessed even when residents are on rotations outside the main hospital and can be used to send emails to groups of residents based on the current rotation schedule. Residents can be polled on important topics by using the survey feature. The discussion forum can be used to stimulate conversation on controversial topics. Journal clubs can be managed using this software, as the articles in previous sessions can be easily archived. Articles for current sessions can be circulated easily using email communication. Registration for meetings can be conducted electronically. A growing number of residency programs (e.g., Duke University, Boston University, and Yale University) are integrating this technology into their resident education programs. The content varies depending on the institution. *Blackboard* and *WebCT* are the two leading course-management systems in use today. The merger of the two companies recently resulted in their supporting more than 3650 clients in close to 60 countries worldwide. *Moodle*, a free open-source course-management system, is also gaining popularity among educators. The material on these sites can be password protected and individualized to each rotation.

The learning-management systems have some drawbacks that must be weighed against their advantages. Although they are often viewed as being the focal point of an e-learning program, much of the learning that takes place in medical education programs occurs in informal settings, and interaction with experienced practitioners remains an essential part of the learning process. Social tools such as networking and interactions between the learners and teachers are essential components of the entire learning experience, and *blogs* and *wikis* can be used to augment the learning experience. Use of a learning-management system is ideal when content delivery is important. Web conferencing, workshops, or discussion forums are better options when the study of a topic requires hands-on application or expert opinion. In short, for optimum results, the tools used should match the outcome desired and the material being taught.

Personal Digital Assistants

In most cases, traditional methods of learning such as textbooks and journals cannot be relied upon to provide information at the point of care. As a result, two-thirds of questions that arise in clinical practice are never answered, and resulting medical errors put an enormous burden on the healthcare industry. One method by which to deliver information for reference at the point of care is the personal digital assistant (PDA), and these devices have become ubiquitous in the medical field within the past decade. Critical information such as anesthetic implications of certain rare conditions and interactions of drugs with anesthetics are immediately available. PDA versions of textbooks such as *Clinical Anesthesia* and *The Manual of Anesthesia Practice* are available for ready reference. With the advance of wireless computing technologies, PDAs can be used to access the Internet from within the OR and make available the vast collection of resources on the Web. Services such as *Avantgo* (http://www.avantgo.com) deliver personalized content and applications to the PDA. Many residents use programs such as *ePocrates* (http://www.epocrates.com) as a reference tool for pharmaceutical agents. *Unbound Central* (http://www.unbound-medicine.com) is another commercial enterprise that has a comprehensive wireless product (Anesthesia Central) for anesthesiologists, which comprises the *Manual of Anesthesia Practice, Pocket ICU Management, Davis's Drug Guide, Pocket Guide to Diagnostic Tests*, and Medline. The Medline feature allows the user to track topics of interest in leading journals and to search the medical literature from a PDA. *The Journal Browser* delivers tables of contents and abstracts from the latest journal issues to a handheld device on synchronization. It is also possible to sync to the full-text article if it is of interest. It allows search of the database of 11 million journal articles at the bedside. With each of these resources, attention must be paid to their instructions for download and their system requirements for optimal function.

The World Wide Web and Quality Control

The World Wide Web has had a major impact on access to information.[10] More and more physicians are turning to the Web for medical information, especially with their limited time. Search engines (e.g., Google and Yahoo!) are being used by both physicians and patients to search for information. According to the Pew Internet American Life project, 80% of Americans who access the Internet (113 million people) look for health and medical information, and 66% of European adults turn to the Internet for health advice.[11] It has been reported that eight million American adults searched for information on at least one health topic on a typical day, a finding that places health searches at the same level of popularity as paying bills online, reading blogs, or searching for phone numbers or addresses. Worrisome, however, is that most of these individuals do not check the source or date of the health information that they find.[12,13]

Quality control of the information that is available on the Internet is a major concern, as the lay public and, to some extent, medical professionals assume that any information placed there is valid and accurate. With more than 100,000 health-related Web sites, the quality of information available varies greatly. Information sources range from peer-reviewed medical journals and not-for-profit physician organizations to commercial sites, Web blogs, and Wikipedia entries. The real problem is that anyone with access to a Web server can add content to the Internet, without peer review to filter out inaccurate information. In an observational study that assessed a medical librarian's search of the World Wide Web to find Web sites applicable to a clinical question, 69% of retrieved Web pages did not indicate an author and 80% did not give the authors' credentials.[14] While Internet search engines are easy and convenient to use, they are probably not the best place for clinicians to seek medical information. A wide range of tools has been developed to assist site developers to produce good-quality sites and to help consumers to assess the quality of sites. These tools usually look at the codes of conduct, quality labels, user guides, filters, and third-party certifications.[15] Filtering tools such as OMNI provide a gateway to evaluated, quality resources in health and medicine. Third-party certification is the most advanced approach for quality rating because a third party provides a label as a result of its own investigation and certifies that the site complies with quality criteria. Such organizations as *Medcertain* (http://www.medcertain.org) and URAC (Utilization Review Accreditation Commission, http://www.urac.org) are running pilot programs for formal accreditation of Web sites.[15] Rating sites such as *Netscoring* evaluate Internet medical Web sites and include scores for transparency, design, and accuracy of the medical content.[16,17] Residents should be educated regarding the pitfalls of accessing information from unreliable sources and should be given the tools to formulate good search strategies and critically evaluate the information that is available on the Internet.

Podcasting

Podcasting is gaining popularity as a media for distributing information, and physicians are rapidly adopting this technology as a means of staying current with CME while they are on the go. Podcasts of medical information allow busy physicians to listen to materials of interest while they exercise, perform household chores, and even drive (while observing traffic rules, of course!). A *podcast* is a media file that is distributed over the Internet using syndication feeds for playback on computers or mobile audio players. The term is an amalgamation of two words: *iPod*, the ubiquitous Apple MP3 audio file player, and *broadcasting*. The term is misleading, as an iPod is not required to listen to these files; they can be heard on any mobile audio player or even a computer. In 2005, the *Oxford American English Dictionary* proclaimed *podcasting* its Word of the Year. The host or author of a program is commonly called a *podcaster*.

A podcast can be created with the use of a computer and a high-quality microphone. The content provider posts the feed on a Web server. The user, with the help of software known as an *aggregator* (e.g., iTunes), copies the link to an RSS (Really Simple Syndication) feed, and the podcast is then downloaded to a personal computer or mobile player. Subscribing to podcasts allows one to collect programs from a variety of sources for listening or viewing offline at a convenient time and place. The podcaster chooses which program files to offer; the subscriber chooses among them based on her interests and preferences. The podcast is then saved to a portable device and can be listened to at any time.

Schools and colleges use podcasts to deliver lectures to their students; podcasts are also used for audio tours at museums, distribution of public-safety messages, self-guided walking tours at places of interest, and as part of interactive multimedia files for teaching. This technology allows learners to set their own pace for learning. In anesthesia residencies, lectures and other educational content lend themselves to being converted to audio files. Podcasts also allow repetition of materials for study and allow learners to individualize the learning process. Video podcasts can be used for lectures associated with visual material. The Web site of the University of St. Louis contains educational material for anesthesia residents (http://www.anesthesiapodcast.com), allowing students to view the material at a time and place of their choosing rather than at a scheduled lecture. A number of medical journals, including the *New England Journal of Medicine*, the *Journal of the American Medical Association*, and *The Lancet*, provide podcasts of summaries of major articles in each issue. Subscriptions to most of these podcasts are free through the iTunes Web site. A number of commercial products such as *Digiscript* (http://www.digiscript.com) allow audio and video files to be captured, transcribed, and delivered for on-demand learning.

Discussion Groups

Global sharing of knowledge is also possible by participation in *discussion groups*, also called *discussion boards* (e.g., the Anesthesiology Discussion group), which provide interactive informal platforms for discussing current relevant topics.[18] Increasing numbers of educational courses at all levels (formal and informal, graduate, undergraduate, and even high school and elementary school) revolve around

Web-based discussion groups. Content development is the most labor-intensive part of designing a course. Conservative estimates of the time required to develop rich, multimedia-based content ranges from 30 to 100 hours for 1 hour of material. Hundreds of teachers in different parts of the world are "reinventing the wheel" each day by producing curricula and content that are shared by their own students only. Global sharing of content should be encouraged, and free flow of information will allow students around the world to access material that they would otherwise not have. It is essential to comply with applicable copyright laws and to credit sources when sharing programs that are created by multiple individuals. A new world of cooperative enterprise and mass innovation can be a reality if all teachers work with the common goal of creating an appropriate multisensory environment for learners.

Topics in these discussion boards include questions and comments about scientific, clinical, administrative, and regulatory issues, and different approaches to a problem in different places can be discussed. These groups also allow people with similar interests in different and possibly remote locations to partner in research, education, and administrative initiatives. With specialists in diverse topics in different parts of the world, discussion boards can cut across time zones and international boundaries. Knowledge sharing is easier and more convenient if participants can contribute at times that are most convenient to their schedules. Information from discussion groups should be used with caution when making decisions that affect patient care because these discussions are not peer reviewed and represent opinions of individual healthcare providers.

"Virtual meetings" are now common and relatively inexpensive to hold. Software such as *Microsoft NetMeeting* can be used to allow one or more participants in remote locations to communicate, attend case conferences, and share expert opinions and information with developing nations.[19] Internet-based CME courses are gaining popularity due to the advantages of convenience and lower cost. They are becoming more interactive, with multimedia formats being used to suit individual preferences. With the ubiquitous use of computers and availability of the Internet, the use of this forum will grow, and it may become an important medium of communication between different areas of the world.

Library Liaisons

Medical professionals are not formally educated in information-seeking strategies that optimize their ability to obtain relevant information. For anesthesiologists, as for other specialties, finding relevant, accurate, and timely information is important. Increasingly, hospitals are turning to medical librarians to fill this gap. Librarians have traditionally been regarded as the experts in information access and retrieval, and they help clinicians to navigate the multitude of electronic resources available to them. More and more libraries now have liaisons to different hospital departments. Clinical medical librarian programs began 30 years ago to meet the need for clinicians to keep pace with new technology and sophisticated means of information transfer in an effort to provide the best possible care to their patients. Today, clinical medical librarians collaborate with clinical teams to promote problem-based learning and evidence-based medical training,[20] improve patient care,[21] and promote time saving for the healthcare team.[22] No other specialty in medicine is so intertwined with technology as the specialty of anesthesia. Having a librarian available to the perioperative team can be beneficial in dealing with problems of "information overload" and navigating the numerous electronic and other resources.[13]

Librarians in the perioperative setting can work with clinical teams and train them to use information sources and other information-management software. Information retrieval requires knowledge of how information is indexed within various databases. Training residents in strategies for searching databases and the proper use of use bibliographic citation management software can result in a tremendous saving of time and effort. Librarians can also serve as a resource in educating medical students/residents by making them aware of new education resources (e.g., course-management programs such as Blackboard) and new social networking tools (e.g., podcasting) and helping them to set up discussion boards or forums and collaborative work tools. In some institutions, librarians collaborate with anesthesiologists to create customized Web sites and other types of information resources designed specifically for their needs.[13]

Librarians are trained to work with information vendors to arrange for trials of useful resources and databases and customize these resources to best suit the needs of the clinical teams with whom they work. They can also spend time negotiating licenses for these products and handle login and access issues to streamline their use by physicians and staff. Familiarity with the use of saving search strategies and organizing RSS feeds and email alerting services on topics of interest help to keep anesthesiologists up to date. Residency programs must take appropriate steps to raise the awareness of sources of evidence, direct users to the best resources for their information needs, help them critically appraise the literature, inform them regarding intellectual property issues, and supply them with appropriate copyright information.[23,24]

Over the last 15 years, American schools have increased spending on classroom technology to more than $5 billion annually. Several organizations (e.g., Edutopia, The North Central Educational Lab) are documenting research that links technology to increases in academic achievement. Medical schools spend considerable amounts of their budget on information technology. According to a 2002 survey of the Association of American Medical Colleges, the median expenditure at a medical school on information technology was $5.5 million. A survey of these schools in 2006 showed that more than 90% of them had wireless access and used online course material and online teaching evaluations in their medical education. Most medical schools have the infrastructure and support, but residency programs are underutilizing these resources. Both in the US and UK, regular Internet use by physicians has increased exponentially. Traditionally, textbooks, journals, and discussions with colleagues were used to gain information at the point of care. Currently, the Internet is used to access information, and the MEDLINE and Cochrane databases and others are used to answer clinical questions by residents and faculty alike.

In the developing world, students had largely been disadvantaged due to the prohibitive high price of computers and software. However, laptops that cost less than $100 each have now been released in the developing world. They can be powered by numerous alternative power sources, including a pull cord, solar panel, or solar-powered multibattery charger. They use less than 1 W of power when in use as an e-book and can operate for more than 12 hours on their batteries. Most of them have been sold with either Linux-type, open-source operating systems, or a free Linux operating system can be downloaded onto them.

Conclusion

Computers and computer-based education continue to innovate the way we teach and learn, and information technology continues to gain predominance in clinical medicine. Although academic medicine adopted the rapidly changing technology fairly quickly to improve patient care in the clinical arena, the field had not done so with the same flexibility and passion in the area of medical education. The learners who have grown up with computers are comfortable with and proficient in using them; however, most teachers are not as computer savvy. This divide must be bridged so that those doing the teaching and evaluating can attain the same proficiency as the learners and understand and utilize methods that they use. Well-designed studies should be conducted with these novel methods of instruction to scientifically ascertain whether their use is effective and efficient for medical education. If so, the goal should be to create the optimal environment in which learners can explore and assimilate relevant information and grow into enthusiastic lifelong self-learners.

In addition to the resources already mentioned, readers are referred to the following very useful educational sites (a) http://www.theanswerpage.com, (b) http://www.mypatient.com, (c) http://www.nysora.com, and (d) http://www.anesthesiapodcast.com.

Key Points

- With the rapidly growing volume of medical information and the increasing complexity of the medical environment, physicians must adapt new strategies to keep pace with the information they need to provide the best clinical care.
- Residents and young physicians use different learning strategies than older physicians. Didactic teaching is not the most efficient method of transferring information to this group.
- E-learning is the use of Internet technology to enhance the teaching experience. Each participant determines his own goals and the structure and pace of the lesson.

- Course-management software can be used to create lessons, post a syllabus, and administer tests. The use of Web-based software allows physicians to participate even when they are assigned to outside clinics or hospitals.
- E-learning must be interactive to be effective. Blogs and wikis can be used to provide social interaction and allow teachers and learners to share ideas.
- PDAs can be used to carry information to the point of care. Various types of software and textbooks are commercially available for PDAs.
- Information found on the Internet should not be assumed to be accurate until its source is verified. Like all other medical literature, information from Web sites should be evaluated and compared to prior knowledge, new studies, and current recommendations.
- Podcasting refers to the practice of using RSS to "broadcast" audio or video files from Web sites to portable players, allowing physicians to access educational materials at their convenience.
- Library liaisons are librarians with specialized interest who can help physicians find information that they need in the clinical setting. Library liaisons understand the unique demands of the clinical environment and can aid physicians in finding critical information at the moment that it is needed.

References

1. Taekman J. Educational technology 2002. ASA Newsletter, May 2002
2. Lauritsen J, Moller AM. Clinical relevance in anesthesia journals. Curr Opin Anaesthesiol 2006; 19(2):166–70
3. Jonas S. The case for change in medical education in the United States. Lancet 1984; 2(8400):452–4
4. Davis D, O'Brien MA, Freemantle N, et al. Impact of formal continuing medical education: Do conferences, workshops, rounds, and other traditional continuing education activities change physician behavior or healthcare outcomes? JAMA 1999; 282(9):867–74
5. Swanson AG. Anderson, MB. Educating medical students. Assessing change in medical education— the road to implementation. Acad Med 1993; 68(6 Suppl):S1–46
6. Sajeva M. E-learning: Web-based education. Curr Opin Anaesthesiol 2006; 19(6):645–9
7. Ruiz JG, Mintzer MJ, Leipzig RM. The impact of E-learning in medical education. Acad Med 2006; 81(3):207–12
8. Clark D. Psychological myths in e-learning. Med Teach 2002; 24(6):598–604
9. Baker R, Dwyer F. A meta-analytic assessment of the effect of visualized instruction. Int J Instruct Media 2000; 27:417–26
10. Cohen JJ. Educating physicians in cyberspace. Acad Med 1995; 70(8):698
11. Sillence E, Briggs P, Harris PR, et al. How do patients evaluate and make use of online health information? Soc Sci Med 2007; 64(9):1853–62
12. McMullan M. Patients using the Internet to obtain health information: How this affects the patient–health professional relationship. Patient Educ Couns 2006; 63(1–2):24–8
13. Kurup V, Hersey D. The perioperative librarian: Luxury or necessity? Curr Opin Anaesthesiol 2007; 20(6):585–9
14. Hersh WR, Gorman PN, Sacherek LS. Applicability and quality of information for answering clinical questions on the Web. JAMA 1998; 280(15):1307–8
15. Wilson P. How to find the good and avoid the bad or ugly: A short guide to tools for rating quality of health information on the Internet. Br Med J 2002; 324(7337):598–602

16. Caron S, Berton J, Beydon L. Quality of anaesthesia-related information accessed via Internet searches. Br J Anaesth 2007; 99(2):195–201
17. Ruskin K. Information services and the Internet. J Clin Monit Comput 1999; 15(7–8): 419–20
18. Ruskin KJ, Kofke WA, Turndorf H. The anesthesiology discussion group: Development of a new method of communication between anesthesiologists. Anesth Analg 1995; 81(1):163–6
19. Ruskin KJ. How to get the most out of the Internet for your clinical practice. Int Anesthesiol Clin 2000; 38(4):115–25
20. Earl MF, Neutens JA. Evidence-based medicine training for residents and students at a teaching hospital: The library's role in turning evidence into action. Bull Med Libr Assoc 1999; 87(2):211–4
21. Cimpl K. Clinical medical librarianship: A review of the literature. Bull Med Libr Assoc 1985; 73(1):21–8
22. Cimpl K. Evaluating the effectiveness of clinical medical librarian programs: A systematic review of the literature. J Med Libr Assoc 2004; 92(1):14–33
23. Knight T, Brice A. Librarians, surgeons, and knowledge. Surg Clin North Am 2006; 86(1):71–90, viii–ix
24. Oliver KB, Roderer NK. Working towards the informationist. Health Informatics J 2006; 12(1):41–8

Chapter 21
Handheld Devices

Ravindra Prasad

The latter part of the twentieth century brought the world firmly into the information age. Whereas improved mechanization and industrial technologic development previously drove the economy, now information and related technologies are preeminent. Information technology companies such as Microsoft and Google are now market leaders, joining the ranks of the companies that traditionally prevailed as leaders (e.g., steel manufacturing, automobile production, and retailing). During this time, our primary methods of communicating and disseminating information have changed as well, from printed (books, newspaper or journal articles), to broadcast (radio, television), to electronic (email, Internet). With these changes has come a concurrent explosion in the amount of available information; in fact, companies are quite successful simply by specializing in tools to filter for *relevant* information (e.g., search tools from Yahoo! and Google, spam-filtering software for email). The new, interactive electronic media formats have particular advantages in medicine: improved ability to find information that specifically addresses the needs of individuals, the ability to combine media formats (text, audio, visual) to meet a variety of learning styles, support for information on demand, and increased ability to disseminate information to both physicians and patients.[1] As the population has aged, the acuity of surgical patients has increased as well. With continued pressure on healthcare facilities to perform and provide better care with fewer resources, average patient loads have also increased. The need for information at the point of care has, therefore, never been higher. Handheld computers give physicians access to this information, specific to the needs of individual patients, where and when they need it most: at the patient bedside.

Early History

Handheld computer devices were mentioned in popular literature as early as 1956, when they were simply portable terminals accessing larger, more powerful central computers.[2] Similar portable electronic devices did not begin to be available to consumers, however, until the mid-to-late 1970s. Initially, these had only limited functionality (calendars, notepads, language translation), but their usability and

J. Stonemetz, K. Ruskin (eds.) *Anesthesia Informatics*,
© Springer Science+Business Media, LLC 2008

reliability improved with technologic development. The first widely accepted incarnation of what is now viewed as a "handheld computer" was the Palm Pilot, released in 1996 by Palm, Inc. Handheld computers, often called personal digital assistants (PDAs), have grown in complexity but generally share several important defining characteristics: these electronic devices are small (hand-sized) and self-powered, designed to be usable within seconds of power-up, have a touchscreen display, offer handwriting recognition and/or a small integrated keyboard (virtual or real), can connect wirelessly with other handhelds or computers (infrared, Bluetooth, and/or wireless network/Internet), have built-in personal information management (PIM) tools (such as address books and appointment books) and the ability to expand functionality through add-on hardware (e.g., memory, keyboard, networking) and software, and can share information with desktop/laptop computers for "synchronization" (data backup, PIM software). Modern PDAs often add other feature, as well (e.g., memory cards, cameras, telephony).

As handheld devices have gained power and usability, a concurrent evolution in computers has also occurred. From large mainframes occupying rooms of space, to desktop PCs, to laptops, computers have become both smaller and more powerful. In 2002, Microsoft introduced the Tablet PC, a computer with a larger (paper-sized) screen that can run typical desktop operating systems (Windows) and applications—an arm-held computer. Further miniaturization brought the "palmtop" computer. On March 13, 2006, Microsoft announced the "Origami Project," a code name for a small touchscreen PC designed for use in a variety of settings.[3] An early example of these "Ultra-Mobile PC" (UMPC) devices was the OQO, a book-sized (4.9 in × 3.4 in × 0.9 in, 14 oz) computer running Windows XP.[4] Other manufacturers later offered their own version of the UMPC: devices packing the full power of desktop computers into a much smaller package. However, these devices initially suffered from relatively poor battery life, poor screen resolution, and user interface difficulties despite a somewhat high price tag (hundreds of dollars more than PDAs). With no clearly defined target audience and no "killer application" (a "must-have" program, highlighting the key advantages of the platform), the long-term success of the UMPC is unclear at this writing. In any case, discussion of these types of computers is outside the scope of this chapter.

The early handheld computers (mid-1970s) were simply calculators with advanced functions (programmability, timers, alarms). In 1978, Toshiba introduced the LC-836 Memo Note 30, which added phone number and memo storage to its calculator functions. Additional development resulted in portable devices with more computing power, allowing them to run other applications, connect via modems to other devices, and function as terminals to larger computers. The PF-8000, released in 1980, even had some handwriting recognition. In 1984, Psion introduced its Organizer, which included a simple database, a calculator, a clock, and removable storage. Hewlett-Packard's HP-18C (1986) offered infrared connections to peripherals. Sharp's Wizard (1988) could be connected to PCs and had more PDA functionality (e.g., memos, phone numbers, alarms). Sony's PalmTop, with handwriting recognition, became available in 1990. However, it was not until 1992 that Apple Computer CEO John Sculley coined the term "personal digital assistant" and introduced the Newton, beginning the modern phase of PDA development.[5]

In 1993, the Newton became the first commercially released keyboardless handheld computer. It had limited desktop connectivity and PIM software, and the handwriting recognition was far from perfect. Nevertheless, several versions were developed (e.g., ruggedized models for field work), and medical applications also became available. While the Newton popularized the idea of PDAs, the devices themselves were too large, handwriting recognition too poor, and desktop connectivity too inadequate for widespread acceptance. At about the same time, Jeff Hawkins was instrumental in the development and release of Tandy's and Casio's ZOOMER. The ZOOMER devices, introduced in 1992, had an infrared transceiver, speaker and headphone jack, and memory card slot, and they were a bit smaller (at 1 in × 4.2 in × 6.8 in). While a commercial flop due to its size, weight (16 oz), slow speed, cost, and poor handwriting recognition,[6] the process of developing the ZOOMER resulted in Jeff Hawkins founding Palm Computing in 1994.[7] Palm Computing's Palm Pilot, released in 1995, was the first commercially *successful* handheld computer. It was simpler than the Newton, used primarily for organizer (PIM) functions, and had limited data storage and a smaller screen, but it had excellent desktop connectivity. In fact, it was marketed as a "connected organizer" rather than a "PDA." Its battery life was excellent, and its handwriting recognition system was more robust and reliable than earlier handhelds. Windows CE, an operating system adapted from Windows 95, was released in 1996. Although it had a poor interface for handheld computers, it was revised in 2000 to Pocket PC to focus more specifically on Palm-sized devices.[8] It has since become one of the major competitors in the PDA market.

In 1993, BellSouth released the Simon smartphone, developed by IBM. "Smart" phones are combination devices: mobile phones with PDA functions. The Simon was large (8 in × 2.5 in × 1.5 in) and heavy (18 oz) but could perform several functions, including traditional PDA applications (e.g., PIM, calculator), email, faxing and paging, and cellular telephony.[5,9] Smartphones are now pocket sized. While some are simply mobile phones with a few additional features, many others offer full-featured PDA functions; they are the latest incarnation of the handheld computer. In fact, with continued technologic advancement, the distinction between phone and PDA continues to blur: many handheld devices now include traditional PDA functions, telephony, and a host of other applications.

Functionality

Today, PDAs and smartphones have a variety of applications available right out of the box. They almost universally include basic PIM tools (address books, calendars with alarms, note-taking applications, task lists) that are integrated ("synchronized") with desktop applications. Most also include calculators, clocks, and games. Smartphones, of course, add telephony to the package. Many PDAs also include word-processing and spreadsheet tools, email readers, Web browsers, and audio/ video playback software. Some also provide microphones and cameras for audio and video capture. In addition, most PDAs can work with customized hardware to provide specialized functions. For example, PDAs can be integrated with barcode readers to facilitate inventory tracking, or with GPS receivers and mapping software to help with navigation. The ability to carry large amounts of information in an easily searchable format makes PDAs especially useful as repositories for references (e.g., dictionaries, textbooks). Furthermore, thousands of software applications that support a diverse range of functions are available, e.g., e-book readers, specialized calculators, portfolio managers, budget planners, shopping tools, calorie counters, and universal remote controls. Databases and programming tools are also available, allowing users to easily create applications specific to their personal needs.

Handheld Devices in Medicine

Needing to access large amounts of information while traveling from patient to patient throughout the day, physicians were early adopters of PDAs. However, even the simple applications provided in the most basic of PDAs can help physicians to manage their busy clinical schedules more easily. For example, task lists can be used as reminders to check lab results or return phone calls. Calendars can be used to schedule patient appointments or professional meetings. Note-taking applications allow users to quickly jot down information that can be easily located later. Local protocols can be saved for easy reference.

Slightly more advanced PDAs often include other applications that can be particularly useful to physicians. These might include, for example, PDA versions of word processors such as Microsoft Word, file readers such as Adobe Reader, presentation tools such as Microsoft PowerPoint, and Web browsers. Word processors can be used to easily access large volumes of local information such as hospital procedures and residency training manuals, and even to modify or edit them to meet individual needs. They can improve note taking or can be used to create patient letters or notifications to be printed and mailed (or emailed) later. Portable document format (PDF) readers can be used to access a personally created library of journal articles, commonly available in Adobe's PDF format, or other documents converted to PDF format. Physicians can create or edit lectures and presentations using the PDA version of PowerPoint; with appropriate hardware, they can give the presentation directly from their PDA. Web browsers allow users to surf the Internet and access medically relevant data such as internal hospital pages or custom-designed departmental Web sites. Some programs (e.g., Microsoft Explorer, Blazer) provide real-time access using a PDA's wireless Internet connection; others (e.g., iSilo, Plucker, AvantGo) use a desktop program to convert Web pages to PDA format and automatically transfer the data to the PDA during synchronization.

As mentioned previously, spreadsheets such as Microsoft Excel or compatible programs allow users to create and use their own customized data tables to meet individual needs, e.g., searchable indexes of local data (phone numbers, call lists, scheduling information, hospital protocols, etc.) or calculators for specific formulas that may not be available in most medical calculator programs. Database programs are also available for PDAs (e.g., SmartListToGo, HanDBase, Pendragon Forms). Like spreadsheets, databases allow collection of related data. However, databases can organize data into related tables and allow users to make queries that automatically search subsets of the data. An example query would be: how many interscalene blocks were performed last year, and what was the complication rate? These PDA database programs allow users to easily develop robust data tables and interfaces to facilitate rapid data entry. For example, they could be used to summarize information such as institutional drug regimens or protocols, maintain personal case and procedure logs, or collect research data. Database programs require more expertise to design and maintain than typical spreadsheets. Fortunately, most of them are available for limited use on a trial basis. Important features that the customer should look for when choosing a specific program include availability of the program for his specific PDA, price, ease of development and use, flexibility, power (compared with "flat file" databases, "relational" databases are generally more powerful and allow creation of more complicated data tables but require more work to design and maintain), and support—most people will eventually need some help in designing or using a database.

Typically, bundled software applications can help physicians in a variety of settings, but PDAs can become exceptionally useful when applications are developed specifically for medicine. Early medical applications for the Newton included a variety of reference texts and handbooks converted to electronic format. For example, many of the popular *Current Clinical Strategies* handbooks and Ferri's *Practical Guide to the Medical Patient*, both of which students and residents have carried with them for decades, were available in Newton format.[10] Drug databases, medical calculators, patient charting, and record-keeping software were also developed.[11] The first study to test the effectiveness of PDAs in medicine, the Constellation Project, used the Apple Newton shortly after its introduction. It was conducted by K2 Consultants with Harvard Medical School, Massachusetts General Hospital, and Brigham and Women's Hospital and provided medical residents with Newtons that were loaded with medical knowledge self-assessment software, a drug database, the hospital medical resident handbooks, a medical calculator, and other medical reference texts. They found that handheld devices could significantly enhance medical practice and improve patient care.[12] K2 Consultants developed many devices; the company eventually evolved into Skyscape.com, a major provider of medical applications for handheld computers.[13]

Medical software initially consisted mainly of electronic versions of standard reference books; these continue to be available (e.g., *Harrison's Manual of Medicine*, *Stedman's Medical Dictionary*,[14] *Taber's Cyclopedic Medical Dictionary*,[15] *Griffith's 5-Minute Clinical Consult*[16]). PDA-based references are modified for ease of use in the small format and take advantage of devices' computing power and ability to search for specific information. Just as with textbooks, the choice of which application(s) to purchase is a personal one based on preference and cost. In addition to standard texts, current literature is easily accessible through Internet connectivity in smartphones or network-enabled PDAs, which provide access to mobile versions of PubMed to conduct literature searches and to evidence-based medicine guides (Info-POEMS). Several applications also offer clinicians opportunities to earn continuing medical education credit through portable topic reviews and study guides.

Several drug databases are also available, e.g., ePocrates,[17] Davis' Drug Guide,[18] Lexi-Drugs.[19] Again, these were initially just electronic versions of previously published drug lists. Later versions of these references took greater advantage of the mobile computer platform by adding features such as cross-referencing of medical conditions, diagnostic aids, integrated drug-dose calculators, drug-interaction checkers, electronic prescription-writing tools, automatic updating of drug information, and notification of medical alerts and warnings. One survey (with analysis of synchronization data) after 4 weeks of physician use of a clinical reference application (including a pharmacopeia, infectious disease reference, diagnostic and therapeutic data) found that 39% of participants reported using the software during more than half of their patient encounters and 61% believed that use of the clinical reference prevented adverse drug events or medication errors three or more times during the 4-week study period. Users believed that using the application helped them to improve patient care and was valuable in learning about recent alerts.[20] Choosing which application to use will depend on a variety of questions that must be answered by physicians on an individual basis: How comprehensive do I want the list to be? Does the application include relevant information in my particular area of practice? How much information about each drug do I need? Do I need any extra features (e.g., drug-interaction checking, automatic updating), or is a simple list of drugs and dosing information adequate? Is the application easy to use? How much am I willing to spend? Most programs are available for trial use; physicians should simply try using a variety of programs in clinical practice, then choose the one (or ones) that meet their individual needs.

PDAs also help directly with clinical work. Medical calculators simplify the calculation of clinically useful parameters (e.g., fractional excretion of sodium, alveolar-arterial oxygen gradient). Most of these are designed to be quick and easy to use: formulas have already been preprogrammed, and the clinician simply needs to enter the missing variables (e.g., height, weight) to automatically calculate the parameter (e.g., body mass index). Additional equations are periodically added to the program by its designer; these are either updated automatically (e.g., during periodic wireless updates) or require the user to install newer versions of the program. Some programs may allow users to create their own formulas, although this may require some level of programming expertise. More generic spreadsheet programs such as Microsoft Excel can also be easily adapted to calculate physician-defined formulas. For example, a cardiologist could easily create a spreadsheet on which echocardiographic findings such as valve size, chamber size, and jet velocity could be entered and instantly calculate valve area, ejection fraction, or pressure gradients.

Patient-tracking software (e.g., Patient Tracker,[21] Patient Keeper[22]) can help clinicians to track their patients' histories, problem lists, and laboratory results. Although some of the built-in applications allow these functions at a rudimentary level, programs specifically designed for use by physicians tend to be more powerful, flexible, and easier to use. With infrared communication, these notes can be printed in a legible format for inclusion in the chart. Wireless communication (infrared PDA-to-PDA beaming and/or Internet) supports teamwork by helping clinicians to easily share information (e.g., hospital phone numbers, patient lists, problem lists, task lists) with each other or to send/receive emails.[23] This feature may be especially important when patient care is transferred from one person to another, as when the in-house on-call team assumes care. Electronic transmission of patient data may reduce or eliminate errors of omission or inaccuracy. In addition, compared with paging systems, PDAs with telephony may improve patient care by reducing the risk of medical error or injury due to communication delays.[24]

PDAs have also been used in the education of patients, medical students, and residents. Images and movies catalogued in a data library can be used during patient consultation to enhance inpatient teaching. Images from a specific patient's surgery can be used during that patient's postoperative review.[25] Wayne State University School of Medicine uses wireless Pocket PCs throughout the undergraduate curriculum. They are used in the classroom and lecture hall to document attendance and to facilitate interaction between the lecturer and the students through use of both instant messaging and anonymous, aggregated question-and-answer software. Students can download course content (lectures, audio and visual supplements) directly onto the handhelds. Students on clinical rotations have access to licensed medical references and tools such as those described. PDAs are also used administratively to arrange schedules, complete lecturer and course evaluations, and track patient encounters.[26] PDAs have been used similarly in residency training programs. A survey of family-practice residency program participants in the US found that 67% of respondents reported PDA use within their departments. Over 40% used PDAs to track inpatients and resident procedures completed.[27] One emergency medicine residency successfully used PDAs to track all patient resuscitations and procedures performed by its residents, with 10 of the 11 participating residents preferring the PDA over paper logs.[28] A urology residency used PDAs to document all clinical and academic activities performed by their residents.[29] The latter suggested that PDAs could be used to obtain objective data to assess a program's curriculum and expose weaknesses. By facilitating recording of clinical patient exposure and procedures performed, PDAs can help residents to ensure that they are meeting their training requirements.

PDAs can also facilitate collection of study data. Study subjects report a preference for PDA-based electronic data capture over paper diaries,[30] despite the potential for technical problems, with a reported incidence of 4%–29%.[31,32] PDAs may also improve the quality of study data collection: data-recording protocol compliance is greater (93.6% vs. 10.9%), and with software-controlled elimination of retrospective fabrication of data (75%–80% incidence with paper diaries), collected data are more accurate.[30,33] Furthermore, having data already in electronic format may reduce or eliminate errors that result from transcription and conversion of paper data forms. A recent review concluded that handheld computers potentially offer great advantages in data collection and handling.[34] Subjects generally preferred them to paper, which could result in improved adherence to data-collection protocols. Technical design can reduce or eliminate errors in data collection and accuracy, although when compared to current well-performing paper methods, handheld computers have generally performed similarly.

Finally, applications can be written specifically for a user or a department. Some of the database programs mentioned previously (e.g., HanDBase, Pendragon Forms) can be used to design data-intensive applications that both can be used on PDAs and can transfer data automatically with desktop applications such as Microsoft Access. These might be useful, for example, to collect case-log data for all residents in the department or to facilitate pain management round charting and data collection. These databases require some level of programming knowledge and expertise but are generally approachable even with only basic background knowledge. However, if more computer programming expertise is available, anything is possible. Typical desktop programming languages and environments, such as BASIC, Microsoft Visual Basic, and C, are all available for PDAs; these can be used to create any application a user or a department may desire. Developing customized solutions, however, requires a significantly higher level of expertise. They may be slower to implement, depending on programming resources. Customized programs also put a significant maintenance burden on computer-support personnel. As PDAs are upgraded, program functionality must be maintained, and if individuals use different platforms (e.g., Windows, Palm OS, Blackberry), rewriting programs for each platform may be necessary. However, if this option is available, it provides the greatest flexibility, allowing design of a solution to the particular problems and needs of a department or institution.

Handheld Devices in Anesthesia

Unlike physicians in many other specialties, anesthesiologists often spend much of their day in the OR at the patient bedside. Access to clinically relevant information at the point of care can, therefore, be especially helpful. The most commonly used applications are likely the same as for other physicians: drug databases and medical references. In addition to the general medical applications, a growing library of software designed specifically for anesthesiologists is available. For example, several popular anesthesia texts and handbooks are available for PDAs (e.g., *Handbook of Clinical Anesthesia, Yao and Artusio's Anesthesiology*,[35] *Clinical Anesthesia Procedures of the Massachusetts General Hospital*[36]). Other references have been designed specifically for PDAs (e.g., *Strategies in Pediatric Anesthesia Practice*,[37] *The Biochemical Origin of Pain*[38]). In addition, drug references that focus specifically on anesthetic drugs (*Sota Omoigui's Anesthesia Drugs Handbook*[39]) and pain medications (*Sota Omoigui's Pain Drug Handbook*[40]) are available. However, currently, only a few applications written specifically for anesthesiology are commercially available. Anesthesia Stat Tracker is a case-tracking program, but it was last updated in 2001 and may not run on modern devices.[41] ZapBill Anesthesia is a Palm OS application designed to facilitate charge capture, but it has not been widely promulgated.[42] Some large-scale systems used by the main hospital infrastructure can also use a PDA as an interface (e.g., Advanced MD, a billing system for non-anesthesiology offices[43]; Typhon Group, a quality assurance software package[44]). Several shareware database tools are also available, but these are not complete, polished applications.

While there may be a dearth of commercial anesthesiology programs, several groups have developed their own software. One group reported on their development of a wireless PDA-based preoperative assessment tool that allowed an assessment that was more comprehensive than traditional pen-and-paper methods.[45] Another group developed a case-logging application to monitor trainee exposure to types of surgeries and anesthetics, patient demographics (age, ASA-PS classification), and types and numbers of critical incidents. They were able to document adequacy of training and analyze procedure performance over time, enabling early identification of trainees who needed intervention.[46] Freestone et al. used the same application to examine PDA-based critical-incident reporting, comparing it with their usual methods. They determined the true incidence of events by examining multiple sources (e.g., morbidity and mortality conferences, retrospective case note reviews, Australian Incident Monitoring Study reports). They found that participants who used PDAs reported as many as 98% of the critical incidents that actually occurred—much more often than the 16.3%–61.7% incidence of cases self-reported when traditional paper-based measures were used.[47,48] Others have reported on the early stages of development of custom-designed PDA systems to capture comprehensive data (from the preoperative assessment, through the intraoperative course, to postoperative morbidity information) with interaction and data exchange with a central database, hospital information system, or AIMS.[49,50] As noted, custom solutions allow the greatest flexibility in designing a program for a specific department's needs. They do, however, require a greater commitment of resources for design and maintenance. In addition, when they are used to collect data of any sort, it may be more difficult to pool data with other institutions that use their own custom-designed programs.

Choosing a Handheld Device

Two factors must be considered when purchasing a device. One important consideration is the combination of features that will be necessary during daily use, i.e., *what can the device do?* As devices continue to evolve, a wide range of functions will become integrated into handheld computers; devices at varying price ranges will offer specific subsets of these functions. A needs assessment must be conducted to determine which subset is necessary for each user. Most handhelds and smartphones will provide the usual PIM tools. Simple PDAs will usually be able to accommodate medical references and the other applications mentioned previously. More fully featured devices may add wireless connectivity, audio and video recording and playback, and telephony. PDA functions can likely be extended even further through hardware add-ons.

The other important consideration is usability, i.e., *how easy is the device to use*? In other words, *can it do what it does well*? If a device is powerful but slow or difficult to use, it will simply sit on the desk collecting dust. Ease of use is determined both by the hardware design and features and by software—the operating system that runs the device and the applications available. From a hardware standpoint, the device should be small and lightweight, convenient to carry, have a long battery life, and yet have a display that is large enough and with high enough brightness and resolution to be read easily in various light conditions. It should power-up quickly and allow use with a minimum of key presses, button clicks, or delays. From a software standpoint, the device should already have available all of the different types of the necessary applications, or it should allow easy development (programming) of custom applications. Currently, two main groups of PDAs exist for medical use: those running the Palm OS and those running Windows Mobile (previously Pocket PC). Other operating systems, such as Linux, Symbian, and Blackberry, are also available. Some examples of current handheld computers are discussed later; others will be developed with advances in technology. Regardless of the operating system, the main considerations are power and ease of use. These can best be assessed with a hands-on approach, i.e., using the devices on a trial basis in the clinical setting.

Blackberry

Research In Motion (RIM) introduced two-way paging in 1996. In 1998, they introduced the Blackberry, a device that included basic PIM functions but was best known for tight integration with email and corporate data. With a paid subscription, these data (e.g., customer details, pricing and inventory information, and other enterprise applications) are automatically synchronized between corporate computers and handheld computers in real time. Blackberries have continued to gain features, now including telephony and Internet connectivity. Despite their widespread presence in the corporate world, Blackberries are much less common in healthcare: email is a less important means of daily communication, and much less software is available (despite recent significant increases in availability).

Linux

The UNIX operating system is an open-source system in which users can add features and correct bugs; all additions are available to users at large. Compared to other operating systems, UNIX is thought to have better security, and it is completely free. Several versions of UNIX are now available to users. Apple's Mac OS is based on UNIX, and Linux, one of the most common versions of UNIX, already runs on many desktop computers. Linux also powered 14% of smartphones shipped worldwide in the first quarter of 2005, which represented a gain of 412% from the first quarter of 2004 and was three times greater than the number of Windows Mobile phones in the same period.[51] By 2012, a version of Linux is expected to be running in 203 million phones.[52] Palm, already offering devices that run Palm OS and Windows Mobile, plans to release a Linux-powered device in 2007 or 2008.[53] However, while Linux PDAs and smartphones will likely become more prevalent and important in the future, the medical software currently available for these devices is very limited.

Symbian

Most PDA operating systems were designed to drive small handheld computing devices; the voice and data features were only added later. However, Symbian was designed specifically to address the needs of smartphones.[54] Symbian licensees accounted for >85% of worldwide mobile phone sales in 2003[55] and >90% of smartphones shipped in Europe in the first quarter of 2004.[56] However, the Symbian operating system has a relatively small presence in the US. Symbian has also been customized by several manufacturers, so that many mutually incompatible versions are now available. Finally, medical software is fairly limited. Therefore, although Symbian devices may be more important in the future, they are currently not a viable choice for most anesthesiologists.

Palm OS and Windows Mobile

Initially a PDA company, Palm entered the smartphone market when it acquired Handspring. Other Palm OS phones are available, but Palm's presence in this market is largely driven by its flagship product, the Treo. The Treo provides full-featured mobile phone services, email, PIM functions, Web support, an MP3 player, video capture and playback, and wireless connectivity. Additional software can give Treos the capability to push email (a mail delivery system with real-time capability to "push" email through to the client as soon as it arrives, rather than requiring the client to poll and collect or "pull" mail manually), a feature that is similar to that found in the Blackberry. In a December 2005 report by Strategy Analytics, the Treo 650 was the highest-rated converged device in the US.[57] In January 2006, Palm introduced the Treo 700w, which runs under the Windows Mobile operating system. Other non-Treo handheld computers, with or without telephony and wireless connectivity, are also available for both Palm and Windows Mobile OS.

Both Palm and Windows Mobile operating systems have been available and actively developed for over 10 years. They support devices with similar features, and important software is usually available for both operating system platforms. Palm OS devices tend to be smaller in size, faster, and easier to use. They also have more applications (commercial, freeware, and shareware) and tend to have better battery life. Windows devices tend to have larger screens, more built-in memory, support multitasking better (able to run multiple applications at once), and may interact (synchronize) with desktop Windows applications better. Anesthesiologists will currently benefit most by using these handheld computers rather than other operating systems. Choosing between them largely depends on individual preferences and specific software application needs.

Handheld devices will continue to evolve. New devices will come to market with features that have not been created or even considered as of today. When trying to choose one of these devices, one must consider several questions: Which features are required for the expected user? For example, are PIM tools, reference texts, and security controls all necessary? Are those features available for the device in question? Is the device easy to use or will it necessitate extensive training? Will users use the device as intended? For example, if battery life is limited or the device is large or heavy or responsiveness is poor, will users simply not use the device? Will the device support future growth in user needs? For example, can customized hardware and/or software be created, or is the device expandability limited? Is support for the device available when unexpected problems occur? Answering these questions should help to narrow the choices of handheld computers down to a manageable level and allow the user to select the best device for his specific needs.

Conclusion

In his State of the Union Address on January 20, 2004, President George W. Bush outlined his Health Information Technology Plan. Citing several concerns, from healthcare costs to medical errors to quality of patient care, the Plan calls for the establishment of EMRs within 10 years. A preliminary step in the Plan is to adopt a common health information standard, to facilitate communication of medical information between different systems and locations.[58] In 2006, the US Department of Health and Human Services issued regulations to encourage healthcare providers to adopt (using standards recognized by the Secretary of Health and Human Services) interoperable health information technologies. These and other measures resulted in the delivery of several prototype architectures for a Nationwide Health Information Network in 2007.[59] The EMR will not be limited to basic information such as medical histories, allergies, and the like. Electronic anesthesia record keepers have been available in some form since at least as early as 1987.[60] Growing evidence suggests that these, too, improve patient safety and quality of care.[61,62] Today, a variety of vendors offer sophisticated systems that record not only the intraoperative data (vitals, medications, etc.) but also the preoperative evaluations and postoperative care information. An increasing number of institutions are evaluating or implementing these systems.

As EMRs become widespread through clinics, hospitals, and ORs, physicians' access to these records must become widespread as well. However, access will likely be obtained primarily through desktop or laptop computers rather than through handheld computers. With a full-sized keyboard and trackpad or mouse, compared to a handheld device, a desktop computer is simply a more efficient interface with which to collect, visualize, and process data. Furthermore, computers that are tightly integrated with monitoring equipment and anesthesia delivery systems will be able to provide decision support in real time, potentially improving quality of care and patient safety. As access to PCs improves, in the OR and beyond, the importance of handheld devices will likely diminish. Although they may continue to be useful in themselves, they may also be used simply to feed information to a central system. For example, PDAs have been used during preoperative evaluations to collect information, which was then fed to the AIMS.[45,49] PDAs are excellent mobile references for pharmacopoeia and medical synopses, and they are flexible in running a variety of other applications. Converged devices can also help physicians to communicate with each other. However, as they proliferate, they may assume some or all these functions. We may, then, return full circle to that first description of handheld computers—when they served primarily as an interface to a centralized, powerful, computing system.[2]

Key Points

- Initially described in the literature simply as access points to powerful central computers, handheld computers actually developed from simple tools into powerful, fully functional computers that could be used independently and could interface with desktop computers.
- Modern handheld devices include both basic management tools for personal information and a variety of software applications commonly seen on desktop computers (e.g., word processors, spreadsheets, databases).
- Recent development has seen a merging of a variety of functions on portable devices. Handheld devices now commonly support audio (e.g., music) and video (e.g., cameras, movies) applications, as well as telephony.
- PDAs are particularly useful in medicine. They can provide access to large amounts of information (e.g., medical references, drug databases) to the mobile physician, allow academic work (e.g., writing or editing lectures or papers) to be done while away from a desk, and support evaluation and decision making with simple tools (e.g., medical calculators, literature searches). They can also improve documentation through the use of patient-tracking and encounter-charting software. In addition, PDAs can facilitate communication both with patients, using pictures and movies as teaching tools, and with other physicians, through telephony and email.

- PDAs may be especially beneficial to anesthesiologists, who spend much of the day at the patient bedside and away from desktop computers. They can function both as information repositories (e.g., reference textbooks, local protocols) and as data-collection tools (e.g., facilitate data collection during preoperative evaluations).
- When choosing a handheld computer, the most important factors are deciding on which functions are required (and whether the software is currently available and will continue to be supported) and evaluating the usability of the device being considered (best answered with a hands-on trial and assessment). Some popular devices operate under the Blackberry, Palm OS, and Windows Mobile operating systems. Linux and Symbian devices may become more important in the future.
- The future will see a shift to EMRs throughout the American healthcare system. As computers necessarily become more widespread to support these hospital-based systems, the importance of handheld computers as stand-alone devices may diminish.

References

1. Robinson TN, Patrick K, Eng TR, et al. An evidence-based approach to interactive health communication: A challenge to medicine in the information age. JAMA 1998; 280:1264–9
2. Asimov I. The last question. Science Fiction Quarterly 1956; Nov:7–15
3. Origami Project. http://origamiproject.com/. Accessed July 20, 2007
4. OQO Model 2. http://www.oqo.com/. Accessed July 20, 2007
5. Koblentz E. The Evolution of the PDA: 1975–1995. May 2005. http://www.snarc.net/pda/pda-treatise.htm. Accessed May 18, 2007
6. Brooks C. A Look Back at the History of Palm. Posted June 4, 2004. http://www.palmloyal.com/addons.php?name=News&file=article&sid=1672. Accessed May 18, 2007. Based on Butter A, Pogue D. *Piloting Palm: The Inside Story of Palm, Handspring, and the Birth of the Billion Dollar Handheld Industry*. New York: Wiley, 2002
7. Company information, Palm, Inc. Management Team. http://www.palm.com/us/company/corporate/executive.html#jeff. Accessed May 18, 2007
8. The History of Windows CE. February 18, 2001. http://www.hpcfactor.com/support/windowsce/. Accessed May 18, 2007
9. Graychase N. Today's PDAs & smartphones—new devices for our organizational arsenal. First Glimpse 2006; 3(6):40–2
10. Current Clinical Strategies Publishing. http://www.ccspublishing.com/ccs/. Accessed May 18, 2007
11. Newton Reference: A list of medical applications; most links are no longer functional. http://www.panix.com/~clay/newton/query.cgi?medical+index. Accessed May 18, 2007
12. Labkoff SE, Shah S, Bormel J, et al. The Constellation Project: Experience and evaluation of personal digital assistants in the clinical environment. In: Gardner RM, ed. *Proceedings of the 19th Annual Symposium on Computer Applications in Medical Care*. Bethesda, MD: American Medical Informatics Association, 1995:678–82
13. Skyscape.com press releases, July 13, 2000. http://www.skyscape.com/company/PressRelease.aspx?id=30. Accessed May 18, 2007
14. *Stedman's Medical Dictionary for Health Professions & Nursing*. http://www.stedmans.com/product.cfm/507/215. Accessed July 20, 2007

15. *Taber's Cyclopedic Medical Dictionary*. Philadelphia: FA Davis Company. http://www.fadavis.com/tabers/. Accessed July 20, 2007

16. *The 5-Minute Clinical Consult*. http://www.5mcc.com/. Accessed July 20, 2007

17. Epocrates. http://www.epocrates.com/. Accessed May 18, 2007

18. *Davis' Drug Guide*. Philadelphia: FA Davis Company. http://www.drugguide.com/. Accessed July 20, 2007

19. Lexi-Comp. http://www.lexi.com. Accessed July 20, 2007

20. Rothschild JM, Fang E, Liu V, et al. Use and perceived benefits of handheld computer-based clinical references. J Am Med Inform Assoc 2006; 13:619–26

21. Patient Tracker. http://www.patienttracker.com/. Accessed May 18, 2007

22. Patient Keeper. http://www.patientkeeper.com/. Accessed May 18, 2007

23. Mohammad A. Handheld computers. Br Med J 2004; 328:1181–4

24. Soto RG, Chu LF, Goldman JM, et al. Communication in critical care environments: Mobile telephones improve patient care. Anesth Analg 2006; 102:535–41

25. Adam M. Handheld computers in clinical practice are useful in informing and educating patients. Br Med J 2004; 328:1565

26. Jackson M, Ganger AC, Bridge PD, et al. Wireless handheld computers in the undergraduate medical curriculum. Med Educ Online [serial online] 2005; 10:5. http://www.med-ed-online.org. Accessed May 18, 2007

27. Criswell DF, Parchman ML. Handheld computer use in US family practice residency programs. J Am Med Inform Assoc 2002; 9:80–6

28. Bird SB, Land DR. House officer procedure documentation using a personal digital assistant: A longitudinal study. BMC Med Inform Decis Mak 2006; 6:5

29. MacNeily AE, Nguan C, Haden K, et al. Implementation of a PDA-based program to quantify urology resident in-training experience. Can J Urol 2003; 10(3):1885–90

30. Gaertner J, Elsner F, Pollmann-Dahmen K, et al. Electronic pain diary: A randomized cross-over study. J Pain Symptom Manage 2004; 28:259–67

31. Tiplady B, Crompton GK, Dewar MH, et al. The use of electronic diaries in respiratory studies. Drug Inf J 1997; 31:759–64

32. Lauritsen K, Degl'Innocenti A, Hendel L, et al. Symptom recording in a randomised clinical trial: Paper diaries vs. electronic or telephone data capture. Control Clin Trials 2004; 25:585–97

33. Stone AA, Shiffman S, Schwartz JE, et al. Patient compliance with paper and electronic diaries. Control Clin Trials 2003; 24:182–99

34. Lane SJ, Heddle NM, Arnold E, et al. A review of randomized controlled trials comparing the effectiveness of hand held computers with paper methods for data collection. BMC Med Inform Decis Mak 2006; 6:23

35. Skyscape.com. *Yao and Artusio's Anesthesiology: Problem-Oriented Patient Management*. http://www.skyscape.com/estore/ProductDetail.aspx?ProductId=1073. Accessed July 20, 2007

36. Skyscape.com. *Clinical Anesthesia Procedures of the Massachusetts General Hospital*. http://www.skyscape.com/EStore/ProductDetail.aspx?ProductID=1136. Accessed July 20, 2007

37. PocketMedicine.com. *Strategies in Pediatric Anesthesia Practice*. http://www.pocket-medicine.com/pdaorder/-/005242001112/item?oec-catalog-item-id=1242. Accessed July 20, 2007

38. Skyscape.com. *The Biochemical Origin of Pain*. http://www.skyscape.com/estore/productdetail.aspx?productid=962. Accessed July 20, 2007

39. Skyscape.com. *Sota Omoigui's Anesthesia Drugs Handbook*. http://www.skyscape.com/estore/ProductDetail.aspx?ProductId=321. Accessed July 20, 2007

40. Skyscape.com. *Sota Omoigui's Pain Drug Handbook*. http://www.skyscape.com/estore/ProductDetail.aspx?ProductId=972. Accessed July 20, 2007

41. Medical Toolbox Software. Anesthesia StatTracker. http://www.medicaltoolbox.com/products/AnesStatTrk/index.html. Accessed July 20, 2007

42. ZapMed. http://www.zapmed.com/. Accessed July 20, 2007

43. Advance MD. Billing Service. http://www.advancedmd.com/billing/. Accessed July 20, 2007

44. Typhon Group Healthcare Solutions. Perioperative Performance Measurement—The QUICC System. http://www.typhongroup.com/products/perfmeas.htm. Accessed July 20, 2007

45. Sawa T, Okahara M, Santo M, et al. Preoperative information management system using wireless PDAs. AMIA Annu Symp Proc 2003; 2003:995

46. Bent PD, Bolsin SN, Creati BJ, et al. Professional monitoring and critical incident reporting using personal digital assistants. Med J Aust 2002; 177(9):496–9

47. Freestone L, Bolsin SN, Colson M, et al. Voluntary incident reporting by anaesthetic trainees in an Australian hospital. Int J Qual Health Care 2006; 18(6):452–7

48. Wolff AM, Bourke J, Campbell IA, et al. Detecting and reducing hospital adverse events: Outcomes of the Wimmera clinical risk management program. Med J Aust 2001; 174:621–5

49. Fuchs C, Quinzio L, Benson M, et al. Integration of a handheld based anaesthesia rounding system into an anaesthesia information management system. Int J Med Inform 2006; 75(7):553–63

50. Fu Q, Xue Z, Zhu J, et al. Anaesthesia record system on handheld computers – Pilot experience and uses for quality control and clinical guidelines. Comput Methods Programs Biomed 2005; 77(2):155–63

51. Linux Trounces Windows Mobile in Smart Phone Shipments. PC Magazine, July 20, 2005. http://www.pcmag.com/article2/0,1895,1839158,00.asp. Accessed May 18, 2007

52. Halperin D. 203 million mobile phones will use Linux operating systems by 2012, with 76 million as RTOS replacements. April 3, 2007. http://www.abiresearch.com/abiprdisplay.jsp?pressid=832. Accessed May 18, 2007

53. Palm fesses up to Linux Treo plans. April 10, 2007. http://linuxdevices.com/news/NS5607883840.html. Accessed May 18, 2007

54. Symbian White Paper, 1–10. Symbian smartphones for the enterprise. February 2004. http://www.symbian.com/files/rx/file6382.pdf. Accessed May 18, 2007

55. BNET (Business Wire) news release. "Gartner Says Worldwide Mobile Terminal Market Increased 12 Percent in Second Quarter of 2003." http://findarticles.com/p/articles/mi_m0EIN/is_2003_Sept_2/ai_107180069. Accessed February 14, 2008. Referenced in Symbian news release: "Agile:Insight AS joins Symbian Platinum Program and announces world's first Symbian OSTM firewall solution." October 5, 2004. http://www.symbian.com/news/cn/2004/cn20042578.html. Accessed May 18, 2007

56. Hardy E. U.S. Smartphone Buyers Prefer Palm OS. Brighthand. April 29, 2004. http://www.brighthand.com/default.asp?newsID=10658. Accessed May 18, 2007

57. Palm, Inc., news release. Palm Treo 650 smartphone named best converged device by strategy analytics. December 8, 2005. http://www.palm.com/us/company/pr/2005/120805.html. Accessed May 18, 2007

58. Whitehouse Policy Summary. Transforming Health Care: The President's Health Information Technology Plan. April, 2004. http://www.whitehouse.gov/infocus/technology/economic_policy200404/chap3.html. Accessed May 18, 2007

59. US Department of Health and Human Services. Health Information Technology Initiative Major Accomplishments: 2004–2006. http://www.hhs.gov/healthit/news/Accomplishments2006.html. Accessed May 18, 2007

60. Gravenstein JS, Paulus DA, Eames S, et al. The electronic clipboard: A semiautomatic anesthesia record. Int J Clin Monit Comput 1987; 4(3):153–9

61. O'Reilly M, Talsma A, VanRiper S, et al. An anesthesia information system designed to provide physician-specific feedback improves timely administration of prophylactic antibiotics. Anesth Analg 2006; 103(4):908–12

62. Vigoda MM, Lubarsky DA. The medicolegal importance of enhancing timeliness of documentation when using an anesthesia information system and the response to automated feedback in an academic practice. Anesth Analg 2006; 103(1):131–6

Chapter 22
Wireless Technologies

William D. Ankerstjerne and Mohamed Rehman

Wireless technology is an integral part of everyday life. Most people commonly think of cellular telephones when they speak of wireless communications, but many other wireless technologies are quickly becoming equally as popular, available, and affordable. The result of this increase in both visibility and popularity is that "wireless" is rapidly becoming a consumer-driven technology. Accompanying this trend, consumer demand is driving the development and evolution of applications for these devices. In the past, it was not unusual for a user or business to actually change its workflow to take advantage of wireless applications, with the benefits usually outweighing the inconvenience. Today, the general public is adopting wireless technology in daily life, and manufacturers are moving fast to meet the demand. This phenomenon is similar to the evolution of PCs throughout the 1980s as they migrated out of the offices into people's homes and became indispensable tools for everyday activities.

Leading the charge of wireless technology is wireless Ethernet (802.11). Commonly known as *WiFi*[1] (wireless fidelity, a wireless technology brand owned by the Wi-Fi Alliance) or *WLAN*[2] (wireless local area network), this standard for wireless networking is changing the way many businesses operate today. These applications can be found in such diverse locations as a secure corporate WLAN to a "WiFi Hot Spot" in an airport or café. The technology allows members of the general public to connect laptops to the Internet to check email or browse the Web, or a corporate user to connect wirelessly to a "fixed" asset on the company's secured local area network (servers, printers, email, intranet, etc.) to perform normal business activities formerly reserved for "wired" connections.

Traditionally, once a technologic "problem" was identified in an organization, the IT department would find or create a solution to that problem, implement the chosen solution, and "present" that implemented solution to the customer as their "fix" for the identified problem. It was then up to the customers to integrate this solution into their daily workflow, existing tools, processes, and procedures. With the current state of technology, any well-informed professional can see how a "consumer grade" wireless device such as a Blackberry can enhance service and delivery in almost any market. With healthcare being no exception to this trend, the introduction of consumer-driven wireless products to business-driven needs has created a unique "interactive team environment" in which nontechnical and technical

J. Stonemetz, K. Ruskin (eds.) *Anesthesia Informatics*,
© Springer Science+Business Media, LLC 2008

staff are working together to create a *convergence* of technology and corporate acceptability (security, accessibility, scalability, etc.) to mutually define "clinical wireless solutions."

"Doctors were the first large worker base that started using PDAs on the job," says Ellen Daley, a principal analyst at Forrester Research, Inc. "Here are a bunch of people who have an appetite for carrying PDAs, and here is a cheap way for wirelessly enabling a hospital. Hospitals decided to put the two together to see how they can improve patient care." This marriage of clinicians and wireless mobile devices, accompanied by hospitals moving to deploy WLANs as a cheaper and more effective way to provide high-speed, reliable connectivity in aging buildings, is resulting in the substantial growth of healthcare-specific wireless applications. As the technology becomes more dependable and secure, hospitals are leveraging the advantages of wireless (through the use of both WLANs and cellular-based networks) as the backbone for their present and future technology needs, offering a scalable, cost-effective means by which to extend technology (Mobile/Interactive Charting, Point of Care Collaboration, Instant Lab Results, Direct Prescriber orders to the respective recipient).[3]

One of the most popular "real" adaptations in wireless healthcare technology thus far is the enablement of accessing and updating EMRs at the point of care, thereby allowing positive patient ID and matching of patient wristbands with medication packages, charts, and records. This adaptation of technology allows the clinician to view, review, and update all patient information in real time at the point of care. Utilization of voice-over-WiFi (VoFI; i.e., Vocera badges, Vocera, Cupertino, CA) devices that provide immediate voice communications for paging, consultations, and nurse call can enhance communication with other team members, further improving care through the use of wireless services.[4] These enhancements to a hospital's workflow increase efficiency, enhance patient care, and maximize patient safety.

The standards for wireless technologies and their applicability for data or voice communications are constantly changing and improving. An advantage of this fast-paced change is that the technology manufacturers have grown sensitive to customers' desires and needs to "stay current" and have taken steps to plan and implement their technology solutions to remain consistent with newer technology designed to be compatible with prior generations. This measure allows an institution to avoid the risks inherent in early adoption of untested technology. In short, users are given the advantage of being able to continually upgrade as technology becomes proven without the disadvantage of discovering a new technology's shortcomings due to a premature deployment.

The two most commonly implemented wireless communications networks are the IEEE 802.11 (WiFi) communications standard and the GSM 3G cellular communications standard. A proper survey of the site and well-architected installation of any wireless network is the key to a successful implementation. Implemented properly, a wireless infrastructure can support any device that depends on the deployed technology (802.11 WLAN, for example, with regard to networks), as well as the adaptation of new and future technologies (e.g., as WiFi has evolved from 802.11 to

802.11b to 802.11g, etc.). Backward compatibility of the technology is inherent in the system, and via the infrastructure, upgrades are possible to "modernize" the wireless network's technology as needed. Knowledge regarding these networks is very specialized, and involvement by a specialist in the respective wireless technology and intended field of deployment (e.g., healthcare) is imperative when planning, installing, and implementing these systems. Similar to planning a wired network, the design is based on variables that can be largely applied to most environments. How far can a signal travel? At what speed can information be transferred? How much power is needed? What are the known obstacles, etc.? The common issues experienced when applying these "rules" to a design are complex due to lack of understanding of what is really happening in the environment. No standard recommendations exist regarding coverage and speed in various areas of a hospital. No studies have been conducted to recommend coverage in areas of reduced penetrance such as the radiology suite and the OR. These are the complexities that make wireless networking in the hospital environment so specialized, leading to experience-based and not evidence-based implementation. In addition to complex coverage issues, simple issues may be encountered, e.g., a microwave oven being operated in an adjacent space to that of a critical wireless communications area (microwave ovens operate in the 2.4-GHz frequency range, similar to WiFi).

The obstacles in a healthcare environment that impact wireless design are nearly endless and are largely specific to a facility (requiring case-by-case consideration). Considering the gamut of interference, from that caused by imaging equipment to that caused by lead-lined walls, it is absolutely paramount that a proper wireless survey be conducted before a design is implemented. A properly executed survey of the facility for which the network is being designed will ensure that the intended results are achieved, maximum performance is obtained, and the best return on investment is realized. Eliminating the need to immediately repair the wireless network to address unexpected performance and coverage issues that are discovered after deployment can mean the difference between a deployment being cost effective and a full success, and one that has a significant budget overrun for a network that does not meet the needs of its users—and hence, a failed implementation. For an organization that is small and/or does not have any dedicated wireless networking resources, engaging a consultant who specializes in the wireless technology intended to be deployed is a reasonable alternative. As proper design and deployment are the paramount factors that affect the overall performance and, ultimately, return on investment, the use of an outside consultant to achieve immediate wireless objectives is a cost-effective means to success. Once a wireless "foundation" has been properly implemented, the operation and maintenance of that system can generally be incorporated into an organization's networking maintenance strategy. With specific wireless administration classes and vendor support broadly available, if the foundation is properly implemented, a smaller organization can concentrate on operation and administration rather than on providing its own expert resources for remediation, troubleshooting, and design modifications solely in efforts to "make it work."

An Overview of 802.11 and Cellular Network Basics

802.11 WiFi

802.11, also known by the brand name *WiFi*, denotes a set of WLAN standards developed by working group 11 of the Institute of Electrical and Electronics Engineers (IEEE), which serves as the "standards body" for many electronics and communications platforms, including 802.11.[5] Governing the policies, standards, development, and "certification" (industry acceptance), IEEE unifies manufacturers to ensure that a device that is branded (in this case) as "WiFi" is fully compatible with those from other manufacturers that produce WiFi devices. To put this into perspective, if a user needs a USB (universal serial bus) cable for the computer (USB is also governed by IEEE), he simply goes to a store and purchases the appropriate length of cable for the application because all that he needs to know is that a USB cable is needed. If not for the IEEE, any manufacturer could refer to its cable as a "USB cable" but could present its own types of plug, cable, application, etc., associated with that reference.

The 802.11 standard appears in various forms, each representing a subsequent "improvement" to the previous technology (Table 22.1). As a direct result of IEEE's efforts, all ensuing releases under the "802.11 standard" will be compatible with all preceding versions. Currently, the 802.11 standard includes "a," "b," and "g" versions, with an "n" version still in development. (Note: some products are being shipped with the yet-to-be ratified standard of "n"; however, they are not referred to as "802.11" devices at this time, as the standard has not been finalized.) As with the instance of the current evaluation of 802.11n by the IEEE committee, if a manufac-

Table 22.1 The key capabilities of 802.11 variations

Protocol	Release date	Operation frequency (GHz)	Throughput (type) (Mbit/s^{-1})	Data rate (max) (Mbit/s^{-1})	Range (indoor) (m)	Range (outdoor) (m)
Legacy	1997	2.4–2.5	0.7	2	Depends on walls	~75
802.11a	1999	5.15–5.25/ 5.25–5.35/ 5.49–5.71/ 5.745–5.825	23	54	~30	~100
802.11b	1999	2.4–2.5	4	11	~35	~110
802.11g	2003	2.4–2.5	19	54	~35	~110
802.11y	March 2008 (estimated)	3.65–3.7	23	54	~32	~5,000
802.11n	Sept 2008 (estimated)	2.4 and/or 5	74	248 = 2 × 2 ant	~70	~160

Mbit megabit—a unit of information or computer storage

turer chooses to take advantage of the available technology advancement prior to IEEE approval, it may market what is referred to as a "pre-n" device. It is important to note that if this device is stated to be WiFi compliant, it is compatible with older WiFi technology—in this case, 802.11g—and while misleading, calling the device "pre-n" does not indicate that it has been approved by any WiFi-certifying agency for the unapproved standard. In this sense, the situation is very similar to "high-definition-ready" televisions being made commercially available before high-definition technology was even released in the marketplace.

It remains a clear constant that consumers want the best technology as soon as possible and are willing to take certain risks that are associated with obtaining that technology. Therefore, the careful check and balance of the IEEE, combined professional/end-user evaluation committees (IT and medical teams), and steering committees that are ultimately responsible for evaluating the various recommendations, risk/benefit analyses, and cost benefits maintain a well-balanced playing field between the users who want the best technology immediately and the technologists who want, in many cases, an unreasonable amount of assurances before adopting something new.

Applied to the "pre-n" example given earlier, manufacturers will proactively create "prestandard" devices that meet all known requirements defined by the IEEE at the time of manufacture (e.g., backward compatibility), as well as all aspects that they "believe" will be included in the final "n" standard. The product is based on the manufacturer's interpretation of what the final standard will be, and it is often not guaranteed to have any interoperability with products other than those of the same manufacturer. While prestandard equipment may satisfy short-term goals (it may offer applications speed, perceived reliability, etc.), it is important to consider that prestandard technology will almost always be a dead-end product, often having a very short support life cycle after the "standard" has been ratified. Typically, no cost-effective upgrade path is available for these products; device and application support is limited, as it is solely at the manufacturer's discretion, and repair and replacement parts typically do not exist. Other than for the purposes of getting ahead of the technology curve and performing a controlled proof of concept (intended to evaluate the technology, not the application of the technology), adoption of prestandard technology in advance of final approval by the IEEE is not recommended.

The 802.11 wireless network infrastructure includes a combination of access points (APs), WLAN controllers (WLCs), antennas, a point of presence (POP) to the LAN or Internet, and wireless end-point devices, including wireless network interface cards (NICs), wireless phones with voice-over-Internet protocol (VoIP), wireless location devices (IP–RFID, Internet protocol–radio-frequency identification), and specialty application devices (CPE, customer premises equipment). In the simplest terms, once implemented, a WLAN is nothing more than an untethered connection to the LAN. Consequently, if properly designed and implemented, any application that can be supported over the LAN can be connected wirelessly and securely. Because healthcare personnel are by nature mobile, wireless technology is indispensable in a healthcare environment. Typical applications employed across an 802.11 network include Ethernet-based wireless devices such as laptops, PDAs, RFID devices, and VoIP devices.

As the technology continues to evolve and mature in parallel with improvements in wireless speed, reliability, security, cost, and availability, more devices will be capable of leveraging a wireless infrastructure. With these devices becoming more common, more dependable, and less expensive, devices and applications that leverage these wireless networks will become more popular, some capable of supporting an institution's needs right out of the box. To put this into perspective, when a consumer purchased a cellular telephone 3 years ago, she considered the cost of the calling plans, the coverage maps compared to where she frequently traveled, and then the cost of the device that would deliver the services desired with the cellular phone. Today, that same consumer typically does not worry about the brand of phone, the technology it uses, where it will and will not work, or even its hardware (the carrier it is working on, whether it uses EDGE or EVDO, etc.); she simply considers the device's ease of use, appearance, and cost. Because the technology has come so far and the "carriers" are so competitive, the consumer assumes that a device being offered by her carrier of choice will work where she wants it to, when she wants it to, and based on her purchase, do what the carrier says it will do. Cellular is now largely a commonplace technology, well integrated into most people's lives; it is a foregone conclusion that a wireless phone will work everywhere (within reason), every time, all the time.

The evolution of WiFi is right behind this trend, quickly becoming a commonplace technology. As this evolution continues, it is believed that personal computing devices will become similar to cell phones with regard to wireless. When purchasing, it will not be a question of whether wireless is desired, but which wireless technology and which wireless hardware is preferred [wireless wide area network, WWAN (e.g., cellular), or WiFi (e.g., WLAN)]. The technology on the device side will continue to become more transparent to the customer who is working anywhere where wireless connection (WWAN or WiFi) is available.

It is important to note that wireless technology is becoming a commonplace application in most professional environments. The demand continues to increase, forcing manufacturers to become more competitive. Greater speeds and performance are offered on a continual basis, and the cost to deploy these systems has significantly decreased. As wireless data volume increases, more applications will become supportable over a common wireless infrastructure. For example, just a few years ago, with an 802.11b deployment (which was cutting edge at the time), having multiple laptop connections and a simultaneous voice call to a single AP was not possible. Today, with 802.11g, it is common to facilitate many connections, both voice and data, over a single AP. Properly implemented, a "g" network may facilitate as many as six voice connections, multiple high-speed laptop connections, and report upon the location of numerous active RFID tags from a single AP. Up from an approximate maximum devices connected to a "b" network AP of six (with serious connectivity reliability issues), it is not uncommon to see greater than 20 simultaneous connections to an AP at any given time on a "g" network, depending on the mix of technologies accessing that AP.

When deploying WiFi technology, numerous steps must be followed to ensure that the infrastructure will be effective in the delivery of the quality of service that today's businesses demand. Performing a site survey is imperative; AP installation locations must be properly identified to ensure that coverage is consistent throughout the intended area of usage. Locations that have dead spots where mobile telephones do not work limit the ability of VoIP devices to place or receive calls, and laptops cannot access vital network resources—these are unacceptable conditions in a critical care environment.

Many hospitals are implementing 802.11 WiFi technologies to support a variety of applications. The innovation of wireless communication is that it has the potential to provide reliable "connectivity" to areas otherwise unable to be connected (i.e., where wired connections are cost prohibitive or otherwise impossible). Some uses of this technology are obvious, e.g., it allows a clinician to connect his laptop or portable computing device to the institution's systems anywhere, anytime, seamlessly, to send emails, place orders for patients, etc. Not quite so obvious is the enabling of instant, on-demand communication between any caregiver anywhere in the coverage area to whatever resources are required in order to facilitate the care and safety of a patient. This linkage is made possible without having to recable a facility to keep up with the demand of an ever-changing topology (what was once a single-patient room may now hold multiple beds or may be a "reading room"). Limiting the clinicians to areas where they can "plug in" and must therefore remain stationary until they complete their task is no longer an acceptable alternative.

Cellular Technologies

Industry consolidation has reduced the number of choices of cell-based providers to a small number of carriers that offer nationwide or regional service. Through their consolidations, carriers have dramatically improved upon their coverage areas, allowing cellular to provide almost ubiquitous coverage nationwide. Cellular telephones, once a luxury item that only wealthy executives could afford, are now common, affordable, reliable communications. Many parents have even equipped their children with these devices for safety, instant communication, and to track their location using advanced cellular global-positioning technology (typically free to users). Cellular technology will continue to evolve, making phones more affordable, accessible, and practical, and making their usage more likely by otherwise disinterested consumers. The technology has simply become so much a part of our lives that some do without home phones altogether and simply use a portable cellular telephone. Cellular service providers have taken notice of this trend and are encouraging usage through calling plans geared toward these specific targeted consumers.

Depending on the service provider and technology in use, cellular telephones generally operate in two different radio-frequency spectrums/technologies: global system for mobile communication (GSM; operates in 900- and 1800-MHz frequency bands) and code division multiple access (CDMA; operates in both the 800- and 1900-MHz frequency bands).[1] Carriers such as Verizon and Sprint have generally implemented CDMA cellular networks, while AT&T and T-Mobile have largely adopted the GSM standard, the technology that is used almost exclusively outside the US.

While GSM and several other current cellular technologies are technically "narrowband" time division multiple access (TDMA) systems, "TDMA-only" systems are in operation in a very limited capacity in both the US and Canada by "legacy" and small cellular providers. The technology is not referenced specifically, as it is generally considered to be at the end of its life and no longer in use by major cellular providers. Each of these technologies has advantages and disadvantages. For example, third-generation (3G) GSM networks allow for simultaneous voice and data connections that enable a user to send a text message during a voice conversation. Most 3G CDMA implementations require separate equipment within the networks to allow for the same simultaneous voice and data connection functionality. In most cases, this equipment is transparent to the end user; however, it has notable differences in technology and implementation.

The applicability of using cell-based services in the professional environment does transcend a variety of possibilities. Some of the uses of cellular phone technology may seem obvious. The ability to communicate a patient's needs, either verbally or via an electronic record transfer, to the caregiver at the point of care can be indispensable. Logistics must be considered when attempting to take advantage of this technology, as implementation can be very challenging. The design of hospitals, in particular, makes it difficult to provide dense cellular service due to the vast amount of electrical interference, physical barriers (lead-lined walls, etc.), and the geographic design of most facilities (through renovations and additions, outside walls often become inside walls, once large open spaces become inhabited, and space is always at a premium, making installation difficult). Additionally, without specialized installations, cellular services almost always provide "outside-in" coverage (the signal is being transmitted from outside the building to devices inside), leading to "reliability issues" whereby the devices may not connect, may stay connected consistently, or may be intermittent. In the healthcare setting, this situation is unacceptable as it creates an unstable platform for reliable communications.

To mitigate these problems, solutions are available that work in conjunction with cellular radio technology, which can largely reduce coverage issues within the confines of a facility. Commonly referred to as a "DAS" (distributed antenna system), a network of in-building antennae can be installed for the specific purpose of facilitating the propagation of the radio-frequency signal into spaces that the cell carriers cannot penetrate through conventional means, including areas such as ORs, underground areas (e.g., parking garages), and places that may have metal-lined walls such as radiology or MRI suites. To accomplish this level of coverage, antennae are placed in strategic locations throughout the complex and a signal from the cellular carrier is then broadcast over the "antenna network," as opposed to transmitting "outside in," thus creating a reliable signal, regardless of where the client is located. This type of coverage is important for a number of reasons: connectivity is improved, cell-phone battery life is substantially increased, and potential interference to sensitive medical equipment is substantially decreased (the phone operates at a significantly reduced power setting in the presence of a DAS).

Although these types of antenna systems can be expensive, must be meticulously designed to provide coverage for their intended use (cellular, two-way radio, paging, etc.), and require well-planned implementation, the realized beneficial results when the systems are implemented properly are unsurpassed by any other solution currently available.

VoFI and VoIP Technology

As a true convergence of the two technologies discussed above (WiFi and cellular), VoIP and VoFI are communication mechanisms that can provide a low-cost, reliable, facility-wide common communications platform. Both technologies have existed for some time. VoIP telephony services are commercially marketed by Vonage and Voice Wing (Verizon), and VoFI simply uses them via a wireless network such as Skype (owned by Ebay). Corporate adoption of IP voice communications is slow. Using wireless infrastructure to take advantage of these technologies can significantly reduce communications costs and dramatically increase reliability. To that end, the next evolution of cellular telephones, for example, will have the ability to automatically stop using their cellular signal when entering a VoFI-supported building and start using the facility's network for voice calls. The intent is for the device to automatically use the strongest, most reliable signal for communications at all times.

VoIP/VoFI is a voice communications media that is delivered via a corporate wireless Ethernet network, resulting in available telephone coverage wherever wireless Ethernet is available. From a speed and availability perspective, a properly implemented wireless infrastructure can far surpass the coverage capabilities that any cellular service provider could offer. In addition to this coverage advantage, a facility has the distinct advantage to tie its communication network directly to its clinical communications systems, such as the corporate directory, nurse call system, house phone/PBX, internal calling plans, and call-forwarding programs. The convergence of these two communications technologies in healthcare is revolutionizing the caregiving capability.

Radio-Frequency Identification Technology

Radio-frequency identification (RFID) is a generic term for technologies that use radio waves to automatically identify objects. RFID technologies are being used by companies such as Wal-Mart to track inventory and EZ Pass (toll roads in the northeastern US from Maine to Virginia) to track vehicle toll service. Several hospitals are now using this technology to identify patients, medications, and equipment. RFID data can be tagged as a client on an 802.11 network (similar to tagging a laptop or PDA), enabling every object that must be identified to be identified. An RFID tag offers the ability to electronically assign a unique identity, which can be in the form of a serial number, social security number, case number, etc. to any device otherwise not able to have an electronic presence. For example, a patient wearing an RFID bracelet can be located anywhere in the hospital. Moreover, an alarm may sound if an incompatible unit of RFID-labeled blood is brought into the same OR as that patient. These data reside on a microchip that is attached to an antenna. This chip with the antenna is called an *RFID transponder* or an *RFID tag*. The antenna enables the chip to transmit the identification information to a reader, where it can then be stored, displayed, or processed by an application.

Two types of RFID tags are available: an *active tag* contains a battery to power the microchip's circuitry and "actively" broadcasts a signal to the reader (e.g., tracking patients in the hospital before and after surgery to improve OR efficiency). A *passive tag* is a tag that contains no battery and draws its power from the RFID reader. Although *semipassive tags* use a battery to run the microchip, they are classified as passive because they still draw power from the reader to communicate and do not broadcast information. Passive tags are commonly used in applications such as medication labeling to reduce dispensing errors, as a physical component is still required in "scanning" the tag. The best way to differentiate the two technologies is to note that an active tag offers the data contained on it to any prescribed reading device, whereas a passive tag releases those data when specifically "asked" via the manual process of scanning (similar to barcode technology).

Wireless technologies and their applications continue to increase in number, and daily advances in communication technologies will continue to improve patient safety, professional collaborations, and personnel productivity. As we are living the "evolution of wireless" through the true convergence of all technologies mentioned, we are faced with the opportunity to actually define what communications technology means to patient care, safety, accuracy, and service.

Following is a typical scenario that would be possible in an institution that is equipped with RFID technology:

Mr. George enters an ED with abdominal pain. During triage, a nurse assigns Mr. George an RFID bracelet and enters his demographic information into the hospital's records and admissions system. From there, Mr. George is taken to the exam room. During the exam, Dr. Johns takes out her wireless tablet and scans the patient's ID; she is presented with the patient's EMR and the intake report. When Dr. Paul saw Mr. George 3 days ago, he had similar complaints. With a touch on the tablet, Dr. Johns is connected to Dr. Paul for a consult. She then updates the records, orders an ultrasound, and scans the patient out of her care, which alerts the ED that Mr. George is now ready to go to ultrasound (his records were all updated in real time by Dr. Johns) and that arrangements should be made for transport. Upon arrival, the transport team scans Mr. George's RFID wristband and selects "in transit" to ultrasound; this action notifies radiology that Mr. George is in route. After the ultrasound, Mr. George needs surgery on an emergent basis. The OR tracks Mr. George in real time, thus reducing miscommunication about patient location. Upon arrival in the OR, the RFID band helps with the time-out procedure by displaying the patient's name and surgical site on the display terminals. All of these functions can be seamlessly implemented with a good wireless infrastructure.

Any new installation of wireless, cellular, and/or DAS networks in a facility must be positioned to take advantage of what the technology can do tomorrow—not what is needed today. Properly designed, a network can answer today's needs automatically. By defining what is best for a given institution during the course of present and future installations, it will be possible to lay a foundation of wireless technology that will be a hub of communication.

The healthcare industry has been concerned about the reliability and safety of using cell phones and wireless networks in critical care areas for some time. Fueled by the dramatic trend of increased consumer usage of these devices (cellular phones, in particular), facilities with such sensitive equipment as mechanical ventilators, electrocardiographic monitors, and other critical life-saving equipment have questioned the pervasive effect of interference from wireless devices used in close proximity to these machines. Studies conducted at the Mayo Clinic and several other centers have shown no significant interference with OR equipment if wireless devices are used appropriately. Many of the studies conclude that use of wireless devices at a distance of one meter or greater from sensitive equipment all but eliminates the chance of the potential negative effects of electromagnetic interference.[6,7] Emerging data show that the appropriate use of a cell phone and/or other wireless technologies may in fact improve upon patient safety as opposed to impeding it.[7] Indeed, appropriately used wireless technology in an anesthesia and critical care setting has great potential to improve communication, efficiency, accuracy, and patient safety.

Conclusion

Technology that is state of the art today is old by tomorrow. *Convergence* continues to be the hot topic when it comes to wireless technology. It is only a question of time when we will be able to carry one piece of communication equipment that will work on cellular and wireless networks flawlessly and will also serve as a PDA. Scientific data and experience are minimal regarding the implementation of wireless networks in the perioperative and intensive care environments. Investing funds during the design phase to engage a consultant with experience in this field will pay dividends in improving functionality and, hence, end-user acceptance and utilization of technology. A well-planned wireless infrastructure today should be ready to accept the newer technologies of tomorrow with minimal manipulation.

Many of the enhancements that the "future" of wireless is going to yield are already present in today's products. This is an exciting prospect, as we can see, touch, and feel the technology that will ultimately make our communications more accessible, reliable, and cost effective. Convergence is the piece of the puzzle yet to be fully defined; the demand as set by the daily use of devices such as laptop computers and cellular phones will ultimately define what "convergence" means to the future of wireless mobility.

Key Points

- Future handheld devices will have the capability of seamlessly switching between WiFi and cellular, based on speed, signal strength, and network availability. Users will not have to interact with the device to make a "connectivity" selection, enabling operations such as phone calls and Internet sessions to go uninterrupted as the user traverses between an office WiFi network and a cellular connection.

- The healthcare community will see "converged" devices in the form of a "Tablet PC," for example, that allow communications from a single device with applications, Internet, and voice simultaneously virtually anywhere that cellular connectivity or a WLAN is available. Devices of this nature will bring the functionality of full-featured laptops together with cell phones, PDAs, and specialty devices such as telemetry monitors or electronic charts.

- *Presence-based communications* will be available through a single device that will integrate paging, applications integration (e.g., corporate directory or nurse call), and virtual office connectivity. A user will enter his office or hospital, and the system will recognize his "presence" (i.e., recognize her device being on-site) and facilitate all communications via that device, thereby eliminating the need for multiple phone numbers and devices that act as interactive pagers (two-way), office phones, location identifiers, and immediate-response voice devices (Vocera, or two-way radio-like functionality).

- The possibilities of wireless technology will be virtually limitless. The convergence of any of the devices that are currently employed with one another is within the realm of reality. The demand for such device functionality will drive what technology converges with what devices, and availability will be dictated by the need within any particular industry.

References

1. http://en.wikipedia.org/wiki/Wi-Fi
2. http://en.wikipedia.org/wiki/Wireless_LAN
3. Rehman M, Shwartz RE. Wireless local area networks (WLAN) for anesthesia record keeping. Abstract, Society for Technology in Anesthesia, Miami, FL, 2005
4. "Badge" that enables staff communication. Br J Healthcare Comput Inform Manage 2006 (May); 23(4). http://www.bjhcim.co.uk/news/industry/2006/ind605003.htm. Accessed February 11, 2008
5. http://standards.ieee.org/wireless/overview.html. Accessed February 8, 2008
6. Wallin MK, Marve T, Hakansson PK. Modern wireless telecommunication technologies and their electromagnetic compatibility with life-supporting equipment. Anesth Analg 2005; 101(5):1393–400
7. Soto RG, Chu LF, Goldman JM, et al. Communication in critical care environments: Mobile telephones improve patient care. Anesth Analg 2006; 102(2):535–41

Chapter 23
Security of Health Information

Gordon Gibby and Keith J. Ruskin

Electronic generation, transmission, and storage of health data have transformed patient care by making it easy to acquire, search, manipulate, and distribute large amounts of information. An electronic workflow facilitates direct patient care and can be used for purposes such as quality assurance and submission of health insurance claims. Information in the health record is also used for purposes not directly related to patient care, including insurance qualification, law enforcement, and litigation. Health information can, subject to specific safeguards, also be used for clinical research and for projects that improve public health. Systematic collection and storage of EMRs imposes the responsibility of protecting health information from unauthorized use, and patients and providers have legitimate concerns regarding the protection of their information.

The organization, delivery, and financing of modern healthcare require the aggregation and storage of personal health information. Privacy and security of health information are therefore crucial to the widespread adoption of electronic health records. The EMR contains intimate details about a person's physical and mental health. Unauthorized access to this information can have devastating consequences for both healthcare providers and their patients. Unintentional release of information about disease processes, medication use, or visits to healthcare providers can result in stigmatization, difficulty in obtaining credit or employment, or disruption of friendships or family relationships. Most importantly, unintended release of information can result in a breach of trust between patient and physician. In response to these concerns, the European Union, United States, Australia, and Japan have all enacted stringent regulations that address the sharing and protection of health information. Compliance with these laws requires sophisticated information-management technologies. Information security encompasses physical protection of hardware, access control, data authentication, and encryption of sensitive information. This chapter discusses the privacy and security of the EMR and proposes strategies for protecting this valuable repository of information.

J. Stonemetz, K. Ruskin (eds.) *Anesthesia Informatics,*
© Springer Science + Business Media, LLC 2008

Privacy

A recent survey reported that 75% of polled American consumers were concerned that sensitive health information might leak because of weak data security.[1] Patients expect that their medical records will remain confidential. Government regulations as well as ethical obligations require that patients' health information be protected whenever it is aggregated, stored, or transmitted. Most of the requirements for storage and transmission of medical records are covered under the HIPAA of 1996. These requirements extend beyond health professionals who collect information. Any person/entity that provides services to a healthcare organization and handles protected health information (PHI) is bound by HIPAA to defend the security of medical records. If, for example, a physician in solo practice collects information that is forwarded to a billing service, that billing service must comply with HIPAA privacy rules. Patients must give their consent to the use of PHI, although HIPAA consents can be interpreted broadly. For example, a surgeon may include as part of a consent a statement about using the consenting patient's PHI for fundraising purposes. In another instance, PHI has been deidentified and used to train insurance claims agents.[2]

When a patient provides personal information, he is entering into a contract that specifies how that information will be stored and used. EMRs should be designed to allow policies to be created and then changed over time. If information is shared with another entity, the policies should be included with it and remain enforceable. At present, policies are governed by clauses in contracts that describe the business relationship. However, as interoperable EMRs become commonplace, it may ultimately be possible for the healthcare provider or the patient to determine how confidential information is used.[3]

Healthcare organizations must (a) limit disclosure of health information to the minimum necessary to achieve the goals of the disclosure, (b) create policies that define which personnel have access to information and how that information may be used, (c) designate a privacy officer who is responsible for enforcing policies and procedures, and (d) train members of the workforce and adopt written policies that describe which personnel have access to information and include procedures for using it.

HIPAA regulations mandate both physical and electronic protection of health records. The requirements for EMRs are more stringent than those for paper records and are applied to information that resides in a single computer or on a server or that is transmitted across a network. The regulations also apply to letters, laboratory results, and even telephone conversations. Health information must therefore be encrypted before it is transmitted over public networks. It is also the responsibility of healthcare workers who are discussing a patient over the telephone to verify the identity of all participants in the conversation.[4]

The right to privacy must be balanced with the potential benefits of sharing portions of the medical record. Obvious examples include prevention of serious threats to health or safety and oversight of the healthcare system.[5] Healthcare providers in the US are required to obtain a patient's written consent prior to disclosure of health information for routine treatment, payment, or oversight operations such as utilization review or quality assurance. However, some experts do not consider the consent to be truly informed, because the eventual contents of the record are unknown at the beginning of treatment, and the record will change over time. Moreover, most patients do not have a clear idea of where the information will go or how it will be used. Although the individual may request that certain restrictions be placed on the use of her information, the healthcare provider is not obliged to comply with the request.[6]

Research is widely accepted to be in the public interest and frequently requires disclosure of selected healthcare information. Federal regulations known as the *Common Rule* apply to federally funded studies and research conducted for the Food and Drug Administration.[7] All research is subject to rigorous scientific and ethical review, which now includes policies for disclosure and use of confidential health information. Although the Common Rule requires approval by an institutional review board, it does not explicitly state requirements for confidentiality. Rather, it requires that adequate provisions be made to protect the privacy of the patient. It also requires that investigators provide subjects with a statement that describes the extent to which confidentiality of identifying information will be maintained.

HIPAA includes regulations that cover privacy in research that is based on review of medical records. A covered entity may use or disclose PHI for research without obtaining prior permission from the patient if it has obtained a waiver from an institutional review board or privacy board. The privacy board is defined under HIPAA and must include people of varying backgrounds, including one member who is not affiliated with the research sponsor or investigator. Requirements for waiver criteria include provisions that state that the use or disclosure involves minimal risk, that the research could not be conducted without the waiver, and that the privacy risks are reasonable when compared to the benefits of the research. The research protocol must also include a plan to deidentify the information unless there is a justification for not doing so, and the investigator must provide a written assurance that the information will not be disclosed to outside parties, except for research oversight or additional research.

Many researchers assume that patient confidentiality will be protected by simply deidentifying information contained within an EMR. Typical approaches usually involve removing the patient name, address, telephone number, and medical record number from the record. Information that has been protected in this fashion is prone to "linkage attacks" in which information in the health record is combined with other publicly identifiable information to reidentify the data subjects. For example, it would be possible to reidentify the health information of a 26-year-old male medical student by looking at the class directories of medical schools in or near the zip code contained in the record. Other approaches to anonymization involve data scrambling or data swapping, which preserves anonymity but changes the information in the data set.[8] A technique called *k-anonymization* renders each record in a data set indistinguishable from at least $k - 1$ other records. This technique involves data suppression (e.g., removing the patient's name and address) and generalization (replacing a specific value with more general values) and offers greater privacy protection at the cost of slightly less specific data.[3]

Email

Email is an effective tool that permits rapid distribution of information and allows images and other attachments to be exchanged easily. Important messages can be saved for future reference. Its asynchronous nature allows busy healthcare professionals to exchange information without having to find each other on the telephone. Physicians routinely use email to communicate with each other and with their patients. In 2006, 17% of physicians routinely used email to communicate with their patients, and more than two-thirds of physicians used email to communicate with other physicians.[9] As physicians become increasingly comfortable with information technology, it is likely that the number of physicians who use email to communicate will increase. One study found that only 1.6% of the physicians surveyed who used email adhered to published guidelines, which include printing email correspondence and placing it into the patient's chart.[9] Only one-third of physicians who used email informed patients about privacy issues. The use of email can enhance the patient–physician relationship by making the physician more accessible but raises concerns about both privacy and security.

Many of the problems that arise during email communication are caused by the fact that it is difficult to positively identify the true author of the message. Unencrypted email may be intercepted during transmission or if the mail server at either end of the transaction is compromised. Email messages can also be intercepted if either the patient's or physician's computer is lost or stolen or if an email account is compromised. Many physicians assume that patients are telling the truth about their identities and diagnoses, but it is relatively easy to impersonate another individual by registering an email address similar to that of the intended victim. Eysenbach sent email to the owners of medical Web sites while posing as a fictitious patient with a dermatologic lesion. While 93% of physicians who responded recommended that the patient see a physician, over half mentioned a specific diagnosis in their response.[10]

As a result of the potential problems delineated, the American Medical Informatics Association developed guidelines for the use of email by physicians and patients. These guidelines recommend obtaining informed consent prior to using email to communicate, prohibiting the forwarding of email without consent, explaining and using security mechanisms such as encryption, avoiding references to third parties, and informing patients who have access to email communications that these communications may become a part of their EMR. The recommendations also include simple tasks such as double-checking all "To" fields before sending messages and printing paper copies of messages and replies to place in the patient's chart.[11] Taking these relatively straightforward precautions will enhance the use of email while minimizing security risks.

HIPAA

Specific requirements for privacy and security of EMR systems were mandated by HIPAA. When Congress failed to pass the required regulations for the specifics of privacy and security, the US Department of Health and Human Services (HHS), as required by the Act, proposed for comment, and eventually adopted, specific regulations. The *Privacy Rule* was proposed in November 1999, and the *Final Rule for Privacy* was published in the Federal Register on December 28, 2000. Compliance by all but small healthcare plans was required by April 14, 2003. The primary impact of the Privacy Rule on the development of pre-anesthetic evaluation systems was to require user identification and authentication, the logging of everyone who accesses the EMR, and making available to the patient a list of all personnel who had accessed the record.

After a review of comments received on the initial proposal, the HIPAA Security Final Rule was published in the Federal Register of February 20, 2003. Most covered entries had until April 21, 2005, to comply with these regulations. Small healthcare plans were given additional time and were not required to implement the necessary changes until April 21, 2006. An unofficial version of the Regulations for both Privacy and Security is maintained by HHS on its Web site, which includes updates and amendments. The Security Rule has had a significant impact on the design and usage of preanesthetic evaluation systems. The Rule requires careful thought, documentation, and implementation of a wide range of procedures to achieve security of medical records systems.

Medical groups that are considering the purchase of an AIMS should be familiar with the HIPAA privacy regulations and coordinate the security aspects of their anesthesia-related medical systems with those of the larger systems in place at the institution. Addenda to the security documentation of the institution may suffice, or a special section may be written to accommodate the anesthesia system. The vendor or manufacturer may have boilerplate procedures and documentation, but one of the first tasks required by the Security Rule is a careful analysis of risks at the institution. Prior to purchasing a system, institutions should carefully evaluate the requirements of the Rule and how they will be satisfied at their facility. Compliance will generally be to the advantage of the anesthesia system, as it will prevent or mitigate many information-related disasters.

The requirements of the HIPAA Security Rule are categorized into *Administrative Safeguards*, *Physical Safeguards*, and *Technical Safeguards*. Further categorizations were denoted by HHS as *Required* (R) or *Addressable* (A). A Required section must be met as described. An Addressable section may not completely apply to a smaller system, e.g., an AIMS, but this must be discussed in writing in the institution's policy documentation. Many groups have published detailed discussions of compliance methods for the Security requirements. The Workgroup for Electronic Data Interchange (Reston, VA) has a very complete discussion. The individual requirements are briefly discussed below.

Administrative Safeguards

Risk Analysis

The most basic and perhaps most arduous requirement imposed by HIPAA is a comprehensive risk analysis. Security threats may be caused by inadvertent release of information to an unauthorized individual but can also result from social or business espionage. Preoperative assessment systems and automated record-keeping systems contain significant sensitive medical and social information, and their vulnerabilities will be system dependent. As a result, the person responsible for the security analysis must create documentation that specifies who is in charge of performing risk analysis and timelines or events that will trigger re-analysis. The analysis must include the specific information that is collected, potential ways in which the security of that information may be compromised, and the consequences of a security breach. The analysis should also document the losses that could result from inappropriate usage or disclosure of information or loss of data integrity. After the risk analysis has been completed, it is necessary to document security measures that have been implemented to reduce to a reasonable level the risks and vulnerabilities that have been identified.

Authorization and Supervision

Access to PHI must be limited to those personnel who require access to perform their duties. So-called role-based policies grant only limited access to personnel who are not directly involved in healthcare delivery and grant increasing access to those with increasing healthcare responsibility. Areas to be considered include requests for access and policy-based authorization. After approval, user IDs and passwords must be transferred to the individual in a secure manner. Furthermore, review (whether periodic or based on an event), modification, and documentation of history of access must be established. It is also important to develop procedures for terminating access should employees change positions or leave the system. HIPAA also requires covered entities to document the ways in which security procedures will be taught to the workforce. The content and training intervals should be commensurate with the level of access provided.

Sanction Policy

Appropriate policies ensure that PHI is used properly. Sanctions must be defined and documented. A range of sanctions should be created and determined by the nature of the infraction by workforce members (including employees, volunteers, trainees, and others under the control of the entity, whether paid or not).

Information System Activity Review

HIPAA requires that procedures be developed that ensure regular review of information system activity, and these procedures must be documented. Suggested tools include audit logs, access reports, and security-incident tracking reports. HIPAA requires documentation of all personnel authorized to access protected information in a very small organization (i.e., one or two healthcare personnel). In large organizations, the documentation requirements include personnel who determine which employees are authorized to access information and the method used to grant access. Security audits must also be documented, and the most commonly chosen methods are electronic and automatic (e.g., access audit trails).

Assigned Security Responsibility

One person, perhaps with multiple workers assisting, must be designated as responsible for developing, implementing, and maintaining security. (This person may also be the person responsible for Privacy, if so desired.) If role-based clearance is chosen, which "roles" have what level of access should be determined and documented.

The *isolating healthcare clearinghouse function* is required (R) if an organization serves as a healthcare clearinghouse (i.e., a repricing company, billing service, community health management information system) in addition to providing healthcare delivery. As much as possible, such entities should use completely separate email, computer, and information systems. Where business or information technology constraints require that both operations occur in close proximity, documentation of policies that ensure physical, technical, and administrative separation is required. For example, server administrators who have access to all information must have the minimum access necessary to perform their jobs. Entities should also determine which systems, policies, and training will be used to reduce the impact of malicious software such as viruses or keystroke loggers; possible strategies include installation of antivirus programs, prohibitions against downloading software to computers used to access PHI, and carrying disks from one computer to another.

A comprehensive security plan should also include password management policies that address how passwords are created, changed, and protected. This security plan should be augmented with a login-monitoring policy that creates a procedure for monitoring access to PHI and detection of unusual patterns. It is also important to educate all employees about these procedures. *Security incidents* must be defined, and the workforce should be educated to report incidents. A response plan must be documented (and followed during actual events), and the outcome of each reported incident must be documented. HHS estimated 50 such incidents per entity per year, with 8 hours of effort expended to deal with each incident, meaning that individual healthcare facilities should plan to spend ~400 hours per year per entity.

HIPAA requires the creation of contingency plans that specify how information will be protected during information system failures. Contingency plans are required for emergencies such as fire, vandalism, system failure, or natural disaster. HIPAA also requires creation of an "exact copy" of all PHI. It is not necessary to backup other information (e.g., email), but planning must allow for business to continue as usual in the event of an emergency. Specifically, the security of electronic PHI must be protected during the emergency, meaning that provisions must be made to allow critical business processes that protect the electronic PHI to continue. A disaster recovery plan must also be in place that documents procedures to restore any lost data after events such as fire, vandalism, natural disaster, or system failure. Note that regular testing of the data restoration process is necessary to ensure that the system works after an emergency. Periodic testing and revision of contingency plans must be planned and carried out.

Based on underlying risk analysis, the relative criticality of various applications and data must be analyzed, with periodic evaluation of how well the security policies and procedures meet all of the requirements set forth, in light of additions, modifications to systems, or other changes. HIPAA regulations also require documentation that states that any business associate of the entity that will be allowed to create, receive, maintain, or transmit electronic PHI will maintain appropriate safeguards.

Physical Safeguards

In the following selected list of HIPAA safeguards, R = Required and A = Addressable. As stated above, those requirements designated as "R" must be met as described. Those designated as "A" may not completely apply to smaller systems.

Facility Access Controls 164.310(a)(1)

Contingency operations (A). Address control of access to the facility during disaster recovery or emergency mode operations, including tasking a person to determine who is allowed to access the facility and how authorized personnel will prove their identity prior to access.

Facility security plan (A). Address the physical security of the facility and its network connections. Considerations might include human threats, such as vandals, burglars, and terrorists, as well as natural threats, such as fire, flood, earthquakes, and storms.

Access control and validation procedures (A). Address how access to the facility by staff and visitors will be controlled.

Maintenance records (A). Plan ongoing maintenance of the physical plant and security systems.

Workstation Use 164.310(b) (R)

Workstations include both fixed and portable electronic devices that access PHI. Documentation must describe how these workstations are to be used and in what physical settings they may be used.

Workstation Security 164.310(c) (R)

Implement physical safeguards to protect the physical workstation (fixed or portable computer) from natural and environmental hazards and unauthorized access. Consider locked areas, covers or enclosures to block unauthorized viewing, and guards.

Device and Media Controls 164.310(d)(1)

Disposal (R). Document how hardware and electronic media that store PHI will be disposed in such a manner that PHI is not disclosed. Three recognized methods are repeated overwriting of the data, degaussing (destruction of the magnetic fields), and physical destruction.

Media reuse (R). Document how media that contain PHI will have that PHI removed prior to being made available for reuse.

Accountability (A). Address measures to keep track of hardware and electronic media used to store PHI, based on the risk assessment.

Data backup and storage (A). Address measures to backup and create copies of PHI and systems software; examples include mirrored hard drives in servers and synchronized servers.

Technical Safeguards

Access Control 164.312(a)(1)

Unique-user identification (R). A unique-user identification system must allow for usage tracking. Methods of creation and use must be documented. Each individual must be granted access to specific software applications.

Emergency access procedure (R). A process must be documented for gaining emergency access, for discontinuation of access, and for a process to audit individual access policies.

Automatic logoff (A). Based on risk assessment, the necessity for automatic logoff must be evaluated; if it is found to be necessary, a method of implementation must be documented, e.g., how inactivity is measured and assessed.

Encryption and decryption (A). Based on the risk assessment, necessity for encryption and decryption must be evaluated; if found necessary, the method of implementation must be documented.

Audit controls 164.312(b) (R). A wide array of logs of events and activities is possible, including logging user login, failed user login, user software access, user record access, administrator activity, equipment location and movement, software installation and software changes, unusual user activity patterns, malicious software attack attempts, and network transmission breaches and errors. Based on the risk analysis, the facility must document the level of audit controls enacted, how and when reviewed, and by whom.

Integrity 164.312(c)(1)

Mechanism to authenticate electronic PHI (A). Integrity controls protect against unauthorized alteration, loss, or creation of both PHI and system software and files. Such controls may utilize checksums, message authentication codes, digital signatures, hash totals, and other methods to detect loss of integrity. Address the methods used and how failed data or software can be corrected. Also address software and methods used to protect against viruses and errors in newly updated software or systems.

Person or entity authentication 164.312(d) (R). Authentication means proving that the person or entity who is attempting access is the one claimed. HIPAA requires at least one method, and more than one method may be used. Typical methods are based on either secret information such as a password, secret, or cryptographic key; an item in physical possession such as a key or a magnetic card; or biometric information such as a retinal scan or fingerprint. Additionally, different entities communicating electronically must prove their identity to each other before exchanging PHI. If passwords are used, procedures must be carefully designed to maintain security. Specifically, passwords must not be shared, must not be common words, and must be known only to the individual user. A "dictionary check" can be used to prevent users from selecting passwords that can easily be guessed. Procedures must also be created to monitor misuse of passwords.

Transmission Security 164.312(e)(1)

Integrity controls (A). The covered entity should address whether the network communications are guaranteed accurate; if not, a digital signature involving the encryption of a message digest with the sender's key can be utilized to prove the accuracy.

Encryption (A). Vulnerable networks may allow unauthorized access or diversion of network traffic. Entity should address whether the network is vulnerable and, if so, the fact that it requires encryption of communications.

Multiple Authorship of Medical Records

It is possible for a single individual to create an anesthetic record by gathering and summarizing previous medical records; collecting a current review of systems, medications, allergies; examining the patient; measuring vital signs; and acquiring laboratory information. In such a case, user identification and authentication unarguably documents who created the entries and therefore takes responsibility for them. Most large practices use a preoperative testing clinic to streamline the process of gathering the information necessary to safely provide anesthesia to patients. This process involves various specialists, all of whom contribute to the final document. For example, a technician may gather vital-sign data, while a nurse may obtain medication and allergies; a nurse practitioner or physician may add additional review of systems and physical examination data. All of these people should individually identify and authenticate themselves, and the document should reflect the authorship of each portion. It is likely that many systems in use today do not meet this standard. The situation becomes more complicated if prior medical records are incorporated into a new document. If the medical practitioner summarizes prior history, she becomes the author of the new document, but this summarization is error prone, time consuming, and therefore, expensive. Anyone familiar with a word processor will immediately question why a "cut-and-paste" operation cannot be performed to select relevant portions of past electronic documents (e.g., a CT scan report or a complicated description of an intraoperative difficulty encountered in a previous anesthetic) and insert that information into the current evaluation. To correctly attribute the authorship of such insertions requires the ability to document the authorship of single sections, even portions of sentences, and it may require that the authorship be a property of the "objects" in the previous document. Displaying the authorship may be difficult. Sections may have to be color coded or have the ability to demonstrate borders on request, with indications of ownership of the data within the borders.

System Maintenance

Like all computerized EMRs, AIMS will require technical upkeep and advancement such as replacement of servers, ongoing improvements in security systems (e.g., adding encryption to network communications), and addition of external communications methods. However, the medical information contained within the system also requires upkeep. New drugs become available and commonplace in the population; new diseases and treatments are discovered; new understandings of the measurement of risk of a disease (such as coronary atherosclerosis) emerge. Many medical record systems are but thin veneers that serve as interfaces to database servers and often have a blocky spreadsheet-like user interface. Such systems usually include methods for changing the text of questions about the patient's health and sometimes for adding or deleting questions. Should treatment guidelines of a particular illness change dramatically, a completely new approach to a section of the preanesthetic interview may be warranted. Medical oversight and upkeep are necessary, and the ability of some systems to accept completely new pathways may be limited.

Perhaps the most significant difficulty in upgrading an AIMS occurs when it is time to completely replace one computerized system with another. Although most systems store their data in relational databases that are technically compatible, great difficulty may arise in moving huge numbers of old patient records into a new system. The fields contained within the new commercial system are highly unlikely to match the structured fields of the previous system. At least one hospital decided to simply lose the previous structured records of over 100,000 patients when it was faced with the complexity of matching 100 or more fields from one system with another. In that case, textual records with little structure had been created for many of the records. Anesthesiologists must be able to make a convincing case for retaining structured records. Individual databases may have limitations and configurations (e.g., a limit on the number of characters in one type of field) that may not match the offerings of various anesthesia applications. Hospital administrators may view preanesthetic evaluation systems as of secondary importance, believing that most of the important information is contained in textual paragraphs of prior surgical H&Ps or in internal medical admission notes. When faced with an upgrade, anesthesiologists should begin from the start to request that all previous data not be lost and that consideration be given to the important process of moving the old data to the new system.

Barriers to Implementation

The two major barriers to implementation of AIMS are the purchase cost and the ongoing effort required to use and maintain them. It is possible that a well-designed and well-implemented system can provide a significant return on investment over its useful life—advantages that include improved scheduling efficiency and charge capture, among others.

From the standpoint of the users, the much larger cost is the difficulty of using these systems. The human–computer interface remains primarily that of mouse and keyboard. Preconfigured "canned" text and algorithms can reduce the tediousness of data entry, but they also reduce the feeling of individualism and professionalism of the users. As demographics increase the seriousness of patient illnesses, more careful and precise documentation of the patient condition is required, which is not always aided by preconfigured, static text. Not all physicians enjoy the keyboard interface, and this may seriously reduce their proficiency.

The costs of a comprehensive EMR system may be prohibitive, while the benefits are frequently intangible, which can lead many physicians to question their advantages. For many purposes, a simple electronic scan of a paper record suffices for adequate medical care documentation. As a result, some medical groups may simply scan handwritten preanesthetic evaluations into an EMR system. Better human interfaces must be created before professionals will widely prefer computer entry over handwriting. Progress in this area will continue.

Cryptography

Cryptography is the science of using mathematics to protect information, and it is essential to information security. Cryptographic techniques are used to protect confidentiality, to authenticate healthcare workers who access the medical record, and to protect information as it is transmitted from one location to another. Cryptographic techniques render information unintelligible to anyone who is not authorized to receive it and have become an integral component of the modern economy. Anyone who has used a secure Web site to purchase an airline ticket or pay a bill has taken advantage of the security provided by modern cryptographic techniques.

A cryptographic algorithm is a mathematic function that uses a key, which may be a word, a number, or a phrase, to render confidential information unintelligible. The recipient then uses a key in conjunction with a different mathematic algorithm to convert the encrypted information back into its original form. Julius Caesar is credited with being the first person to use a cipher to secure information. Caesar invented a simple *substitution cipher*, in which each letter in his message was shifted three positions to the left.

X|Y|Z|A|B|C|D|E|F|G|H|I|J|K|L|M|N|O|P|Q|R|S|T|U|V|W|X|Y|Z

After encryption with the Caesar shift, ATTACK AT DAWN would read as XQQXZH XQ AXTK. If an enemy intercepted the encrypted message, it would appear to be a random string of letters. Only Caesar and his generals knew the algorithm and could return the message to its original, intelligible form.

Because of their simplicity and predictability, ciphers like the Caesar shift are vulnerable to easy interpretation. Given a sufficiently large sample of text, each letter in the alphabet will occur at a known relative frequency. It is therefore possible to match letters in encrypted text with the letter that occurs at the expected rate. Guessing a few letters allows short words to be found, which in turn, may provide clues to the identity of other letters. This strategy requires only a pencil and paper; simple ciphers can sometimes even be found in Sunday newspapers next to the cross-word puzzle. More advanced ciphers may be resistant to casual attacks, but with the wide availability of high-speed computers, many ciphers can be solved relatively quickly.

Modern cryptographic techniques are designed to be resistant to attacks using supercomputers. *Strong cryptography* is used to describe encoding techniques that are nearly impossible to decipher without possession of the correct decoding tools. Demonstrating resistance to attack is a complicated process and ideally involves testing in a public forum. A good cryptographic algorithm is obviously required, but the algorithm must reside on a computer that is physically secure and that has a secure operating system. Subject to these limitations, most modern cryptosystems are impenetrable even to resources possessed by the governments of large nations. As a result, they are sufficiently secure to comply with current privacy and security regulations and are widely used for healthcare applications.

Symmetric Key Cryptosystems

Cryptosystems can be broadly divided into *symmetric key systems*, which use a single key, and *public key systems*, which use more than one key. Symmetric key systems use trivially related keys for encryption and decryption. The key may be a single key that is shared between sender and recipient, or a simple mathematic transformation may prepare the key for encryption or decryption. Symmetric key systems are fast and secure and have many applications. The Data Encryption Standard (DES) is a symmetric key system that was initially developed by the International Business Machines Corporation (IBM) and the US government. Its primary flaw is that its key length is only 56 bits, making it susceptible to attack with currently available computers. Although DES is no longer considered to be a strong cryptosystem, a variant of DES (Triple DES) is still used to secure financial information.

Symmetric key cryptosystems require that the sender and the recipient share a single, secret key. Every party who will send or receive information must therefore know the key before the cipher can be used. This protocol requires a secure method of transmitting the key, which may involve transporting a disk, sending the key through a secure telecommunication channel, or agreeing upon a mutually trusted third party to transfer the key. If the key is intercepted, the privacy of any information that has been encrypted with that key is compromised. A stolen key can be used to encrypt a fraudulent document. If the recipient is unaware that the key has been intercepted, he will assume that the document is authentic.

Asymmetric Cryptography

Public key encryption (PKE), also known as *asymmetric cryptography*, allows users to communicate securely without the prior need to exchange a key. This encryption technique uses two separate keys and a "one-way" mathematic algorithm. The system is based on the fact that multiplication of very large integers is a simple operation, but finding the prime factors of an extremely large number can be very difficult. Information that has been encrypted with one of the keys in the pair can then only be decrypted with the other key. Even though the keys are related, it is impossible to deduce one key from the other. In most applications, one key is made public and one key is known only to its owner, allowing information to be shared between people without a preexisting security arrangement. A person wishing to send a confidential document uses the public key to encrypt the document. Once encrypted, the document cannot be decoded with the public key; only the private key will work. The public key is available to anyone and can be distributed in many ways. Public key registries allow a person who wishes to send a confidential document to look up a public key by name or institution. Some people link to them on email signatures, staff directories, or institutional Web pages. Although PKE is highly secure, it is relatively slow due to the large number of mathematic calculations it requires. Most PKE systems are ~1000 times slower than conventional encryption.

Pretty Good Privacy (PGP) is a widely used cryptosystem that takes advantage of a hybrid technology to provide both high security and rapid encryption and decryption. When PGP is used to encrypt data, the data are first compressed, which decreases the size of the file and makes it more difficult to spot patterns that an unauthorized interceptor can use to break the encryption. PGP then creates a "session key," a single-use secret key, to encrypt the data. In most computers, the session key is a random number that is generated by monitoring keystrokes and mouse movements. The session key is then encrypted using the recipient's public key and is transmitted along with the encrypted data. To decrypt the data, the recipient's private key is used to decrypt the session key, which is then used to decrypt the information. PGP has been recommended as a technique to provide data security for health information.[12] The Radiological Society of Germany has adopted PGP as its technique for encryption and has developed a public key infrastructure for all radiologists in Germany, allowing German radiologists to exchange patient information in a secure, authenticated fashion.[13]

Hash Functions

Hash functions are widely used for data authentication. A hash is a mathematic method of creating a number that is reproducible and is essentially a digital "fingerprint" of the data. If the hash functions of two documents are different, then the documents are different in some way. If they are the same, the likelihood is strong (but not absolute) that the documents are identical. Most hash functions are designed to be "one way." In other words, it is impossible to predict an input that would yield the same hash function as another document. Once the hash is created, the document's owner then encrypts that value with a private key. In addition to information about the document, the hash function should also contain a date and time stamp, thus verifying the specific time at which the document was created or modified. Anyone with access to the signer's public key can then decrypt the hash function. Passing the document through the hash algorithm should then yield the same hash that was encrypted and stored with the original document.

Digital Certificates

When confidential information is encrypted with a public key, the owner of the corresponding private key will have full access to that information. For this reason, many applications, especially in finance and healthcare, require positive identification of all parties to a transaction. *Digital certificates* are the "photo identification" of the digital world and ensure that the true owner of a specific key pair is known. A certification authority (e.g., Verisign) is a trusted third party that verifies the identity of the owner of a given key pair and issues digital certificates. Identification may be done in person, using a photographic identification such as a driver's license or passport. Major certification authorities do not usually issue certificates to individuals. Instead, they issue certificates to institutions, which in turn, sign the key pairs of their employees.

A digital certificate consists of three things: a public key, the identity of the key's owner, and a digital signature. The certification authority digitally signs the public key with its own private key, attesting to the fact that the identity of the owner has been verified. Digital signatures rely on strong encryption techniques to create a digital "certificate" that could only have been affixed by the person who owns it.[14] The techniques in most common use take advantage of PKE, which uses two separate keys: a public key and a private key.[15] Typically, the signer creates a "hash" function, or a digital fingerprint of the document. A trusted third party, an entity whom both parties trust to verify the authenticity of a signature, encrypts the hash with its private key. The ability to decrypt and verify the hash using that third party's public key proves that the certificate is valid.

Authentication, Data Integrity, and Digital Signatures

One of the most important features of the EMR is the ability to share information between all persons involved with patient care. Trust and security are essential to effective patient care. As a result, it is imperative that any member of the healthcare team who makes an entry into the EMR be able to be uniquely identified. The paradigm with the paper medical record is the signature affixed by each person who makes a notation. This signature absolutely and irrevocably identifies the person who makes the entry. In the EMR, digital signatures replace the traditional handwritten signature and allow anyone with access to the record to identify personnel who have made additions or changes to it.

The EMR must be preserved for at least the lifetime of the patient, and sometimes even longer. As more powerful computers are developed, their greatly improved processing power may enable them "break" the encryption, making forgery possible. In contrast, most certification authorities place a limit of 1–2 years on the lifespan of certificates based on a 1024-bit key pair. Also, the information necessary to verify digital signatures, such as certificate chains and certificate revocation, may not be available in the distant future. Even the trusted third party may have ceased to exist or may no longer fulfill the necessary requirements.[16] As a result, both encryption schemes and digital signatures must periodically be updated. For this reason, the hash must be periodically re-encrypted by a trusted party.[15] In addition to privacy and access control, it is critical to preserve the integrity and verifiability of the EMR. Issues to be considered include central archiving, ownership of the record, tampering with communication channels, and repudiation of entries.

Modern encryption technology also allows digital time stamping of information. Time stamp provides important information about entries in the EMR, such as the time and location of entries into the record, which can be used to determine the time of specific occurrences during the patient's interaction with the healthcare system. Time stamps become especially important when the healthcare record is used for purposes such as enforcement or quality assurance.[17] The technology provides the ability to trace and audit changes to a record and allows relatively secure and irrefutable identification.

Digital images represent another challenge, but new technologies may help to preserve both the integrity and privacy of medical imaging studies. *Digital watermarking* is the process of imperceptibly modifying an image in order to add information to it. This information can be retrieved with the proper key if the watermarking system is known. Information that might be attached to a medical image includes patient identifiers and a description of the examination. Different keys might be used to encode specific information, so that varying levels of access may be granted.[18] Such a system can be used to document the authenticity of the image and to determine whether it has been modified. Digital watermarks can also facilitate research. Images can be deidentified and distributed while privacy is maintained, as the identifying information is irretrievable without the proper key. Digital watermarks can also be used to detect tampering, in that modification of the image destroys the watermark.[19]

Smart Cards

One potential solution that may be used to ensure privacy and security of digital information is to encrypt the EMR. A "smart card" carried by the patient would contain a key that permits access to the medical record. Providing the smart card would allow access to specific areas of the record for a defined period of time, as defined by the type of encounter. Under such a system, a clinical laboratory worker might be granted one-time, write-only access to the record, unless a specific test required additional privileges. If the patient is admitted to the hospital, read-and-write access would be granted to authorized personnel for the duration of the patient's stay. A primary care provider could be granted unlimited read-and-write access for the duration of her relationship with the patient. Records of encounters with mental health professionals would be in a separate, highly confidential category and would require specific permission to access. The patient could also choose to restrict access to specific portions of the EMR. In the event of a medical emergency, information would be made available to the clinician through the use of a third key that would be administered by a regional or national agency. Taiwan is one of the first countries to implement the use of smart cards as part of a national health system. Although implementation of the system was complicated by problems with the card readers and lack of familiarity with the system, most hospitals in Taiwan were satisfied with smart cards as a way to gain access to patient records.[20]

Telephone calls and consultations are now widely used by both physicians and patients in the healthcare setting and pose a different set of problems. However, this practice can lead to a breach of patient confidentiality. Healthcare workers rarely, if ever, ask a caller to prove his identity before releasing information.[4] Curious friends or relatives, attorneys, or other parties may potentially call and lie about their identities to gain access to confidential information.[21] Even staff members who claim that they can recognize a patient's voice can be fooled: the acoustic properties of the voice are modified during transmission over the telephone network, making it possible for another person to impersonate the patient. To alleviate this problem, Sokol and Car[4] have recommended the use of a password authentication system; prior to discussing health information on the telephone, the caller is required to provide a password. In this way, the patient or an authorized representative can easily identify himself.

Information Security

Health information is collected from a variety of sources and must be integrated, managed, and secured. For example, physicians frequently carry patient information on handheld computers, laptop computers, memory sticks, and CDs. No technology is currently available for securing information or enforcing disclosure policies on these devices. Loss or theft of a personal device could have devastating consequences for patients whose information was stored on them. For example, a laptop computer that contained the names of every pilot with a mailing address in Florida was stolen from a car belonging to a government employee who had legitimate access to that information. This event placed thousands of people at risk for identity theft.[22] Information that is no longer needed must be identified and removed, along with persistent data that may allow recreation of the deleted information.

Attacks on personal computers in the form of viruses, keystroke loggers, and "phishing" attacks are a growing threat and have the potential to interfere with patient care. Hundreds of viruses are released everyday. Many healthcare applications rely on Intel-based computers running the Microsoft Windows operating system. As a result, they are vulnerable to the same kinds of viruses that affect home and office computers. Some experts have suggested that terrorists may specifically target the information infrastructure in hospitals and clinics to increase the number of casualties during an attack. In addition to rendering a computer unreliable, viruses and worms can compromise or destroy health information. Information networks are part of the critical infrastructure of most healthcare institutions and should therefore be protected. Fortunately, electronic and physical protection of critical infrastructure is a mature industry, and most healthcare institutions have taken the necessary steps to secure their data.

Most computer users are aware of *viruses*, which are small programs that are attached to email messages or disguised as useful programs that, once activated, can destroy information or simply slow down the computer as they send copies of themselves to thousands of other computers. The most common purpose of a virus is to turn the victim's computer into a "zombie," allowing it to be controlled over the Internet. Access to groups of zombie computers is bought and sold through underground Web sites. Such computers can be turned into pornography Web sites, made to pose as financial Web sites to collect credit card information, or used to distribute unsolicited commercial email.

Adware and *spyware* are programs that are usually installed along with other, marginally useful software such as a screen-saver or file-sharing program. Once installed, these programs monitor computer usage and report back to a central site. They may generate pop-up windows with advertisements or redirect Web searches to a preferred site. They also cause the infected computer to slow down and may make it unstable, causing it to crash and lose valuable information. A *keystroke logger* is a variant of spyware that is usually distributed as an email attachment through a malicious Web site or as the payload of a virus. This program automatically installs itself and waits for the victim to log into a bank or credit card site, at which point all identifying information is relayed to the scammers. Keystroke loggers can compromise the security of an individual health record or that of an entire system if a user ID and password are stolen.

A few simple precautions, combined with common sense, can minimize the risk of information theft or damage. All access to Web sites, especially those of financial institutions, must be protected by a carefully chosen password, which should ideally consist of a series of letters, numerals, and punctuation marks. A good password is easy for its owner to remember but should be difficult for anyone else to guess. Passwords, especially bank or credit card PINs, should never be given to anyone else, sent by email, or posted on a Web page. Remote access to home computers that may not have the latest security updates should be allowed only when necessary.

Hardware and software tools decrease the probability that a computer will be infected by a virus, be compromised by a hacker, or become a "zombie." Antivirus programs marketed by Symantec and McAffee, among others, are essential tools that should be installed on every computer. It is important to update the programs frequently, as new viruses are released everyday. Most of these programs also protect against keystroke loggers and Trojan horses.

Firewalls determine whether information traveling across a network should be allowed to continue. *Software firewalls* prevent unauthorized programs from using an Internet connection. Specific programs (e.g., a Web client) are permitted to send information to a location on the Internet. If an unknown program attempts to establish a connection, a software firewall blocks the connection until the user grants access. By limiting the programs that can send information to external computers, software firewalls prevent information from being stolen by spyware or adware. A *hardware firewall* is a piece of equipment that is installed between a home or office network and a cable or DSL (digital subscriber line) modem and helps to protect against attacks from outside computers. Hardware firewalls guard an entire network against an outside attack but usually permit any computer on the local network to establish a connection.

As a result, hardware firewalls do not protect against programs that harvest information. A hardware firewall has an added benefit: it allows an Internet connection to be shared between several computers. Ideally, protection of computers on a network should involve a comprehensive approach that includes both hardware and software firewalls, antivirus software, and frequent security analyses.

Conclusion

The widespread adoption of EMR systems and the electronic exchange of PHI combined with the adoption of HIPAA and similar laws around the world have necessitated that medical groups develop and implement comprehensive information-security programs that must comply with all applicable regulations and include methods for maintaining confidentiality in the collection, storage, and transmission of PHI. Protecting the privacy of health information has value—patients are more likely to reveal information that may affect healthcare decisions when they know that their physicians are taking appropriate steps to safeguard that information. Physicians and other healthcare providers can also highlight their security programs as proof that they value their patients' privacy. The importance of information security will continue to grow in proportion with the increasing amount of PHI that is collected and stored electronically, requiring that all physicians have at least a basic understanding of this important topic.

Key Points

- Privacy and security of health information are essential components of the modern medical practice environment.
- HIPAA in the US and numerous international regulations mandate the protection of health information, which requires a partnership between healthcare providers and information technology specialists.
- Disclosure of PHI must be limited to those with a need to know, including healthcare professionals, allied health professionals, and billing and insurance companies.
- The use of email for sharing of PHI requires positive identification of all parties, prior consent from the patient, and reasonable steps (such as encryption) to ensure confidentiality. Email messages that concern a specific patient should be printed and placed in that patient's chart.
- HIPAA requires numerous safeguards to protect patient information. The steps taken should be documented as part of an institution's policies and procedures.
- Modern cryptographic software tools are relatively inexpensive and easy to implement; they can provide extensive protection and aid compliance with HIPAA mandates.
- Digital signatures can be used to verify authenticity and completeness of patient records.

References

1. Electronic Privacy Information Center. Medical Privacy Public Opinion Polls. http://www. epic.org/privacy/medical/polls.html. Accessed November 15, 2007
2. The new threat to your medical privacy. Consum Rep 2006; 71(3):39–42
3. Agrawal R, Johnson C. Securing electronic health records without impeding the flow of information. Int J Med Inform 2007; 76(5–6):471–9
4. Sokol DK, Car J. Patient confidentiality and telephone consultations: Time for a password. J Med Ethics 2006; 32(12):688–9
5. Gostin LO. National health information privacy: Regulations under the Health Insurance Portability and Accountability Act. JAMA 2001; 285(23):3015–21
6. Gostin LO. Public health law in a new century. Part III. Public health regulation: A systematic evaluation. JAMA 2000; 283(23):3118–22
7. Protection of Human Subjects, 56 Federal Register 28003 (1991) 45 CFR §46
8. Samarati P, Sweeney L. Generalizing data to provide anonymity when disclosing information. In: *Proceedings of the 17th ACM SIGMOD–SIGACT–SIGART Symposium on the Principles of Database Systems*. New York: Association for Advanced Computing Machinery, 1988:188
9. Brooks RG, Menachemi N. Physicians' use of email with patients: Factors influencing electronic communication and adherence to best practices. J Med Internet Res 2006; 8(1):e2
10. Eysenbach G, Diepgen TL. Responses to unsolicited patient e-mail requests for medical advice on the World Wide Web. JAMA 1998; 280(15):1333–5
11. Kane B, Sands DZ. Guidelines for the clinical use of electronic mail with patients. The AMIA Internet Working Group, Task Force on Guidelines for the Use of Clinic-Patient Electronic Mail. J Am Med Inform Assoc 1998; 5(1):104–11
12. Kelly G, McKenzie B. Security, privacy, and confidentiality issues on the Internet. J Med Internet Res 2002; 4(2):E12
13. Schütze B, Kämmerer M, Klos G, et al. The public-key infrastructure of the Radiological Society of Germany. Eur J Radiol 2006; 57(3):323–8
14. Schneier B. *Applied Cryptography: Protocols, Algorithms, and Source Code in C*, 2nd ed. Hoboken, NJ: Wiley, 1995:784
15. Pharow P, Blobel B. Electronic signatures for long-lasting storage purposes in electronic archives. Int J Med Inform 2005; 74(2–4):279–87
16. Lekkas D, Gritzalis D. Long-term verifiability of the electronic healthcare records' authenticity. Int J Med Inform 2007; 76(5–6):442–8
17. Pharow P, Blobel B. Time stamp services for trustworthy health communications. Stud Health Technol Inform 2002; 90:118–22
18. Hartung F, Kutter M. Multimedia watermarking techniques. Proc IEEE 2006; 87(7):1079–107
19. Giakoumaki A, Pavlopoulos S, et al. Multiple image watermarking applied to health information management. IEEE Trans Inf Technol Biomed 2006; 10(4):722–32
20. Liu CT, Yang PT, Yeh YT, Wang BL. The impacts of smart cards on hospital information systems—An investigation of the first phase of the national health insurance smart card project in Taiwan. Int J Med Inform 2006; 75(2):173–81
21. Sokol DK, Car J. Protecting patient confidentiality in telephone consultations in general practice. Br J Gen Pract 2006; 56:384–5
22. Yen H. IDs of active military personnel on stolen laptop. Associated Press, June 4, 2006. http://www.heraldtribune.com/apps/pbcs.dll/article?AID=/20060604/BREAKING/60604004. Accessed December 20, 2007

Chapter 24
Simulation-Based Learning as an Educational Tool

Ruth Fanning and David Gaba

Simulation-based education in healthcare owes its origins mainly to the discipline of anesthesia. The practice of anesthesia has often been likened to the dynamic environment of aviation, where the stakes are high and safety is of paramount importance. In recent decades, a number of innovative and forward-thinking individuals have developed the discipline to a point where simulation-based education is an integral part of medical training in a wide array of medical disciplines, involving individual and team training, at both the undergraduate and postgraduate levels.

Definition of Simulation

Simulation may be defined as an imitation of some real thing, state of affairs, or process. The act of simulating something generally entails representing certain key characteristics or behaviors of a selected physical or abstract system.[1] Simulation as a generic concept refers to the artificial replication of sufficient components of a real-world situation to achieve specific goals.[2] The term *simulation* encompasses areas as diverse as the modeling of natural or human physiologic systems, technologic reproductions of equipment and environments, or entire cyber worlds of computer-generated environments in which individuals can interact. Children emulate or model adult behavior and actions to learn how to interact with the world about them. If we broaden the definition of simulation to include rehearsal for activities or roles, we see evidence of role-playing in many cultures over the centuries.[3] Role-playing and theatrics are used not only as ways of trying new activities, but also of learning behaviors, operating as a team, and interacting socially.

The incorporation of technology into simulation also has historic roots. Throughout history, the military has led the way in applying technology to simulation. In Roman times, a "quintain"—a device that crudely simulated the behavior of an opponent during sword fighting—was an example of a primitive simulator.[4] The military has continued its role in the development of simulators in modern times, both on land and in the air. It is probably the area of aviation,

J. Stonemetz, K. Ruskin (eds.) *Anesthesia Informatics*,
© Springer Science + Business Media, LLC 2008

both civilian and naval, that has contributed most significantly to the development of simulation and its public exposure and recognition. Simulation in this arena has become a combination, not only of advanced technologies, but also of educational, communication, and team-building models that have made it what it is today. The development of such models with the widespread availability of technology has made simulation a practical and financial possibility across a wide range of disciplines, from high-hazard industries, to transportation, healthcare, and beyond.[5-7]

Finally, simulation is a series of techniques, not simply an array of technologies, which when incorporated into a structured educational curriculum provides a teaching tool or, perhaps more accurately, a learning tool that is particularly well suited to learning in dynamic and challenging environments.

Simulation as a Form of Experiential Learning: Theories Behind Simulation as a Learning Tool

As children, we learn naturally by imitating or modeling activities, but as adults, we often have a reluctance to immerse ourselves in "playful" activities, even if they have an educational component. Most educational research is based on children and how they best learn.[8] Increasingly, with advancements in technology, changes in the working environment and a greater degree of mobility in the workforce, the area of adult education has become more relevant and important. All areas of the workforce face challenges; but healthcare, with its rapidly advancing techniques, technologies, procedures, and ever-increasing treatment options, is particularly affected.

Adult learning provides many challenges not seen in the typical student population. Adults arrive complete with a set of previous life experiences and frames (knowledge, assumptions, feelings), ingrained personality traits, and relationship patterns that drive their actions.[9] Adult learners become more self-directed as they mature. They like their learning to be problem centered and meaningful to their life situation, and they learn best when they can immediately apply what they have learned.[10] Their attitudes toward any specific learning opportunity will vary, depending on factors such as their motivation for attending training, whether the learning is voluntary or mandatory, and whether participation is linked directly to recertification or job retention.

Adults learn best when they are actively engaged in the process, participate, or play a role—when they experience not only concrete events in a cognitive fashion, but also transact events in an emotional fashion. Each learner must then make sense of the events experienced in terms of his own world. This type of learning is often described as *experiential learning*: learning by doing, thinking about, and assimilating lessons learned into everyday behaviors. The experiential learning cycle has been described as containing four related parts: concrete experience, reflective observation, abstract conceptualization, and active experimentation.[11] Four phases have also been suggested: planning for action, carrying out action, reflecting on action, and creating a theory based on this reflection.[12] Similarly, the experiential learning process has been described as having an experience, thinking about it, identifying learning needs that would improve future practice in the area, planning what learning to undertake, and applying the new learning in practice.[13] Grant and Marsden described the process in relation to teaching doctors in training. The training in this instance was the traditional apprenticeship model: "learning by doing," or "on the job training." This model, though "experiential," relies on an unsystematic or "chance" approach to learning objectives or goals and is thus fraught with problems when the goal is to employ a competency-based curriculum for medical education.

Simulation training sessions, which are structured with specific learning objectives in mind, offer the opportunity to progress through the stages of the experiential cycle in a structured manner and often combine the active experiential component of the simulation exercise itself with a subsequent analysis of, and reflection on, the experience, aiming to facilitate incorporation of changes in practice. Unlike the traditional apprenticeship model, "see one, do one, teach one," the goals of learning are chosen in advance in simulation-based education. Simulation does not rely on chance exposure to rare diagnoses or situations. In essence, this mode of training offers the opportunity of practiced experience in a controlled fashion, which can be reflected upon at leisure. Experiential learning is particularly suited to professional learning, in which integration of theory and practice is pertinent and ongoing.[13]

Experiential Learning and Team Training and Dynamics

Today, healthcare providers increasingly work in teams, and the cohesiveness of the team will determine how effective and timely healthcare is delivered. Simulation, or immersive learning, is particularly suited to team training, giving participants the opportunity to interact, play different roles, and practice team-based activities in real time. Traditional teaching in the form of didactic lectures or noninteractive teaching is poor when the learning objective is to educate a team.

Lewin's work in the area of group dynamics provides an insight into how teams act and learn, introducing the concepts of task interdependence and the interdependence of the group fate. A number of key views that frame the approach to team learning evolved from his work: reflective conversation, the role of leadership, and the experiential learning process as the key to team development.[14] A team can reflect on its experience and develop a shared image of itself through conversation. Often referred to as a "shared mental model," this conversational process allows the team to "be on the same page" and function cohesively, as individual members share the same outlook and goals, a concept particularly relevant in the delivery of acute medical care. Kayes et al.[15] further described experiential learning in teams, concentrating on the fact that individuals have different learning styles and that this impacts differently on the team, as was illustrated when they incorporated the concept of the experiential learning cycle and integrated basic learning styles.

They identified four prevalent learning styles: diverging, assimilating, converging, and accommodating. Participants with *diverging learning styles* use concrete experience and reflective observation to learn. *Assimilating-styled learners* prefer abstract conceptualization and reflective observation. *Converging-styled learners* use abstract conceptualization and active experimentation. *Accommodating-styled learners* use concrete experience and active experimentation. When learning in teams, individuals tend to orientate themselves and contribute to the team learning process by using their individual learning styles to help the team achieve its learning objectives. Highly effective teams tend to possess diverse individuals with a number of different learning styles; thus, pairing appropriate learning-styled individuals may add to the team's performance.

Simulation: Facilitating Learning—The Role of Debriefing

In experiential learning, the experience is used as the major source of learning, but it is not the only one. Both thinking and doing are required and must be related in the minds of the learner.[12] Simply practicing a task or participating in an activity does not guarantee learning. The concept of reflecting on an event or an activity and subsequently analyzing it is the cornerstone of the experiential learning experience. In practice, however, not everyone is naturally capable of analyzing, making sense, and assimilating learning experiences on their own, particularly those included in highly dynamic team-based activities. The attempt to bridge this natural gap between *experiencing* an event and making *sense* of it led to the evolution of the concept of the "postexperience analysis" or *debriefing*.[16]

Historically, debriefing originated in the military, in which the term was used to describe the account individuals gave on returning from a mission.[17] This cognitive reconstruction of events was performed in groups, resulting in a shared meaning of the experience. Another variant of debriefing grew from work among emergency first responders; critical incident stress debriefing is a facilitator-led process designed to review a critical event and reduce stress among those involved.[18] The field of experimental psychology's concept of debriefing describes the means by which participants who have been deceived in some manner as part of a psychology study are informed of the true nature of the experiment.[19] Each of these fields has contributed to the development of debriefing in the experiential learning arena—facilitator-led participatory discussion of events, reflection, and assimilation of activities toward producing long-lasting learning and behavioral changes.

Structural Elements of the Debriefing Process

A fundamental precondition common to all forms of debriefing is the ethical obligation of the facilitator to determine the parameters within which behavior will be analyzed, thereby attempting to protect participants from experiences that might seriously damage their senses of self-worth.[20] To ensure a successful debriefing process and learning experience, the facilitator must provide a supportive climate in which students feel valued, respected, and free to learn in a dignified learning environment.[21] Participants must be able to "share their experiences in a frank, open, and honest manner."[18] Recognition of the vulnerability of the participant is paramount, a concept highlighted by a recent study regarding the barriers to simulation-based learning, in which approximately half of the participants found it a stressful and intimidating environment and a similar proportion cited a fear of the educator and their peers' judgment.[22] It is therefore essential that the facilitator create an environment of trust early on, and this typically occurs during the *prebrief session*. The prebrief period is a time when the facilitator illustrates the purpose of the simulation, the learning objectives, and the process of debriefing and what it entails. It is the period during which the participants learn what is expected of them and the ground rules are set for the simulation-based learning experience.

Debriefings may move through three phases: description, analogy/analysis, and application. However, without a facilitator, participants may have difficulty moving out of the descriptive phase—particularly the active "hot-seat" participant (the participant most involved in the scenario/task), who is emotionally absorbed in the event and is blinkered in her view of what has occurred. The exact level of facilitation and the degree to which the facilitator is involved in the debriefing process can depend on a variety of generic factors:

- The objective of the experiential exercise
- The complexity of the scenarios
- The experience level of the participants as individuals or as a team
- The participants' familiarity with the simulation environment
- The amount of time available
- The role of simulations in the overall curriculum
- Individual personalities and whether the participants know each other

Varying degrees of facilitator input may be employed, depending on the setting. When participants are familiar with simulation-based education and are experienced working in a team situation, the level of facilitator input may be low. Participants in this setting largely debrief themselves while the facilitator outlines the debriefing process and assists by gently guiding the discussion when necessary.[23] In inexperienced groups, the facilitator may need to lead the discussion more actively, asking questions and being directive. In this instance, the facilitator typically confirms statements, recaps and reinforces thoughts and ideas, and often directly answers participants' questions. He may use techniques such as active listening, echoing, and nonverbal encouragement. Most groups fall into an intermediate category, in which the facilitator aids in reaching deeper analysis of the experience, often asking one participant to comment on another and encouraging the entire team to participate. It is probably most beneficial to facilitate at the highest possible level, with the participants independently generating a rich discussion of key issues among themselves.

When multiple debriefers are involved, they may decide to use opposing styles to encourage discussion and cohesiveness within a participant team. A group of debriefers may offer advantages when specific educational or technical points need to be addressed. A subject-matter expert may debrief on these specialized issues and offer increased credibility to the discussion, particularly when dealing with an experienced group of participants. When multiple facilitators are present, their roles must be clearly delineated before debriefing commences to avoid excessive facilitator input.

Other Practical Elements of Debriefing

The physical environment in which debriefing is conducted is also an important factor. For complex debriefings that last more than a few minutes, debriefings often take place in a room separate from the active portion of the simulation to allow diffusion of tension and to provide a setting conducive to reflection. Increasingly, simulations (from the simplest form of role-play and practicing a simple task to more complex team-based exercises and dynamic acute care scenarios) are taking place outside of dedicated "immersive learning sites" in real-world locations. With the wide-scale adoption of simulation for both undergraduate and continuing professional education and the investment in simulation technologies by a large number of healthcare facilities, simulations are now commonly being conducted in the everyday work environment, otherwise known as *in situ simulations*. Many exercises are short, played out in either dedicated time slots or only when opportunities arise. Dedicated facilitation rooms are often not available, and debriefing is often limited by time constraints. In this instance, a simple debriefing may take place "on the spot," and a more in-depth debriefing may occur remotely, either in time or place.

Many educators are nervous concerning the concept of debriefing and may indeed delay the introduction of simulation-based learning at their institutions until they feel "adequately trained" in facilitation. In truth, however, debriefing and facilitated learning occur in clinical practice everyday. Often after adverse events or "near-miss" situations, those involved, if only in an informal manner, discuss the event, reflect on it, and decide on ways to improve practice in the future. They are, in fact, bringing the event through the stages of the experiential learning cycle, with the aim of achieving a learning objective or goal. Adding structure to normal practice can be beneficial in making every experience a learning one.

Simulation: Improving Safety

Current simulation technologies developed mainly in the aviation and military arenas. The modern-day flight simulator owes its origins mainly to the pneumatically driven aircraft simulator patented in 1930 by Edwin Link. His "LINK Trainer" became a standard for instrument flight training before World War II.[24] However, simulation in aviation extends far beyond the technology of simulation and includes not only the technical training of individuals, but also team training, human factors, and safety and organizational practices. Many other disciplines have followed suit, with healthcare initially slow to join the process but currently gaining ground. For a number of reasons, simulation-based training has been embraced by high-hazard industries such as petrochemicals, nuclear energy, and firefighting. Safety is of particular concern for both the workforce and the maintenance of plant and equipment. In an oil refinery, for example, an accident can be fatal and may lead to the destruction of equipment and subsequent loss of production, therefore providing a double incentive to improve safety, often through simulation exercises, to avoid such potential catastrophes. Simulation has been adopted as a valuable tool in what are referred to as *high-reliability organizations*.[25] High-reliability organizations often involve industries that are highly hazardous but, despite this, have a very low accident rate. In their efforts to run a safe operation, they have embedded into their organizational psyche a number of principles, including process auditing, appropriate reward systems, avoiding quality degradation, risk perception, and command and control.[26,27] They also include such features as preoccupation with failure (analyzing near misses), a reluctance to simplify interpretations, sensitivity to operations, commitment to resilience (having staff and equipment that can cross function as required), and deference to expertise rather than rank.[25] Because the concepts of high reliability challenge traditional hierarchical models, intensive training is required to embed such principles into an organization. Simulation-based training is used in these environments to change the culture of an organization. Healthcare can also be viewed as a highly hazardous industry and one that might benefit from the concepts of a high-reliability organization.

The Technology of Simulation in Healthcare

No uniformly accepted classification scheme exists for patient simulators, and any single classification scheme necessarily involves overlaps and gray areas between different devices. As a starting point, a "patient simulator is a system that presents a patient within a clinical environment in so much as the patient can respond appropriately to the clinical actions taken by the clinician undergoing simulation."[2] Classic environments might be the OR, the ICU, the delivery suite, and the ED, but they could also be as diverse as an ambulance or an in-flight transfer, or even a public area where an emergency event could occur. The patient and the environment may be presented in many formats, e.g., in actual reality (defined as a realistic simulator or hands-on simulator), a representation of a part of a patient or partial-task trainer, on a computer screen only, or as a virtual environment or world ("virtual reality"). The evolution and current capabilities of each of these systems are described in detail below.

Mannequin-based Patient Simulators (High-fidelity Simulation)

Anesthesia was considered to be particularly hazardous in the past, which was reflected by the high costs of medicolegal insurance in many jurisdictions. Over time, anesthesia as a discipline has gone from being considered a high-risk specialty to moderate or low risk. This progression is due in part to the increased safety of anesthetic drugs and sophistication of monitoring equipment, but it is also due to the training of anesthesia providers and the paramount role of safety embedded in such training. The entire area of healthcare simulation owes its roots to the discipline of anesthesia, a discipline that has always been highly cognizant of, and at the forefront of, patient safety initiatives. In fact, pioneers in the area of anesthesia from the medical, scientific, and engineering perspectives were responsible for the adoption and incorporation of simulation-based techniques into anesthesia training, and they played an integral role in the development of the technology of healthcare simulation.

The mannequin-based simulators with which we are familiar today owe their origins to developments over the last 40 years. In the late 1960s, an aerospace company working with anesthesiologists at the University of Southern California developed a mannequin-based simulator—Sim-One—heralding the starting point for computer-controlled mannequin simulators.[28,29] However, issues such as cost and a reluctance on the part of the healthcare field to embrace a new paradigm in teaching led to Sim-One being a prototype only. The concept of linking physiologic and pharmacologic models, initially in the form of a screen-only simulator, was the brainchild of Ty Smith and associates at the University of California, San Diego.[30] Another screen-based simulator, developed by Howard Schwid and Daniel O'Donnell and called the Anesthesia Simulator Recorder, evolved into the Anesthesia Simulator Consultant, which was specifically designed for training anesthetists in managing patient care.[31,32] The coupling of such physiologic and pharmacologic models with mannequin-based technology added a level of realism to mannequin-based simulation and allowed a certain degree of automated function.

Mannequin-based simulators grew in fidelity in the 1980s with the development by Gaba and DeAnda of the CASE (Comprehensive Anesthesia Simulation Environment) series of anesthesia simulators, which used commercially available clinical waveform generators to provide signals to actual clinical instruments from equipment and was capable of many functions that emulated the anesthesia environment.[33] A later generation, the CASE 2, incorporated a physiologic model of the cardiovascular system. The virtual Anesthesiology Training Simulator system (later changed to the CAE Patient Simulator) contained complete models of cardiovascular, pulmonary, fluid, acid–base, and thermal physiology, and most importantly, was a mobile device. At the University of Florida, a team led by Good and Gravenstein[4] developed the GAS (Gainesville Anesthesia Simulator), which originally focused on anesthesia-machine fault scenario design. A special programming language was developed to allow clinicians and technicians to quickly program new and more complex events. In the 1990s, a number of European simulator projects were developed, namely, the Leiden Anesthesia Simulator, the Anesthesia Simulator Sophist,[34] and PatSim, developed at Stavanger College, Norway—though none of these models ever became commercially available.[35] However, this earlier research and the individual simulator development projects culminated in a number of the currently commercially available mannequin-based simulators.

A modern patient simulator typically features full-scale mannequin models of adult, child, and baby, as well as mannequins that are produced for particular curricula such as Advanced Life Support. They are capable of spontaneously breathing and being intubated and mechanically ventilated, and they have auscultatory breath sounds, vocal capacity, palpable pulses, and audible heart sounds. They can be defibrillated and paced, and many models allow or have incorporated the capacity to perform procedures, such as pericardiocentesis, insertion of chest drains, or cricothyroidotomy, to name but a few. The operator is capable of producing a wide range of clinical scenarios, either preprogrammed or operator designed. Preprogrammed scenarios often incorporate computerized physiologic models. Simulators come equipped with a simulated patient monitor and allow interfacing with a range of commercially available data systems, including radiology, electro-cardiography, and other data collection systems. Some systems also have the ability to integrate facilitation and debriefing functions. Modern mannequin-based simulators have the added advantage of being highly portable, providing an infinite forum for the development and execution of clinical scenarios in any environment.

Virtual Reality/Virtual Worlds

The concept of *virtual reality* encompasses, in its simplest form, a limited virtual world that is computer screen based with interaction by the participant via mouse, pen, or touchscreen device. In the entertainment world, simple computer games are in this format. The continuum of virtual reality extends to the creation of an environment where the user is literally immersed in a virtual world that is indistinguishable from the real one. To achieve this capacity, the virtual reality must incorporate at least three senses: visual, auditory, and tactile; as such, it is a haptic/kinesthetic system.[2] Some systems replicate fewer senses or have restrictions of interaction with the virtual world. Elements of different systems can be combined to produce their most realistic effects, depending on the goal of the exercise. Some systems can incorporate the physical environment, and virtual reality and virtual worlds are overlain on the physical environment.

Most development in virtual worlds and environments is occurring in the gaming/entertainment industry and, to a lesser extent, in the military. Entire communities have been developed in the gaming world (e.g., *Second Life*).[36] In such worlds, "avatars" represent people and are "human" in appearance and behaviors. They have virtual lives, work at virtual jobs, exist in virtual environments, and can perform activities as directed by the operator. Others systems involve games, often in a team structure, in which avatars may be animal, human, or indeed, superhuman.

In the simplest forms, these virtual worlds exist on a single computer screen in a single physical space, but an ever-increasing number are Web based and are simultaneously accessible to vast numbers of players.[37] The incorporation of senses other than visual and auditory to these virtual worlds produces endless possibilities for learning. As we explore how the gaming world has progressed in developing these technologies, it becomes clear how they might be applied to healthcare, in both the teaching and the practice of medicine. Teamwork in a virtual environment—assigning tasks to various players/healthcare providers—has been applied in many virtual clinical situations. Screen-based simulations allow participants to, for example, treat a trauma patient in an ED, resuscitate a patient using the principles of Advanced Cardiac Life Support, or interact with a screen-based standardized patient (SP) in an outpatient department. They may also be used to represent a mass casualty incident in which patients pass through a continuum of care received from many providers acting as a team in a clinical environment.[38] Systems have also been developed for teaching anatomy, either via a virtual tour of the body or through a series of dissection images.[39] Some systems are available at specific learning locations, but in the future, they may be available online. Many systems link the active portion of the exercise to other Web-based tutorials, which can be accessed by the participants as needed. The concept of immersion in a virtual world, particularly with overlay of the virtual world on a physical environment, would enable teams of healthcare workers to actually act out various team roles in major catastrophes (e.g., natural disasters or terrorist attacks) and thus practice for a potential but rare event in a "realistic" manner.

Partial-Task Trainers

Part-task training or *partial-task training* may be defined as *subordinate-skills training* (operations/procedures) that resembles portions, or subtasks, and responses of an actual system operation. A part-task trainer, or partial-task trainer, is any device that permits selected aspects of a task to be practiced independent of other elements of the task. An example of a part-task trainer in its simplest form would be using an orange to practice intramuscular injections or a watermelon to simulate "loss of resistance" when inserting an epidural. From a technologic standpoint, the earliest partial-task trainer was the concept of Michael Gordon. The "Cardiology Patient Simulator," or "Harvey," simulates a number of cardiac conditions.[40] "Harvey" is a full-sized mannequin that was constructed to teach and assess particular cardiac problems and, as such, illustrates the use of a simulator to teach elements or aspects of a chosen curriculum.

Partial-task trainers of every level of sophistication are currently offered, including laparoscopic/endoscopic simulators (some with kinesthetic properties), endovascular simulators, and simpler devices such as simulators that emulate central-line placement, chest-drain insertion, suturing techniques, and physical examinations. Most are capable of interfacing with real-life equipment such as IV catheters, ultrasound devices, and numerous data collection and display systems. Many have feedback functions to enable learners to assess their progress and improve their technical skills. Partial-task trainers are often used by novices to achieve a critical skill level before attempting a procedure in a real patient. They may also be used to train on new equipment or to perform new procedures. Indeed, this pretraining using a partial-task trainer has become a federal requirement for the placement of certain endovascular arterial stents. The scope of partial-task trainers is broad and is currently extending to the "practice of a difficult case" in advance, which may be achieved by preinstalling a patient's data (e.g., radiologic images), allowing for tailoring of the system, and practicing that particular patient's procedure in advance. This technology, when combined with Web-based technology, allows the potential for many operators to "work on the case" using expertise from specialists all over the world.

Standardized Patients

SPs are people who have been trained to accurately portray the role of patients with a specific medical conditions. They may also play the role of family members or any other members of the public. The term *standardized patient* is derived from the fact that these people are specifically trained not only to represent the context of the situation or problem, but also to consistently re-create the same simulation or problem each time they encounter a student. Consequently, each student will see a patient with the same history and physical findings. A variant of this practice was always an important element of medical education in more traditional times, when, in many cases, a patient with an interesting "history" told his story in an auditorium to medical students. The power of storytelling is profound; it has served as a learning tool across many cultures. Interestingly, within the area of high-reliability organizations, storytelling is used to enhance safety culture.[41]

When we think of simulation, we do not instantly consider the role of SP educational programs, but such programs play an integral part in simulation or immersive learning in the broadest sense. In most SP programs, the SP is employed either in teaching sessions or for assessment purposes, be they formative or summative. During teaching sessions, students are given the opportunity to practice their skills and receive feedback on their performance. In formal examinations, SPs both role-play and complete evaluations. SPs are often actors, many professional, and as such, are experts in enabling a story to unfold over time.

Multimodal Modes of Simulation/Interplay

As the world of immersive or simulation-based learning develops, technologies and modalities increasingly overlap. At a curricular level, many programs combine simulation modalities to teach particular subjects or learning objectives. A tutorial may initially be used to teach basic cardiac rhythms and their treatments, followed by screen-based interactive exercises for practicing what has been learned. Training may then progress to a full-scale, mannequin-based simulation that exercises both the technical skills and knowledge necessary to treat the patient and the team skills necessary to ensure that treatment is conducted in a timely and effective manner. For example, a multimodal simulation learning exercise might initially employ an SP to play a patient who subsequently deteriorates clinically to critical status, whereupon a mannequin replaces the SP. As the students effectively treat the mannequin, the SP is reintroduced. The scope for learning in such an environment extends beyond the acute scenario to the chronic care of the SP at the outpatient or ambulatory level.

Simulation-based Education: The Development of New Curricula

The education of medical professionals is currently undergoing change unparalleled since the days of Flexner.[42] Flexner envisioned a curricular change that would encompass the professional elements of medical practice as well as its scientific aspects, but in the intervening years, the emphasis turned mainly toward the accumulation of factual knowledge, which was accompanied by an institutional shift in emphasis from clinical teaching to research productivity.[43] The art of medicine was eclipsed by its science. In an effort to revive the orphaned elements of medical education—namely, professionalism, leadership, and communication—the Accreditation Council for Graduate Medical Education introduced the concept of structuring curricula around a set of core competencies (patient care, medical knowledge, professionalism, practice-based learning and improvement, communication and interpersonal skills, and systems-based practice).[44] Traditional teaching methods and curricula are being challenged by the concepts included in this now well-underway "outcomes project." Whereas patient care and medical knowledge were always incorporated into traditional curricula, the concepts of professionalism, communication, and interpersonal skills have often been left to the auspices of the even more traditional apprenticeship model, often relying on good role models to instill these qualities. The area of systems-based thinking and practice has often been left unaddressed. The new requirements of the Accreditation Council Outcomes Project, coupled with work-hour restrictions and, often, a reduction in training time, have exposed gaps within the traditional apprenticeship education model. Simulation-based education has provided many solutions to this dilemma, having always been at the forefront in addressing holistic professional training.

Since the introduction of formal simulation-based learning in healthcare, medical education has expanded (a) to incorporate the vast array of technologic aids to simulation and its various modalities and (b) to encompass methods or theories of education. Immersive learning derives many of its principles from the concepts of experiential learning theory, but this is not the only source. Simulation-based training also incorporates the concepts of human-factors engineering and ergonomics, i.e., how we as human beings interact with the world around us.[45] Aviation was one of the first disciplines to teach in this fashion. The concept originated at a NASA workshop in 1979 in response to recognition of the role that human error plays in airline accidents.[46] The concept of *crew resource management* can be described as "using all available resources—information, equipment, and people—to achieve safe and efficient flight operations."[47,48] Training in crew resource management involves the experiential component of the exercise, debriefing, and performance assessment. This concept was adapted and incorporated into simulation-based learning in medicine, first in the discipline of anesthesia[49] and then in a number of healthcare disciplines.[50,51] *Crisis resource management*, as it is referred to in this context, highlights teaching skills that are not commonly taught at the undergraduate and postgraduate levels and emphasizes a number of universally applicable concepts that will be useful in a crisis situation irrespective of the nature of the event. While incorporating the medical and technical elements of practice, crisis resource management particularly stresses the importance of cognitive and interpersonal skills. The basic tenets of crisis resource management are:

- Know the environment
- Anticipate and plan
- Call for help early
- Mobilize and use all available resources
- Exercise leadership and followership
- Practice effective communication
- Distribute the workload
- Wisely allocate attention[52]

Education based on the principles of crisis resource management also stresses the importance of systems issues and systems-based thinking in assessing how humans function in their working environment and how examination of such systems and subsequent changes may result in safer work practices. The core tenets of crew resource management are particularly suited to teaching individuals and teams how to function in stressful, highly dynamic environments. Acute-medical-care specialties, of which anesthesia is a classic example, require practitioners to be decisive, multifunctional, effective, and efficient in times of crisis. In addition to skills such as good communication, effective distribution of workload, and competent leadership, a number of other attributes are essential for the practice of anesthesia. In complex, dynamic domains such as anesthesia, many problems require decision making under uncertainty.[53] In such situations, deriving a solution through formal deductive reasoning from "first principles" requires too much time. Experts in these environments use precompiled rules or response plans for dealing with a recognized event, a method referred to as *recognition-primed decision making*.[54,55] In anesthesia, these responses are usually acquired through personal experience alone, although the field is increasingly recognizing that critical-response protocols must be codified explicitly and taught systematically.[56] In conjunction with this rapid-response system, the participant is usually trying to diagnose the problem at hand, thinking about the dilemma, and making sense of it. These cognitive processes have been explored at length in education. The exploration, or thinking about thinking, known as *metacognition*, provides insights into how an individual thinks or uses powers of deduction. Within traditional teaching and assessment methods, little is known about why a particular practitioner behaves in a particular manner during a given crisis situation.[57] Simulation-based education allows for the videotaping of an event and subsequent debriefing of the scenario, providing the opportunity to explore the thought processes involved in the participants' actions, both in hindsight during the debrief and in real time, if students are coached appropriately prior to the simulation session. Teaching participants to "talk aloud" during the scenario allows exploration of thought processes in the "heat of battle"—an invaluable educational tool.

Re-evaluation is another core skill. To cope with rapid changes and the profound diagnostic and therapeutic uncertainties seen during anesthesia, the central process must include repetitive evaluation of the situation. The practice of continually updating the situation assessment and monitoring the efficacy of chosen actions is termed *situation awareness*.[58] Faulty re-evaluation, inadequate plan adaptation, or loss of situation awareness can result in a type of human error called a *fixation error*, which is the persistent failure to revise a diagnosis or plan in the face of evidence that suggests that revision is necessary.[59] This type of error is extremely common in dynamic, challenging situations. During simulation-based exercises, participants can see where they fell victim to fixation errors and can be taught strategies to avoid them, including reappraisal, re-evaluation, considering other possibilities, using all available resources, and most importantly, asking for and receiving help. Debriefing following simulation, particularly if it involves discriminatory use of videotaping, can be a very powerful tool to highlight strengths that can be acknowledged and applauded and deficiencies that can be improved upon, all of which can be assimilated into everyday, real-life situations.

Interfacing Simulation with the Real World

The tools of simulation, the techniques employed, and marrying the virtual/simulated world with the real world to change behaviors have been discussed, but the question remains: how can real-life technologies be married with simulated ones? In this ever-changing and increasingly technologic age, compatibility of equipment in the simulated and real environments poses many challenges.

Most simulation-based scenarios involve the unfolding of a tale. The story weaves about, changing according to how the participant plays or the team acts, just as a game might. Ensuring that the tale is and remains credible is crucial. The concept of realism is particularly pertinent in simulated activities, where buy-in by the participants is essential. To maximize the realism of the activity, initially at the stage of scenario design, the scenario created must tell a believable tale, the story has to fit, and it must unfold realistically and logistically over time. For example, if the patient starts to bleed in the OR or the ED, certain signs should be apparent. The patient's blood pressure should fall, her heart rate should rise, and she should become cool and eventually lose consciousness. To enable this to occur, the technology must simulate real-life physiology. Just as the physical signs should match the patient's condition, the equipment, monitoring systems, and treatments should be as close as possible to what exists in the real-world environment. This realism may involve constructing an ED scene like the ED in the institution and having similar monitors and equipment. Drugs should be the same as those in use, and the physical space should be similar to the ED environment. As equipment and clinical environments have changed over the last few decades, the simulated environment must change with it, e.g., an automated blood pressure monitor rather than a manual one, an electronic thermometer rather than a mercury one. One modern-day example of changing technologies is the way in which patient data are now collected, stored, and retrieved. With the advent of EMRs and their widespread use, it is becoming less credible to provide the participant in a simulation scenario with medical histories, test results, x-rays, blood results, and other patient data in a paper format. In the world of simulation-based learning, this situation has produced a dilemma. What should the simulated EMR look like, and how should an EMR be produced for simulated environments and simulated patients?

During patient-care simulation activities, the clinical arena and the behavior of a patient are re-created over time, necessitating the chronologic unveiling of data about the simulated patient that appropriately match the simulated clinical state. The general issue is essentially the reverse of typical data flows. Typically, patient data are collected and stored in data-management systems from which they are retrieved by clinicians and then archived in data repositories. A simulation may begin with a repository of clinical information about real or created cases, with data unveiled over time to become available to clinicians via different types of interfaces. Ideal electronic tools/systems required for simulation exercises would enable and simplify:

- Collection of actual (deidentified) patient data for use in part or in whole for a simulated patient, including administrative data, data on prior clinic visits or hospital admissions, current history and physical examination(s), notes, and consultations
- Current and past laboratory data and image data (e.g., radiology, pathology)
- Tools for the simulated creation, editing, storage, and retrieval of integrated, multimodality patient data profiles
- Mechanisms to define the temporal availability of data to the clinician in real time, with various types of time compression and ways to feed data to different interfaces for use by, or transmission to, clinicians
- Mechanisms to allow real-time entry of new data or modification of existing profiles, e.g., data-user interface for a simulation operator/instructor to enter or modify a profile or change temporal sequence or availability of data
- Transfer of data from the mathematical models of commercially available simulators in real time, with or without modification
- Mechanisms to include the relevant patient laboratory and image data to the overall record of a given simulation scenario

Benefits

The Benefits of a Realistic Electronic Data System to the Arena of Simulation-based Learning

A realistic EMR would offer a degree of credibility to the simulation scenario. Participants would be more likely to buy into the clinical situation as it unfolds, being in a familiar environment and operating in a familiar manner. In the case of complex scenarios in which participants quickly become overloaded with tasks, they must prioritize tasks and distribute the workload effectively and efficiently between team members. Throughout the exercise, they must interact with data systems to retrieve and update information about their patient. The ease of use of the data systems will determine their usefulness in times of challenging patient care.

The Benefits of the World of Simulation to the Development and Deployment of Electronic Records

Simulation can offer a complete testing of an AIMS, from the point of patient entry into the hospital (represented by an SP), admission, transfer to surgery, and transfer to either postoperative or ICU setting. Systems/design features may be explored in a real-time setting with a simulated patient who may be sick, unstable, or requires transfer. This walk through the AIMS in a simulated clinical scenario could potentially reveal any glitches in the system and allow changes to be made prior to its implementation. Such a preview allows users to conduct real-time trials of the system in stressful situations (e.g., unstable patients or challenging environments), testing its user friendliness. The wealth of information gained is invaluable both to the designers and the operators of such systems because regardless of how impressive an AIMS is in a controlled environment, the true test is how the system functions in complex environments in crisis situations. The results will determine the functionality of a system and the likelihood that users will adopt it.

The EMR is only one example of how technology and informatics in general can benefit from the world of simulation-based learning and vice versa. Just as technologic advancements contribute to the realism of the experience for participants, the simulation environment allows the study of interactions of human beings with equipment. It affords the opportunity to resolve potential glitches in operating systems in a realistic setting without harming patients. Although practitioners currently have an *ethical responsibility* to ensure that systems are explored in advance of real-life "trials on patients," in the future, public and government pressure may increase to *demand* that practitioners ensure that systems are tested both for operational soundness and for their ability to function in realistic environments, taking human factors into account, particularly in crisis settings.

Do We Need Simulation-based Learning, and If So, Why?

Education in healthcare is based on traditional teaching techniques, hierarchical in design, and based largely on an apprenticeship model. "See one, do one, teach one" is no longer an appropriate method for practicing and teaching healthcare in the 21st century—from the perspective of medical practitioners, the public whom they treat, and the federal oversight entities. The association of fatigue and human error in healthcare has led many jurisdictions to reduce work hours for healthcare professionals.[60,61] The subsequent reduction in "training" hours has highlighted the need for other methods of producing competent, effective healthcare workers—in particular, physicians. This reduction in work hours, in combination with a move toward competency-based training and accreditation, challenges the effectiveness of traditional teaching methods. Simulation-based education, due to its cross-disciplinary applicability, its dynamism and innovation, and an ever-increasing array of technologic advancements, provides many solutions for both professional education and improved patient care through safer work practices and systems.

Conclusion

The incorporation of simulation-based education within the healthcare arena originated within the specialty of anesthesia and has grown to include not only acute-care specialties but also every discipline within the healthcare profession. Simulation is a comprehensive teaching tool that consists of a series of pedagogic techniques—not simply an array of technologies—and particularly facilitates learning in dynamic and challenging environments.

Healthcare professionals work in teams, and the cohesiveness of the team determines how well effective and timely healthcare is delivered. Simulation, or immersive learning, is particularly well suited to team training, giving participants the opportunity to interact, play different roles, and practice activities in real time; it has therefore grown to include team training, human-factors concepts, and safety and organizational practices. Simulation has been adopted as a valuable tool in high-reliability organizations, which include industries that are intrinsically hazardous but have a very low accident rate. The concepts of high reliability challenge traditional hierarchical models; thus, intensive training must occur to embed such principles into an organization. Simulation-based training is used in these environments to change the organizational culture.

The wide-scale adoption of simulation for both undergraduate and continuing professional education and the investment in simulation technologies by a large number of healthcare facilities has enabled simulation training to be used in the everyday work environment. Otherwise known as *in situ simulations*, these training sessions provide realistic environments for learning and opportunities to investigate systems that are in place—opportunities to detect flaws or latent errors within a process.

Simulation-based education employs multimodal techniques to achieve learning objectives, from human beings to partial-task trainers to life-sized mannequins to virtual worlds. Future development in the areas of virtual realities, virtual worlds, and online systems will afford the opportunity to expand simulation-based education globally. The capabilities of simulation-based learning are infinite and may lead to interesting developments in the analysis and investigation of healthcare systems and processes in addition to education of healthcare professionals, which leads to the ultimate goal of better, safer, and more globally available patient care.

Key Points

- Simulation may be defined as an imitation of some real thing, state of affairs, or process and consists of techniques that provide a teaching tool that is particularly well suited to dynamic and challenging environments.
- Simulation allows complete testing of any new system or technology, illustrating problems, allowing changes to be made prior to its implementation, and allowing users to perform in real-time trials in stressful situations or environments.
- Adults learn best with experiential learning—learning by doing, thinking about, and assimilating lessons learned into everyday behaviors.
- Simulation training sessions offer the opportunity to progress through the stages of the experiential cycle in a structured manner. In simulation-based education, the goals of learning are chosen in advance and do not rely on chance exposure to rare diagnoses or situations.
- Debriefing plays a critical role in simulator-based education and provides an environment in which supportive and respectful discussion of the simulation can take place. The level of facilitation provided by the debriefer depends on learning objectives, complexity of scenarios, and the level of experience of participants and their familiarity with simulation.
- A patient simulator is generally considered to be any system that presents a clinical environment that responds appropriately to a given clinical event. Tools can include mannequin-based patient simulators, partial-task trainers, virtual reality, and standardized patients.
- *Virtual reality* is defined as a limited virtual world that is computer screen based with interaction by the participant via mouse, pen, or touchscreen device. Screen-based simulations allow participants to, e.g., treat a trauma patient in an ED, resuscitate a patient using principles of Advanced Cardiac Life Support, or interact with a screen-based standardized patient in an outpatient department. Immersion in a virtual world, particularly when overlain on a physical environment, enable teams of healthcare workers to act out various team roles in major catastrophes and thus practice for potential but rare events in a "realistic" manner.
- A partial-task trainer is any device that permits selected aspects of a task to be practiced independent of other elements of the task. Personnel who are learning

a new procedure or piece of equipment may use partial-task trainers to achieve a critical skill level before attempting that procedure in a real patient.

- Standardized patients can consistently recreate the role of a patient with a specific medical condition each time they encounter a student so that each trainee sees a patient with the same history and physical findings.

- Simulation-based learning now incorporates the concepts of human factors and ergonomics. *Crisis resource management* emphasizes the teaching of a number of universally applicable concepts that will be useful in any crisis situation. While incorporating medical and technical elements, it particularly stresses the importance of cognitive and interpersonal skills.

- Simulation-based education, due to its cross-disciplinary applicability, its dynamism and innovation, and an ever-increasing array of technologic advancements provides, many solutions for both professional education and improved patient care through safer work practices and systems.

References

1. http://en.wikipedia.org/wiki/simulation. Accessed March 10, 2007
2. Ehrenwerth J, Eisenkraft J. *Anesthesia Equipment: Principles and Applications*. St. Louis, MO: Mosby-Year Book, 1993
3. Easterling P, Hall E. *Greek and Roman Actors: Aspects of an Ancient Profession*. Cambridge: Cambridge University Press, 2002
4. Good ML, Gravenstein JS. Anesthesia simulators and training devices. Int Anesthesiol Clin 1989; 27:161–66
5. Caro PW. Human factors in aviation. In: Weiner EL, Nagel DC, eds. *Flight Training and Simulation*. San Diego, CA: Academic, 1988:229–60
6. Gaba DM. The future vision of simulation in healthcare. Qual Saf Health Care 2004; 13:i2–i10
7. Sansone S, Aroneo S. New fire simulator at FDNY Training Academy. WNYF (With New York Firefighters) 1987; 48(2):8–11
8. Piaget J. *The Origins of Intelligence in Children*. London: Routledge and Kegan, 1953
9. Rudolph JW, Simon R, Dufresne R, et al . There's no such thing as "nonjudgmental" debriefing: A theory and method for debriefing with good judgment. Simul Healthcare: J Soc Med Simul 2006; 1(1):49–55
10. Knowles M. The modern practice of adult education. In: *Pedagogy to Andragogy*. San Francisco, CA: Jossey-Bass, 1980:44–5
11. Kolb DA. *Experiential Learning: Experience as the Source of Learning and Development*. Englewood Cliffs, NJ: Prentice Hall, 1984
12. Gibbs G. *Learning by Doing: A Guide to Teaching and Learning Methods*. London: Further Education Unit, 1988
13. Grant J, Marsden P. *Training Senior House Officers by Service-Based Training*. London: Joint Centre for Medicine Education, 1992
14. Lewin K. *Field Theory in Social Science*. New York: Harper and Row, 1951
15. Kayes AB, Kayes DC, Kolb DA. Experiential learning in teams. Simul Gaming 2005; 36:330–54
16. Lederman LC. Intercultural communication, simulation, and the cognitive assimilation of experience: An exploration of the post-experience analytic process. Presented at the 3rd Annual Conference of the Speech Communication Association, San Juan, Puerto Rico, December 1–3, 1983

17. Pearson M, Smith D. Debriefing in experience-based learning. Simul Games Learn 1986; 16:155–72
18. Mitchell JT, Everly GS. *Critical Incident Stress Debriefing: An Operations Manual for the Prevention of Traumatic Stress Among Emergency Services and Disaster Workers.* Ellicott City, MD: Chevron, 1993
19. Lederman LC. Debriefing: Toward a systematic assessment of theory and practice. Simul Gaming 1992; 2:145–60
20. Lederman L. Debriefing. A critical reexamination of the postexperience analytic process with implications for its effective use. Simul Gaming 1984; 15:415–31
21. Gibb J. Defensive communication. J Commun 1961; 11:141–48
22. Savoldelli GL, Naik VN, Hamstra SJ, et al. Barriers to the use of simulation-based education. Can J Anaesth 2005; 52:944–50
23. Dismukes R, Smith G. *Facilitation and Debriefing in Aviation Training and Operations.* Aldershot, UK: Ashgate, 2000
24. Rolfe JM, Staple KJ. Flight Simulation. Cambridge: Cambridge University Press, 1986
25. Weick KE, Sutcliffe KM. *Managing the Unexpected.* University of Michigan Business School Management Series. San Francisco, CA: Jossey-Bass, 2001
26. Roberts KH, Bea RG. Must Accidents Happen: Lessons from high-reliability organizations. Acad Manage Exec 2001; 15(3):70–8
27. Roberts KH. HRO has prominent history. APSF Newsletter, Spring 2003
28. Denson JS, Abrahamson S. A computer-controlled patient simulator. JAMA 1969; 208:504–8
29. Carter DF. Man-made man: Anesthesiological medical human simulator. J Assoc Adv Med Instrum 1969; 3:80–86
30. Smith NT, Sebald AV, Wakeland C, et al. Cockpit simulation: Will it be used for training in anesthesia? Anesthesia Simulator Curriculum Conference, Rockville, MD, 1989
31. Schwid HA. A flight simulator for general anesthesia training. Comput Biomed Res 1987; 20:64–75
32. Schwid HA, O'Donnell D. The anesthesia simulator-recorder: A device to train and evaluate anesthesiologists' responses to critical incidents. Anesthesiology 1990; 72:191–7
33. Gaba DM, DeAnda A. A comprehensive anesthesia simulation environment: Re-creating the operating room for research and training, Anesthesiology 1988; 69:387–94
34. Chopra V, Engbers FH, Geerts MJ, et al. The Leiden anaesthesia simulator. Br J Anaesth 1994; 73:287–92
35. Rettedal A, Freier S, Ragna K, et al. PatSim—Simulator for practicing anaesthesia and intensive care. Int J Clin Monit Comput 1996; 13:147–52
36. www.Secondlife.com. Accessed March 12, 2007
37. www.teamwarefare.com. Accessed March 12, 2007
38. Kusumoto L, Heinrichs WL, Dev P, et al. Avatars alive! The integration of physiology models and computer-generated avatars in a multiplayer online simulation. Stud Health Technol Inform 2007; 125:256–8
39. Dev P, Srivastava S, Senger S. Collaborative learning using Internet2 and remote collections of stereo dissection images. Clin Anat 2006; 19:275–83
40. Gordon MS. Cardiology patient simulator: Development of an automated manikin to teach cardiovascular disease. Am J Cardiol 1974; 34:350–55
41. Reid C. A practical approach to developing an HRO culture: A theatrical piece presented at The HRO International Conference 2007, Deauville, France, May 2007
42. Flexner A. *Medical Education in the United States and Canada: A Report to the Carnegie Foundation for the Advancement of Teaching.* New York: The Carnegie Foundation for the Advancement of Teaching, 1910
43. Cooke M, Irby DM, Sullivan W, et al. American medical education 100 years after the Flexner report. N Engl J Med 2006; 355:1339–44
44. ACGME outcome project. http://www.acgme.org/outcome/comp/compFull.asp. Accessed February 2007

45. Salvendy G. *Handbook of Human Factors*. New York: Wiley-Interscience, 1987
46. Cooper GE, White MD, Lauber JK. Resource Management on the Flightdeck: Proceedings of a NASA/Industry Workshop. Moffett Field, CA: NASA Ames Research Center, 1980. NASA Conference Publication No. CP-2120
47. Lauber JK. Cockpit resource management: Background and overview. In: Orlady HW, Foushee HC, eds. *Cockpit Resource Management Training: Proceedings of the NASA/MAC Workshop. Moffett Field, CA: NASA Ames Research Center, 1987*. NASA Conference Publication No. 2455
48. Wiener EL, Kanki BG, Helmreich RL. Cockpit Resource Management. San Diego, CA: Academic, 1993
49. Howard SK, Gaba DM, Fish KJ, et al. Anesthesia crisis resource management training: Teaching anesthesiologists to handle critical incidents. Aviat Space Environ Med 1992; 63:763–70
50. Reznek M, Smith-Coggins R, Howard S, et al. Emergency medicine crisis resource management (EMCRM): Pilot study of a simulation-based crisis management course for emergency medicine. Acad Emerg Med 2003; 10(4):386–9
51. Johannsson H, Ayida G, Sadler C. Faking it? Simulation in the training of obstetricians and gynaecologists. Curr Opin Obstet Gynecol 2005; 17:557–61
52. Rall M, Gaba DM. Patient Simulators. In: *Miller's Anesthesia*. New York: Elsevier, 2004: 3073–103
53. Hall KH. Reviewing intuitive decision making and uncertainty: The implications for medical education. Med Educ 2002; 36:216–24
54. Reason JT. *Human Error*. Cambridge: Cambridge University Press, 1990
55. Klein GA. *A Recognition-Primed Decision (RPD) Model of Rapid Decision Making*. Norwood, NJ: Ablex, 1993:138–47
56. Gaba DM, Fish KJ, Howard SK. *Crisis Management in Anesthesiology*. New York: Churchill Livingstone, 1994
57. Rasmussen J. *Cognitive Control and Human Error Mechanisms*. Chichester, UK: Wiley, 1987
58. Sarter NB, Woods DD. Situation awareness: A critical but ill-defined phenomenon. Int J Aviat Psychol 1991; 1:45–57
59. DeKeyser V, Woods DD. Fixation errors: Failures to revise situation assessment in dynamic and risky systems. In: Colombo AG, Bustamante AS, eds. *Systems Reliability Assessment*. Dordrecht, Germany: Kluwer, 1990
60. Pickersgill T. The European working time directive for doctors in training. Br Med J 2001; 323:1266
61. Sprangers F. The Dutch experience of implementing the European Working Time Directive. BMJ Career Focus 2002; 325:S71

Chapter 25
Future Implications of Simulation in Anesthesia

Laurence C. Torsher*

It is a simplification to view simulators as *the* solution that will address shortcomings in education. Simulation is not the end point; it is only a tool that must be one part of a well-considered and well-executed curriculum. This chapter will discuss some of the forces that are shaping how simulation is currently being used and will speculate on how they may impact the ways in which simulation may be used in the future, both in education and in the clinical setting. Recent technologic advances and how they may impact the use of simulation will be addressed.

Practice, Policy, and Pressures

Many changes have occurred in the medical educational environment in recent years. In response to increased awareness of the errors in medicine, the public has become skeptical of the healthcare system, which has led to growing demands for accountability, safe care, quality care, and demonstration of competency by the individuals and facilities that provide care. Patients are more vocal than ever about their care and are increasingly reluctant to participate in clinical education so that physicians in training can learn their craft, particularly if the physicians are junior learners. In addition, payers are demanding that clinicians produce evidence that they are improving the quality of care that they deliver. These factors frequently collide with the needs of learners in a clinical environment; as mentors carry heavier clinical loads in the face of lower reimbursements, patients become reluctant to have learners involved with their care, and their threshold for acceptance of errors becomes ever lower.

---

* The author has been involved with all aspects of simulation training, including making equipment choice decisions, developing a new simulation center, developing simulation curriculum for multiple audiences, and being involved with professional organizations that are in the process of determining how simulation impacts their membership and how best to serve that membership. Like any forecast, this chapter is primarily the author's speculation on the future of the field.

J. Stonemetz, K. Ruskin (eds.) *Anesthesia Informatics,*   481
© Springer Science+Business Media, LLC 2008

Educational organizations, e.g., the American Council of Graduate Medical Education (ACGME) and its subordinate organizations, have made demands on teaching programs that require innovative solutions. For example, work-hour limitations have limited the exposure of trainees to the breadth of cases that they might otherwise have seen; hence, exposure to uncommon situations is decreased. Educators are struggling to evaluate the effects of work-hour limitations on both clinical care and education.[1] Because of the crushing debt faced by most medical trainees, extending the length of residency is not a popular option. At the same time, various agencies demand documentation of experiences as well as demonstration and documentation of competence in the face of this decreased clinical exposure.

Trainees' expectations are also evolving. As adults, the learning needs of medical students, residents, and allied health trainees are significantly different from the needs of child learners (Table 25.1).[2] The current approach to medical education frequently does not meet those needs. Trainees are far more ready to express

Table 25.1 Principles of adult learning and application to medical education

Needs of adult learners	Actions that should be taken by medical education programs
Adults have accumulated a foundation of life experiences and knowledge	Connect life experiences and prior learning to new information
Adults are autonomous and self-directed	Participants should be involved in the learning process, with the instructor serving as a facilitator and not just a supplier of facts
Adults are goal oriented	Create educational programs that are organized with clearly defined elements that show how the programs will help participants to reach their goals
Adults are relevancy oriented and practical	Help learners to see a reason for learning something by making it applicable to their work or other responsibilities of value to them
Adults need to be respected	Acknowledge the experiences that adult participants bring to the learning environment, allowing for opinions to be voiced freely
Adults are motivated to learn by both intrinsic and extrinsic motivation	Show learners how the learning will benefit them and create a comfortable and appropriately challenging learning environment
Adults learn best when they are active participants in the learning process	Limit lecturing and provide opportunities for sharing of experiences, questions, and exercises that require participants to practice a skill or apply knowledge
Not all adults learn the same way	Accommodate different learning styles by offering a variety of training methods
Adults learn more effectively when given timely and appropriate feedback and reinforcement of learning	Provide opportunity for feedback from self, peers, and instructor
Adults learn better in an environment that is informal and personal	Promote group interaction

Modified from Collins J. Education techniques for lifelong learning—Principles of adult learning. Radiographics 2004; 24:1483–9 dissatisfaction when their needs are not met than were trainees of the past, as the modern trainee likens her relationship with an educational institution to one of a consumer with a market. This open line of communication can be frustrating sometimes, but it does push the educational provider to be responsive to learners' needs, forcing the program to move from a teacher-centered approach to one that is learner centered.

Current educational models are frequently in direct conflict with the pressures of all of the participants in the training process—the credentialing agencies, the trainees, the trainers, i.e., the faculty and their institutions. A simulation-based component to education can address many of these conflicts. By exposing trainees to some of the uncommon events that they may miss as a result of reduced work hours and by providing an opportunity to document the trainees' exposure and management of a gamut of clinical problems in a reproducible manner, simulation-based training addresses many of the ACGME's demands.[3] In ensuring that trainees have an opportunity to "practice" challenging management situations in a simulation center, a healthcare institution can assure the public that their concerns are being addressed. As medical simulation becomes more common and public awareness is heightened, payers, policymakers, trainees, patients, and their advocates will be demanding that it become part of training programs. It is conceivable that a simulation experience will be a part of every training program. Many applicants to residency training programs now commonly ask if a simulation center is available. If a training program does not have a simulation center, its residents will have to be sent to another location for a portion of their training so that they gain these experiences.

The maintenance of competency and demonstration that midcareer practitioners are current in their knowledge and skills have traditionally been relegated to continuing medical education (CME) courses. Unfortunately, traditional CME does a poor job of bringing new clinical concepts into practice. Again, the public, the payers, and the policymakers are increasingly demanding a higher level of demonstration of maintenance of skills. Therefore, time-limited board certification and maintenance-of-competence programs have been introduced, such as the Maintenance of Competence in Anesthesia program offered by the American Board of Anesthesiology and the Maintenance of Certification (MOC) program offered by the Royal College of Physicians and Surgeons of Canada. Traditional CME courses that are lecture based do not meet the needs of the adult learner (see Table 25.1) as effectively as do more active learning models. The American Board of Anesthesiology will include the use of simulation experiences as criteria for fulfillment of the requirements for certification of Maintenance of Competence in Anesthesia.[4] The Canadian MOC program recognizes the value of simulation in ongoing maintenance of skills by providing two credits for each hour of simulation experience in contrast to one credit per hour for traditional CME.[5] The American College of Surgeons (ACS) has embraced simulation as an educational method for their membership, particularly as new surgical techniques and procedures are introduced into practice. Active CME or experiential CME, in which the participant is required to be actively involved in the educational experience rather than snoozing in the back of a lecture theater, will be increasingly common.

Anxiety about one's performance in front of peers and fear of humiliation have been identified as potential barriers to acceptance of simulation in CME in a survey of midcareer anesthesiologists.[6] Credible simulation centers address this issue by maintaining a "safe" environment. In addition, as simulation is potentially a more expensive offering than traditional lecture-based CME, it is incumbent upon simulation centers to provide an experience that is perceived to provide good value for the cost. As more and more trainees who have experienced simulation in their training proceed into practice, these attitudes will change—whether they involve perceptions of the relative value of a simulation experience, anxiety concerns, or even expectations or lack thereof of a simulation experience. In fact, this generation of "simulation-savvy" practitioners will push simulations centers to offer even more high-quality programs.

Currently, most simulation centers emphasize simulation as a tool for education. Although simulation seems attractive as an assessment tool, concerns have been raised because it has not been validated as such. Numerous studies have shown that people who have undergone simulation-based training perform better in simulated crises than do those who have not, but no studies have been conducted to show that this fact translates into better performance in a real clinical setting. However, it is clear that people who do poorly in a simulation exercise perform poorly in clinical practice. Studies that show a correlation between good simulation performance and good clinical care performance are limited. Simulation proponents would argue, though, that neither written nor oral exams have been subjected to the degree of validation as that being demanded of simulation as an assessment tool. In ongoing studies, simulation is being measured for its effectiveness as an educational tool, its impact on clinical practice, its validity as an assessment tool, and its validity as a predictor of clinical competency, with results in some studies being compared to traditional assessment methods such as written and oral examinations.

Despite the concerns regarding lack of validation of simulation in high-stakes examinations, it is being used in some settings as part of a high-stakes assessment process. Using actors as simulated patients, Part 2 of the US Medical Licensing Examination has, since 2004, evaluated candidates in clinical encounters.[7] Candidates travel to one of five sites in the nation and undergo a set of standardized patient encounters. They are evaluated on an Integrated Clinical Encounter component in which they must demonstrate their skills in eliciting findings from the standardized patient by taking a history and performing a clinical exam, based on which they must generate a patient note with pertinent findings, diagnostic impression, and initial workup. They are also evaluated on a Communication and Interpersonal Skills component in which professionalism, questioning skills, and communication skills must be demonstrated. Finally, they must demonstrate facility with the English language in the Spoken English Proficiency component.

The examination to qualify for fellowship in cardiology within the Royal College of Physicians and Surgeons of Canada consists of a written exam and an eight-to-ten station Objective Structured Clinical Examination (OSCE).[8] One of the OSCE stations requires the candidate to examine and describe clinical findings on the Harvey Cardiopulmonary Patient Simulator.[9]

The Israeli Board of Anesthesiology has added a simulation-based OSCE to its traditional written exam.[10] This OSCE consists of five simulation-based stations, including initial trauma management with emphasis on advanced trauma life support, resuscitation with emphasis on advanced cardiac life support, OR crisis management, mechanical ventilation management, and regional anesthesia skills. Since its inception in 2004, this component has evolved from being an adjunct portion of the exam to a "must-pass" portion. Other medical credentialing organizations are studying the role of a simulation-based component in their assessment process as well.

In 2004, the US Food and Drug Administration approved the marketing of a new carotid stent, with the condition that physicians who operate the device must undergo a training and assessment program that uses simulation through task trainers; this was the first time that the Food and Drug Administration had mandated a specific mode of training.[11] With the stroke of a pen, simulation was mandated for all users of a specific medical device. It remains to be seen whether similar requirements will follow as other new medical devices and procedures enter the marketplace.

Simulation began in a limited number of centers, usually staffed by a small cadre of jack-of-all-trades champions who diligently made it work. A community of cooperation and collegiality was built among these early pioneers. As outlined, the demand for simulation-based training is growing rapidly. New simulation centers are opening quickly throughout the world, and it is a challenge to develop and nurture the expertise necessary to offer consistently strong programs at all these simulation centers. In addition, a for-profit model of simulation centers will likely emerge if simulation becomes a mandatory part of recertification or if it becomes required as part of other medical device releases. Will the collegiality of the simulation pioneers be replaced by rivalry? How can users be assured that the experience offered by individual simulation centers is credible?

Many professional organizations have been struggling with these issues. The Society for Simulation in Healthcare faces the challenge of trying to serve a membership that consists of educators and clinicians from multiple specialties and professions within the healthcare system.[12] The ACS has developed the Accredited Education Institute program and promotes educational offerings by simulation centers that have been designated as Accredited Education Institutes.[13] Centers earn this designation by undergoing an extensive review process in which the physical plant, staffing, process of curriculum development and staff development, foundations of funding, and anticipated audiences are reviewed both by application and site visit. The goal of the program, in addition to ensuring a quality simulation-based educational offering for ACS membership, is to foster the growth of a surgical simulation community through research and development.

The ASA has developed an endorsement process that began taking applications from centers in 2007.[6] The goal of the ASA with this initiative is to "foster the access of ASA members to high-quality, simulation-based CME."[14] Simulation centers that apply for endorsement will be reviewed by a Web-based application process and selected site visits, based on examples of educational offerings, curriculum development and assessment process, physical plant and equipment, staffing, credentialing of instructors, and program leadership. Reviewers are looking for evidence of responsiveness to the needs of the learners through course offerings, assessment of course effectiveness, innovative course development that is in keeping with accepted simulation practices, and sensitivity to performance anxiety by participants. The goal is to build a simulation community that will be able to work together to develop effective curriculum, share research proposals, and advance the science of simulation-based education, as well as to provide quality CME offerings to the anesthesia community.

New Practice Trends and Uses of Simulation

In analysis of maloccurrences in the healthcare setting, human factors issues are frequently identified as contributing to the event. Examples include poor handoffs between care teams, poor communication within teams, and poor functioning of teams as groups—even as individuals are trying to do the right thing. Strategies that have developed to address these human factors shortcomings involve changing the culture of the healthcare environment, e.g., development of the reflective practitioner—one who scrutinizes his practice on an ongoing basis—and development and institution of crew resource-management models. Institutions and individuals are struggling with how to introduce these strategies into practice. Simulation-based learning, with people training in the teams in which they work rather than simply with their peers, is an ideal format with which to introduce these strategies. A simulated clinical scenario followed by a thoughtful debriefing with the entire team fosters contemplation as the team members consider their individual performances as well as their performance in functioning as a team. This group reflection provides an opportunity to see the value of some of the strategies and to practice them in a safe environment. As the strategies are embraced, a simulation approach to dissemination is likely.

The simulation center as a "usability lab" in the evaluation of new clinical practices or processes, or in the evaluation of new equipment, is a new role within the clinical community. Industry has utilized usability labs, mockups, and prototypes of equipment or processes for many years.

Better Technology

The technology of simulation is evolving rapidly. Similarities exist between the evolution of the personal computer and the simulation industry. Early adopters in both cases were tech savvy and as committed to tinkering with the intricacies of the technology, troubleshooting, and performing basic development as they were to actually using the technology. As the customer base expanded beyond people fascinated with both technology and education, users were less interested in the depths of the technology but had an expectation that equipment would work consistently, reliably, and reproducibly. At the 2007 meeting of the Society for Simulation in Healthcare, attendees were surveyed as to what frustrations and issues they thought simulation manufacturers should address. Responses included the need for easier programming of the equipment, the need for more robust equipment that is not so fragile and prone to damage, standardized interfaces (both hardware and software) to allow both task trainers and mannequins to work together, open-source software to facilitate innovation, development of a common programming language, and more thorough documentation. Interestingly, many of these comments were similar to those made in the early era of the personal computer. Representatives from the major simulator manufacturers were present at the meeting; it remains to be seen how many of the suggestions will be implemented.

Improved haptic, or tactile, feedback is being developed for many of the task trainers. In addition, improved metrics are being developed and applied to facilitate comparison among learners. These metrics, in conjunction with well-designed courseware, allow independent use of the task trainer as one part of a comprehensive curriculum. As new equipment and techniques are introduced into clinical practice, a task trainer may well be part of the marketing and education process, as occurred by mandate with carotid stents. Task trainers are in development for the robotic surgical systems. As simulation is embraced for skills teaching, low-fidelity models are being rediscovered and can play a role; e.g., basic knot tying can still be practiced on a drape before advancing to laparoscopic suture manipulation in a sophisticated task trainer. In simulation training for the civilian aircraft industry, one of the basic tenets is to use only as much fidelity and sophistication as is necessary to achieve specific training objectives, which makes for a more cost-effective approach to teaching. The benefit to the student is not so much from the simulator itself, as his being part of the paradigm of experiential or "hands-on" learning.

Mannequin simulators are also undergoing exciting changes. The tetherless mannequin—one that is controlled remotely, is battery powered, and requires no external lines—is coming onto the market at this writing. This innovation is exciting because it will facilitate moving simulation experiences out of the simulation center and into the actual clinical setting, which will encourage learners to train as they work and transfer the lessons learned into their daily practice. As mentioned above, demands by some users for increased realism through more supple skin, color changes, realistic movements, etc. must be balanced against the increased cost and the potential for failure associated with more features. As each new feature adds cost and the potential for failure, the user must constantly assess whether the feature truly helps to achieve the objectives of the lesson or experience.

A poor lesson on ultrasophisticated simulation equipment is still a poor lesson. The emphasis must move beyond technical developments in the machinery to the design of good educational material that is facilitated by simulation. Development of educational material is the biggest challenge of new simulation centers. Educational material is currently shared throughout the academic community; however, as commercial vendors of this material are also recognizing that the need exists, one would expect to see them entering the marketplace soon. Curriculum with a simulation component is being developed by many of the professional organizations, e.g., the ASA and the American College of Chest Physicians. Their goal is not only to provide education for their membership on topical issues, but also to act as a kernel for further simulation-based curricular development and to foster the success of simulation centers.

Conclusion

Many forces, including patients, payers, trainees, and professional organizations, are challenging the traditional approach to medical education and making the current model more and more difficult to maintain. Simulation-based education will address some of the shortcomings of the current educational model by providing a safe and documentable experiential approach that can provide the learner with standardized and reproducible experiences. Active learning, with simulation being one example, is becoming increasingly embraced in the CME community. Major professional organizations are setting standards to ensure that their membership is receiving a quality educational experience from simulation education providers. A simulation-based experience may become part of the maintenance-of-competence certification for some professional organizations. Simulation's role in high-stakes assessment is evolving, as a growing number of organizations maximize its potential in this area. Although the sophistication of simulation equipment is increasing, the simulation community is demanding more reliable equipment, standardized interfaces, and most importantly, curriculum development. In the future, vendors will no doubt increase their focus on quality simulation curriculum products.

Key Points

- Simulation can help to address the current demands on medical education by providing a safe, reproducible, and documentable educational experience. It is conceivable that almost any medical education facility will need to provide its learners with simulation experiences.
- Simulation-based CME will become increasingly common.
- Simulation as a component of high-stakes assessments is already in place in some settings and being studied for applicability in others.
- Simulation may become part of the rollout and marketing of new medical equipment and techniques.
- Although the technology of simulation is becoming increasingly sophisticated, without good curriculum it is of marginal benefit. The real focus for the future must be on curriculum development.

References

1. Reed DA, Levine RB, Miller RG, et al. Effect of residency duty hour limits. Arch Intern Med 2007; 167:1487–92
2. Collins J. Education techniques for lifelong learning—Principles of adult learning. Radiographics 2004; 24:1483–9
3. Philbert I. Simulation and rehearsal. ACGME Bull 2005; Dec:1–16
4. Olympio MA. Innovation and the future in continuing medical education. ASA Newsletter, September 2005
5. Maintenance of Competence (MOC) Section Descriptions, Royal College of Physicians and Surgeons of Canada. http://rspsc.medical.org/mainport/index.php. Accessed July 26, 2007
6. Sinz EH. Anesthesiology National CME Program and ASA activities in simulation. Anesthesiol Clin 2007; 25:209–23
7. United States Medical Licensing Examination. 2007 USMLE Step 2 CS Content Description and General Information Booklet. http://www.usmle.org/step2/Step2CS/Step2CS2007GI/description.asp. Accessed July 26, 2007
8. Format of the Comprehensive Objective Examination in Cardiology (adult). The Royal College of Physicians and Surgeons of Canada. http://rcpsc.medical.org/residency/certification/examformats/405a_e.php. Accessed July 26, 2007
9. "All-New Harvey Cardiopulmonary Patient Stimulator." Michael S. Gordon Center for Research in Medical Education. http://www.crme.med.miami.edu/harvey_changes.html. Accessed July 26, 2007
10. Berkenstadt H, Ziv A, Gafni N, et al. Incorporating simulation-based objective structured clinical examination into the Israeli National Board Examination in anesthesiology. Anesth Analg 2005; 102:853–8
11. Gallagher AG, Cates CU. Approval of virtual reality training for carotid stenting. What this means for procedural-based medicine. JAMA 2004; 292:3024–6
12. Society for Simulation in Healthcare. http://www.ssih.org/public/. Accessed July 26, 2007
13. Accredited Education Institutes. Enhancing Patient Safety Through Simulation. American College of Surgeons. http://www.facs.org/education/accreditationprogram/index.html. Accessed July 26, 2007
14. ASA Workgroup on Simulation Education White Paper. ASA Approval of Anesthesiology Simulation Programs. Submitted to the ASA Committee on Outreach Education July 18, 2006, for ASA BOD ACTION. ASASimWhitePaper071806.pdf. Accessed February 7, 2008

Index

Printed in the United States of America